The Extremely Unfortunate
SKULL VALLEY
Incident

Revised and Enlarged

What a seriously concerned citizen needs to know about the tragedy, science, politics, and history of the biological hazards' labyrinth

Includes information on government and government-sponsored biological warfare weapons research in the United States, the former Soviet Union, Japan, Great Britain, Nazi-Germany, and Canada. With special emphasis upon disease entities that have emerged since 1971 and have links to biowar research and deployment, including Marburg Disease (1967); Lassa Fever (1969); Lyme Disease (1975); Ebola Fever (1976); Legionnaires' Disease (1976) ; Adult T-cell leukemia (1977); AIDS (1981); chronic fatigue syndrome (1981); *Eschericia coli* 0157:H7 (1982)

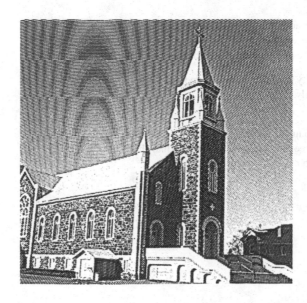

The Chelmsford Publishers,
Box 133, Station B,
Sudbury, CANADA. P3E 4N5

Trafford rev. 10/07/2021

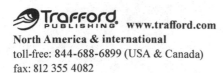 **Trafford** PUBLISHING® **www.trafford.com**
North America & international
toll-free: 844-688-6899 (USA & Canada)
fax: 812 355 4082

Donald W. Scott and William L.C. Scott
dedicate this study to the following persons all of whom are casualties we have encountered in our seven year search to find our way through the labyrinth of the hidden war of biological weapons research.

To Ms. Diane Martel
Representative of all those victims of chronic fatigue syndrome.

and

To Boyd (Ed) Graves
Victim of the laboratory-developed 'biological agent, an agent which does not naturally exist and for which no natural immunity could have been acquired' and all the millions of people who have died and those who are doomed to die from AIDS.

and

To Captain (Retired) Louise Richard, R.N.
and her heroic comrades-in-arms.
Served in the Canadian Navy during the Gulf War,
was critically injured in the line of duty, and was
abandoned by the Canadian Military.

and

To Emily Catherine Ainsworth
"The Awesome Dude"
Who died at the age of ten from a
cancerous brain tumour in 1998.

And to the millions of others who are victims of the neuro/systemic degenerative diseases whose incidence has increased dramatically as a consequence of the weaponizing of the mycoplasma species and which has turned rare and occasional diseases into epidemics: Alzheimer's; amytrophic lateral sclerosis; autism; bi-polar depression; cancer; Creutzfeldt-Jakob disease; diabetes, type one; dystonia; endometriosis; fibromyalgia; Huntington's; inclusion-body miositis; lupus; Lyme disease; multiple sclerosis; Parkinson's; rheumatoid arthritis; schizophrenia; and others.

And
For Cecile Marie Scott
and
Krysten & Alex Scott

With Love

**A history
You might not like hearing...
but one we have to tell.**

Other Books by the Same Author(s)

Donald W. Scott

Hamlet: A Guide to Study (1966; re-issued 1996)
King Lear: A Guide to Study (1966; re-issued 1996)
Paradise Lost: A Guide to Study (1968; re-issued 1996)
Corrupt Decades: American Politics from 1952 to 1976 (1988)
Steve's Dream Catcher (1999)

DRAMA

The Twist (1979)
Celebrating Sudbury: A Chronicle with Music (1983)
The Tragicall Historie of Gertrude Queene of Denmark (1986)

POETRY

Editor: Northern Lights 14 (1983)
Editor: Northern Lights 15 (1984)

Donald W. Scott and William L.C. Scott

The Extremely Unfortunate Skull Valley Incident (1996)
The Brucellosis Triangle (1998)

Works in progress

William L.C. Scott: Watergate: The rest of the stories

CONTENTS

Introduction by Donald W. Scott

I began my study of biological warfare without any idea that was what I was doing. I thought at the time that I was just helping a person who had called me one day in June, 1995 with a request for help.

The call was from a lady who said "Mr. Scott, you don't know me, but I need someone to help me, and a friend referred me to you."

I invited her to my home and asked her to bring any relevant documents with her. When she arrived she told me that she had 'chronic fatigue syndrome'. I had only a passing acquaintance with that illness, so not only was I listening to her as a person, it turned out that I was listening as a novitiate in a new calling. A calling I still pursue: the search for the truth about chronic fatigue syndrome.

I learned from her about the devastating effects of her illness as well as the terrible way that she had been used by her employer, her union, most of her medical doctors and members of Ontario's legal community. But I also learned something else. As a graduate from Guelph University, I knew that with respect to her disease I had to respond as a scientist. I had to collect data; categorize data; formulate hypotheses; design tests of those hypotheses; apply those tests; tabulate results; re-formulate my original hypotheses.

Thus, at the age of 71 I embarked on my new calling: discover the cause of the terrible disease afflicting my caller; and, determine why a person so tragically disabled was being bullied, neglected, denied social benefits, and humiliated in a way few if any other ill persons were used.

I can honestly state that not a single day has gone by since the day I received this cry for help, that I haven't devoted at least some time to the quest. On holidays it may be as little as one or two hours. On social occasions I find myself discussing not just chronic fatigue syndrome, but what I have learned about related diseases such as AIDS, fibromyalgia, multiple sclerosis, Parkinson's, etc. In a few words: the neuro/systemic degenerative diseases. Some days I work 12 to 14 hours.

And I have not only been able to help my original caller, but I have been able to track my way through a labyrinth of scientific research; through government deceit and double-cross; through media psychobabble; to a core of profound evil based upon a complex of political/ military/ industrial/ and pharmaceutical interests, for, the study of health issues today requires as this book will demonstrate the study of biological warfare research and its consequences for humanity.

The goals and methods of the warfare biological researchers are not enunciated to the world. The planning is not haphazard. The methods are not random. But the consequences are all around us and are posing ever-growing threats to the health of humanity.

I have learned over the past six years that there are deliberate efforts being made by certain political persons in the United States, Canada, Great Britain and quite likely other countries to use advanced scientific knowledge about disease; sophisticated psychological understanding of people; compliant and complicit mass media; and the power of crafted social myths to reduce individuals to managed units in the functioning of a single world society.

These efforts have been translated into actual research, various test programs (mostly upon unwitting civilian populations), and deployment of developed pathogenic biological agents by elements of the military establishment in each country cited above and by the various security agencies in such countries. Furthermore, at all levels and since the inception of the enterprise, elements of the federal public health agencies in the United States and Canada have monitored and otherwise co-operated with the political/ military/ security agencies involved.

The burden of researching and publicizing the reality of the neuro/systemic diseases from a medical/ scientific point-of-view was thus made heavier by virtue of the political/ military/ security agencies' roles as noted. This made it necessary for me to recruit the help of my son, William, an Honours graduate in History and Political Science from Laurentian University of Sudbury. Together we have followed where the evidence has led. The trail has not been the open clear highway of scientists and of honest activities by governments and their agents concerned with the health of their citizens. The trail has led through a labyrinth and has been characterized by dishonesty, immorality, and deviousness at the highest levels.

Plain and simply, health for the citizen has not been the focus of much of the medical research and development over the past six decades. For many politicians and the military, the focus has been upon the development of biological weapons which must be tested upon someone, somewhere.

For example, the whole City of Winnipeg was sprayed in 1953 by a United States bomber diffusing a carcinogenic chemical over the unwitting population *with the agreement of the Government of Canada.*

Or, in 1998 the 'Head' of Medical Services for the Canadian Armed Forces, Major Tim Cook, M.D., sent a copy of a Memo he had written for his Commanding Officer to Captain Kenneth Hyams of the United States Naval Research facility in Bethesda, Maryland.

What purpose is served and by what right does a Major in the Canadian Military have to send copies of such Memos to members of another nation's military? When I served in the Canadian Military, this would have been seen as treason.

For the pharmaceutical industry the focus has been to make money. Researchers get grants on the basis of serving the industry, not on the basis of curing the ill.

For governments, much of the focus has been upon serving as handmaidens to the military and to industry. A city is sprayed with a carcinogenic chemical because the military says that it needs to learn what will happen when their new chemical is taken into the lungs of people. Or caring doctors of medicine and other health care providers are harassed and prosecuted if they depart from the party line set by the status quo medical associations.

When I began my quest in 1995, I thought that I was helping one ill person who had a mysterious disease. That was, indeed, where I started. But, step-by-step I and Bill have been led into the labyrinth of biological research that I have spoken of.

We have been given increased motivation to update our original book by the events of September and October, 2001, when suddenly several persons were found to have been exposed to anthrax. Such an eventuality is a natural consequence of the path followed by the United States over the past six decades, for the strain of anthrax identified in Boca Ratan, Florida was already known to us from our research.

The media reports that the strain of anthrax that had killed a photo editor in Florida was a strain developed at Iowa State University College of Agriculture in the early 1950's...and our files contain a United States Senate Report that Iowa State University had received six contracts from the U.S. Department of

Defence in that time frame, to develop biological weapons!

Our files also contain the Riegle Report which reveals that anthrax was sold by the U.S. to Iraq in 1988, for use against Iran. President George Bush Sr. is on the record with the explanation that he saw Saddam Hussein as a 'force for stability in the Middle East'.

In 1996, after our early efforts to research chronic fatigue syndrome, Bill and I as mentioned above, self-published an account under the title of *The Extremely Unfortunate Skull Valley Incident.* We thought at that point we knew something. But, our book drew letters from all over the world from all manner of people and we have learned more and more about just how complex and tragic the biological labyrinth was and undoubtedly still is.

The new information that we have received, plus our continuing research, has now led us to this date of writing in March, 2002, and our dramatic revelation in Chapter 15.

From a quiet weekend in June of 1995 when a lady ill with a mystery disease visited my home to a frantic day of action and confusion in October of 2001 in Senator Thomas A. Daschle's Hart Building Office may seem totally unrelated. But over these seven years, Bill and I have learned that a path that had started in the Senate Office of people like Senator Prescott Bush of Connecticut in 1959, and various of his evil associates such as General William Draper and Allen Dulles, had wandered from Washington to Fort Detrick, Maryland, and to Stanford University of California, through Africa and the U.S. smallpox eradication program to Incline Village, Nevada...leaving a trail of death and disability behind.

And in October, 2001, under the Presidency of Prescott Bush's grandson, the chickens are coming home to roost.

And, we are compelled to believe, there's even greater tragedy yet to come.

So, we start this revised *Skull Valley*, with Diane Martel's original phone call and her visit in June, 1995, and we end it with our terrible discovery of the 'common cause'. Written without rancour or hate, but with a profound sense of sadness about what man can do to man, and with the conviction that the more people know about what has gone on in the name of biological research, the less will they be victimized in the future.

This book is for you, your children and generations yet to come.

"I'm sick and I need help."

"Mr. Scott, you don't know me, but I need someone to help me, and a friend referred me to you."

It was towards the end of the Ontario election campaign in June of 1995 and, as the Provincial Leader and Sudbury candidate for the *Ontario Options Party,* I was receiving many such calls. After all, in a democracy when candidates are looking for the votes of anyone that they can persuade to support them, many constituents use the opportunity to air a grievance, make some proposal for change, or, as with the caller, to ask for assistance.

Rather than discuss her situation on the phone, I suggested that she visit me following the election, and to bring any documents she had which might serve to verify any claims about her situation. I really didn't want to spend time as a sounding board for people who might simply be looking for a sympathetic ear to listen to their real or perceived problems, and I have found by experience that requesting documentation at the outset pares away some of the latter category. Then I added my final condition:

"Would you also take some time over the next few days to summarize in four or five pages the nature of your problem, the principals involved and salient details to date?"

My caller replied that she would do so. All that remained was to set a meeting date and a time.

"How about Saturday at 9:00 am?" I asked, having learned from experience that triflers are not inclined to favour early hour appointments, especially on a weekend. She accepted.

Diane Martel arrived at my apartment at precisely 9:00 am on Saturday, June 10, 1995. She carried a bulging briefcase.

After an exchange of introductions and pleasantries, she opened her brief case and removed a thick pile of papers and we got down to the matter at hand...her problem and what role I might have in helping her with it.

She was a middle aged, attractive-looking and well-groomed lady. She spoke carefully while I made notes. She had brought a neatly written eleven page summary of her situation, which I accepted and told her I would review later after I had made my own summary from our conversation. I asked her to start

at the beginning and to keep things in a chronological order.

"It's Not Board Policy"
An Employer and a Sick Employee

The story she told me was very moving. Diane Martel was suffering from something that she called 'chronic fatigue syndrome'. She had been bullied by her employer, The Sudbury Separate School Board; had been ignored by her union, the Ontario English Catholic Teachers' Federation; and double-dealt with by the Ontario Human Rights Commission. Although unable to work at her job as a teacher, the insurance company that handled the disability plan refused to pay her any benefits. From time-to-time in her narrative she would pause in silent distress, then would compose herself and carry on. I knew from the outset that here was a lady who had suffered greatly and who deserved any help I could give. Although I was moved by her account, I maintained a business-like 'The facts, Ma'am, just the facts' manner, and now and then I would interrupt her to get things straight as to time, or some other detail. Although the interview lasted nearly three hours, I wound up with just six pages of notes.

At the end of the interview I told her that I would review my notes, correlate these with her eleven pages, and read over the thick pile of supporting documentation. I would then call her the next day and let her know what I felt she should do, and what I felt I might be able to do to help her. Then, as a matter of principle, I told her that I would require a ten dollar payment from her to cover any out-of-pocket expenses I might incur as we developed her case. I felt that by asking for such a token payment I put her relationship with me on a more professional footing and would tend to make her feel less like an intruder upon my time.

She paid me the ten dollars and I said, "Okay. Let's get started. From what you tell me you have been very badly used; in fact, I might even say you have been bullied, and I'll do what I can to help you achieve some justice."

At this point, tears welled up in her eyes and she

dabbed at them with a Kleenex. I let on that I hadn't noticed this sign of emotional stress, and said: "I'll call you after dinner, tomorrow."

I put all of her papers away, resolving to start afresh on Sunday morning after I had had a chance to sort out my sense of outrage at the way this sick lady had been abused. After all, I reasoned, perhaps I am missing something in all of this that will become evident only after a period of quiet reflection and detachment.

The next morning, while my wife slept in, I sat down with my notes, Diane's notes, and the pile of files, and began a slow, careful review of her six years of physical and mental distress, often made worse by people with whom she has had to deal who treated her in some cases with rudeness, in other cases with impatience, and in far too many cases with what can only be called cruelty.

Hardly a day has passed since that moment on a Sunday morning when I began to read, that I have not spent some time on Diane Martel, chronic fatigue syndrome and the labyrinth of evil into which it was all to lead. I was to discover that this lady, like so many other victims of CFIDS, was a victim of a crime against humanity. A crime which needed to be placed on public view to achieve justice for all those who suffer from this terrible disease and by having the truth clearly on the record to move towards a cure.

Furthermore, as my research developed, I felt a growing need to help all those family members, friends, employers, legal and union representatives, and even medical doctors of the victims of CFS , to achieve a better understanding of the agony these victims have endured, often in lonely and misunderstood isolation.

Friendless when friends were most needed; alone when their agony was most extreme.

Diane Martel

Born in 1950, and trained as a teacher of French, Diane had worked as a teacher, a real estate agent and as an agent for Air Canada. In 1989 she started to teach full time for the Sudbury Separate (i.e. Roman Catholic) School Board.

In the Fall of that year she found that she had a split schedule. That is, she would teach in the morning at one school, then she would drive a few miles to another school to teach for the afternoon. In nice weather, this regime was not too onerous, but when winter winds were blowing and snow was gusting across the roads the break between the two schools was not at all re-creative.

Besides having to drive in all kinds of weather, Diane had to 'brown-bag' her lunch and eat part of it as she coped with the traffic and the highway.

When she returned from the Summer break in 1990 she was concerned to learn that not only did she still have a split schedule, but she had been assigned to teach at *three* schools! Twice each day, after the challenge of classes, she could not flop into a chair in the staff room, but had to get into her car and drive to another school. Such a drive now and then does not loom large as a problem, but when one has to do it every day of the week in all kinds of weather and regardless of how one feels physically, such a schedule can be exhausting, and towards the end of each day Diane felt completely wrung out. Her only consolation was the fact that she had been given a half hour 'preparation' period each day from 2:00 to 2:30.

Then, in order to accommodate another class, she was informed by her Board that her one and only 'prep time' had been cancelled. When she arrived at her last school each day she would be expected to go directly to her classroom and begin to teach. It was about this point in time that she found herself silently sobbing as her penultimate class of students filed from her room and before the final class for each day had filed in.

She now wonders whether this was the point of on-set for her chronic fatigue syndrome. Whether or not such was the case may be difficult to say with any certainty, but what is not in dispute is the way her employer responded to her plight. I reconstructed the events from her notes and the pile of records she had left with me. It happened like this.

One day before her final class of excited, chattering students arrived, and as she stood in a window looking out over the wind-blown fall fields, with her head bowed and a handkerchief to her eyes, silently sobbing, she was startled by a sympathetic question. "Are you alright?"

It was a fellow teacher who had popped in before the class began. Diane explained that she felt so utterly fatigued, and what with the need to shift schools twice each day, she could hardly meet her final class.

"Have you talked to the Superintendent?" her friend asked.

"No, I feel intimidated by him," she replied.

"Let me call him for you," suggested her colleague, and Diane reluctantly agreed.

When he heard of her problem, Superintendent Mike Csinos was not sympathetic. "We could actually fit in another class for her," he said." There are many redundant teachers." The implication was clear: Diane was lucky to have a job at all so it was best not to complain.

After some urging by her colleague, Diane agreed to visit Dr. Farrell, who it turned out was not able to diagnose a specific disease, but who did agree that her fatigue warranted some prescribed rest. Diane applied for benefits under the Long Term Disability Insurance Plan carried by her employer, and, in January, 1991 began a leave with pay.

By May, 1991, she was feeling somewhat better and she scheduled an appointment with Giselle Brett, a rehabilitation counsellor with her insurance carrier, the Ontario Teachers' Insurance Plan. Ms. Brett agreed that if Ms. Martel was up to it, she should try to return to employment, but she preferred that such a move be a graduated process. Ms. Brett indicated that the OTIP would pay a 50 percent benefit, and suggested that Diane ask the School Board to assign her to a half day time-table at half pay. Thus, she would receive a full day's pay for a half day's work, and she would have each afternoon to recuperate. It seemed to be an arrangement where everyone concerned would win. It would not cost the School Board anything beyond their negotiated pay rates; OTIP would only have to pay out half of what they were currently paying; and Diane would have a phased return to full employment.

Delighted with what seemed to be an ideal way to cope with her situation, Diane took the proposal to Robert Hammond, Superintendent of the English Language section of the Board.

His response was a flat "No." The only explanation he was prepared to offer was: "It is not Board policy."

When she heard of the Board's response to Ms. Martel's request, Ms. Brett intervened directly with Mr. Hammond and received the same "No. It is not Board policy." There was no discussion encouraged about what might be good for a sick employee.

In March, 1992, Diane tried again. She wrote to Hammond with the same proposal. He replied that he would take her back to half time duty, but only on condition that she accepted a modification to her contract which would designate her as 'part-time'. The Ontario English Catholic Teachers' Federation recommended that Diane not accept such a condition since it could jeopardize her future seniority and pension entitlements. After all, if she returned under her present contract status and did a half day's work for a half day's pay the Board would be getting what it was paying for and Diane would be safe-guarding pension rights that so many people, especially women, have in the past unwittingly signed away.

Mr. Hammond was adamant… "No. It is not Board policy."

It was only some time later that Diane Martel learned that at the very time that Mr. Hammond was rationalizing his adamant stand on accommodating her, there were two other employees of the same Board who were working on just such a basis. Apparently it had less to do with 'Board policy' than with Mr. Hammond's attitude to Diane Martel's illness.

By September, 1992, still ill but feeling the pressure caused by her substantial reduction in income, Diane decided to return to work on the Board's terms. She accepted a full-time posting at Our Lady of FatimaSchool. Although she was now spared the ordeal of a split schedule, by noon hour each day she found herself experiencing a 'bone crunching' fatigue. Reluctantly she returned to her disability insurance plan at the end of the month and stayed on until March, 1993, when she returned to work on a graduated rehabilitative plan finally worked out for her between her Board and her union…OECTA.

The Board's letter of March 8, 1993 read more like a schedule prepared for a city bus being shuttled around a route on a fixed schedule than a plan to help a sick employee. No where does it indicate that the schedule was for a living human being whose health status was subject to a variety of factors that 'the flesh is heir to.' Each stage of the 'rehabilitative' plan was given a specific time frame and specific goals were set for Diane's return to good health…

"Step I-Duration- 4 weeks approximately…Step II-Duration- 4 weeks approximately…" etc.

As it turned out Ms. Martel was not able to march steadfastly towards the final goal of 'good health and full-time work' on the Board's carefully scripted schedule.

Not only was the plan of her employer unrealistically specific, but there were other features one would not expect to find in a letter discussing the welfare of a sick employee. For example, Ms. Martel had purchased a hot tub on the recommendation of her doctor. The doctor felt that the heat and massaging effect of the pulsing water would ameliorate her bodily aches that were becoming more prevalent. When the union representative had mentioned that Diane was under financial stress and had accompanied his letter with a summary of her expenses (which showed a payment on the hot tub) Simon Ouellet , Manager, Human Resources, suggested in his reply that "…if Mrs. Martel had financial difficulties, one must question the reasonableness of a $4,600.00 expenditure on a luxury item (i.e. the Hot Tub)".[1]

Furthermore, even though the medical evidence of her condition was being provided by a licensed and fully qualified medical practitioner, Ms. Martel was advised by Mr. Oulette that "…the Board reserves the right, under article 6.06 (10), to have Mrs. Martel examined by a doctor selected by the Board."

At about this point in my reading of her files, I began to puzzle over the nature of Diane Martel's illness. Chronic fatigue syndrome? I had heard very little about the disease, but that wasn't unusual for me since I was not by any stretch of the imagination a 'health buff'. I recalled as I reflected upon what I did know, that once I had heard an interview about chronic fatigue syndrome on the CBC morning show hosted by Peter Czowski. I recalled that his questions were concerned, thoughtful and kind. And I recall that the victim with whom he was talking had recounted how difficult it was to cope with the disease and at the same time try to cope with friends, family and employers who couldn't see any physical signs of illness. I went back to my reading of the files.

At the end of September, 1993, Ms. Martel did not feel up to the "Step" of her 'bus schedule return to health' schedule to which she had been advanced, and she asked to stay on the previous "Step" a while longer. Mr. Oulette would have no such trifling with his time-table for return to health and he advised her abruptly: "There is no space to go back a stage…" Overcome with fatigue, Diane stayed home for a week on the recommendation of her doctor. Then she phoned the Board to say "I'll be back on Monday." Shortly after leaving this message with the Board Secretary, Diane received a message from Mr. Oulette : "Don't report to your school. Report to Simon Oulette at the Board office at 8:30 Monday morning."

As a lady already timid about confronting authority figures, and still suffering from fatigue, Ms. Martel phoned her union and told the representative,

Mr. Robert Kirwan, that she 'felt intimidated' by the message.

When Mr. Kirwan called Mr. Oulette, he was advised that the Board was not going to allow Ms. Martel to return to work until they had a report from a doctor that they would select…who (presumably) would be able to tell them the 'truth' about her condition. Kirwan was told to tell Ms. Martel to await a call as to which doctor she was to attend.

A month went by with no word from Mr. Oulette. Since she was feeling better and wanted to get back to work and to the larger pay cheque that meant, Diane again phoned Robert Kirwan , who took her request to Mr. Hammond. When the latter heard that Ms. Martel had been waiting at home for a month (though for no fault of hers) he was very exercised and demanded that "…she be back in her classroom to-morrow morning."

There was more in the file that reflected the way the Sudbury Separate School Board dealt with their sick employee, Ms. Diane Martel, but I had seen quite enough and I drafted a letter to Mr. Hammond. When he had not replied to any of my concerns, I sent a reminder letter . He then sent me a one sentence reply: "I am not at liberty to respond to your letter of June 13th, 1995, re: Diane Martel."

In my letter I had raised the following five concerns:

i. Although Diane Martel had been told that the 50-50 arrangement proposed by OTIP was not 'our practice', there were two other teachers who were being extended the privilege…

ii. In a Board letter dated October 19, 1992 Hammond had promised a 'formal reply shortly', but no such reply had been received. Had such a letter been sent, and if not, why not?

iii. In a letter of March 8, 1993 he had written: '…we would like at this stage to introduce goals for Mrs. Martel to attain.' I asked:"Is it the policy of your Board to 'set goals' for sick employees 'to attain' and is such goal setting compatible with reasonable medical practice?"

iv. In a letter of November 12,1993 he had stated: "It is therefore expected that Mrs. Martel will be able to undertake Step V on December 1, 1993." I asked: "Did you base the 'expectation' upon a medical prognosis made by a properly qualified medical practitioner?"

v. In a letter of January 27, 1994 he had suggested that if Mrs. Martel does not find her options suitable she can always 'resign'. I asked: "…when dealing with a sick employee…(is) resignation a humane and considered 'option'?"

There were two more questions which I will discuss below when I review the role of the Ontario Human Rights Commission.

As I have mentioned, Mr. Hammond did not feel that he was 'at liberty' to respond to my letter or to answer my questions.

So much for the way one victim of chronic fatigue syndrome had been used by an 'enlightened' and 'Christian' employer.

Diane Martel was the first person I had ever met who to the best of my knowledge, suffered from chronic fatigue syndrome. I was later to learn that there were two others in our family who had been diagnosed with CFIDS. However, they called their condition fibromyalgia, and at the time I had no idea that the latter was but one of a wide spectrum of concomitant diseases and diagnoses which clustered about an equally wide spectrum of symptoms.

My initial concern had been with the way an employer in our society had used a sick employee and I found that there was something very distressing about the manner in which at least one victim of CFIDS had been abused by her employer. I was soon to find that such a response was pretty well the rule and not the exception. And I was also to learn that not only did employers seem to have a mind set which was very callous and even cruel, there were several other persons with whom the CFIDS victim had to cope who for some reason or other, were inclined to treat the sick person with anything from indifference to outright hostility.

People with a leg missing or who need to tap their way along a street with a white cane and a seeing-eye dog are treated by those they encounter with varying degrees of concern, often erring on the side of being overly-helpful. But people who endure a 'bone crunching' fatigue are told: "Well, I'm tired all the time, too, but I still get up and go to work."

Where did this type of response to CFIDS spring from? I was soon to find out, but my route to that knowledge was not to be an easy one to find nor an easy one to follow.

Bureaucrats And Bullies

Question: What is the difference between a bully and a bureaucrat?

Answer: A bully enjoys the misery he inflicts, a bureaucrat just isn't aware of it.

Under the Ontario Human Rights Code, 1981, which is to be enforced by The Human Rights Commission, there are provisions for citizens who have been discriminated against to present their case in a formal and business-like manner and have the merits of their complaint evaluated. If the Commission, depending in large part upon the recommendation of its field investigators, determines that there has been a violation of a person's human rights , the Commission may order that certain actions be taken by the offending party to set right the injustice suffered by the Complainant.

As recounted above, Ms. Diane Martel had been very badly used by her employer, The Sudbury Separate School Board. Ms. Martel was handicapped by an unusual illness, and the Human Rights Code (paragraph 4(1) specifically prohibits discrimination because of *handicap*).

Furthermore, under paragraph 16(1)(1a) Employers are required "to accommodate handicapped employees unless "the needs of the person cannot be accommodated without undue hardship on the person responsible for accommodating those needs, considering the costs, outside sources of funding, if any, and health and safety requirements, if any."

When, as we have seen, Ms. Martel's attempts, with some assistance from her union, had been frustrated by an adamant Board, she had decided to ask the Ontario Human Rights Commission to intercede on her behalf. On February 1, 1993, Diane filed the necessary "Intake Questionnaire", supported by a five page summary of her situation, prepared for her by OECTA. Her 'intake' officer was a Mr. Gilles Lepalme of the Commission who asked all parties to attend a preliminary discussion of the case. At first, the Board representative, Simon Ouellet, (Manager, Human Resources) indicated that he did not plan to attend the meeting!

Mr. Lepalme suggested that such a no-show would reflect poorly upon the Board and would be seen as evidence that the employer was indeed, not willing to work towards the accommodation of the handicapped employee.[2]

The meeting did not get off to an auspicious start since Mr. Ouellet at first denied any need for the Board to accommodate Ms. Martel. He was challenged on this point by union representative, Robert Kirwan and after much "shouting and anger" [3] he agreed that the Board would, indeed, have to accommodate her under the existing legislation.

What struck me as I reviewed the records of this

meeting and the previous correspondence was an apparent inability to treat Ms. Martel as a handicapped employee who should be extended sympathy and should be used in a manner which respected her dignity. Instead, the Board's representatives from Director Robert Hammond on down, seemed to feel that they were engaged in some kind of conflict with Ms. Martel and that they had to fight her every inch of the way.

Why would that be? I puzzled. It would only become evident over the next few months that their attitude as an employer seemed to be the rule and not the exception when dealing with an employee who was the victim of this strange new disease… chronic fatigue syndrome.

When Mr. Ouelette was reconciled to the fact that the Board had to accommodate the handicapped employee, the discussion turned to just what nature such accommodation should take. At this point the union representative produced a carefully thought out plan which was geared to the needs of the employee and which looked forward to helping her return to health. The Board countered with a rigid plan which would "set goals" for the employee "to attain".

Again, as I read over the file, I was mind boggled. How does a bureaucrat set goals for a sick employee to attain? It reminded me of Professor Frank Scott's lines about teachers who:
Make laws for averages and plans for means,
Print one history book for a whole province, and
Let ninety thousand reach page 10 by Tuesday…"[4]

In order to reach an agreement, Ms. Martel, with the encouragement of her union representative, accepted the Board's lock-step plan. At the time, she felt that her union help was not sufficiently assertive, but since it was the only help she had, she felt compelled to accept less than she believed she needed to recuperate. She returned to the classroom "very discouraged and overwhelmed by the fatigue." She barely made it to the end of June, when the summer break gave her a chance to recreate herself. But the psychological warfare against her by the Board continued.

At the beginning of June, and despite the accord previously worked out, Mr. Ouellet's secretary 'phoned her to advise that she was being offered a fifty percent teaching job at two schools several miles apart for the next teaching year!

This was exactly what the Board had originally asked her to accept. Now, after going through the 'Human Relations Code' hoops, and with Ms. Martel again on her own, they were asking her to go back to square one. So much for good faith bargaining. Despite her fatigue and emotional stress, Diane Martel said 'No'. She was sick, but she still had heart.

Then in August she received a 'phone call from Mr. Ouellet, himself. During this conversation he repeatedly asked her to 'skip' over stage four of their lock-step plan and go immediately to a seventy-five percent teaching day. He suggested that if she didn't accept this proposal, she would be removed from the recall list and some other teacher would get the job. He gave her time to 'think over' this Hobson's choice.

The intimidation and uncertainty seemed to aggravate Diane's physical condition. She went back to her doctor who referred her to a cardiologist, who in turn diagnosed 'anginal pectoris' and prescribed nitroglycerine, cardizem, and coated aspirin. At this point her doctor suggested that she revert to the Board's Stage One. In response Mr. Ouellet advised that their 'agreement' did not call for a 'regression of stages.' No hint of concern that he was dealing with a sick human being who did not fit his arbitrary template.

It was shortly afterwards that Ouellet 'phoned to tell Ms. Martel to stay at home until the Board had secured a 'second medical opinion' from a doctor whom they would select. They had never, in fact, bothered to request a *first* opinion, nor had they ever asked Diane's doctor for even a summary of her condition. It seems that there was something about the diagnosis of 'chronic fatigue syndrome' that made such careful and considerate research unnecessary before they took any position in respect to Ms. Martel's health and her job assignments.

After waiting for over a month for Mr. Ouellet to arrange for his 'second' opinion, Ms. Martel, as we noted earlier, 'phoned the Board to enquire about the delay. It was at this point that Robert Hammond, again without any apparent regard for the agreement worked out in February, 1993, ordered her to be 'back in the classroom' the very next morning! Let Ms. Martel tell of her reaction in her own words:

"I (had) expected to have some notice for my re-entry, and I therefore requested a two day notice… The Board refused, stating that I was to be in the classroom the very next morning. This entire episode was highly abusive and placed me into a severe stress level. I returned to work on Tuesday, October 26, 1993 with difficulty. I experienced chest pain, dizziness, and nausea at the school several times, to the point of being hospitalized at Memorial Hospital twice on December 24, 1993 for three days and again on December 31, 1993 for three days…"[5]

At this point Ms. Martel returned to the Human Rights Commission and asked that her case be reactivated. Then a funny thing happened on the way to a Human Rights 'Ruling'.

On December 5, 1994, almost a full year after her first request, the Human Rights Commission wrote to Ms. Martel that her up-dated complaint was being "referred to the Commission for a decision." In the next paragraph was a puzzling reference to the Section 34(1)(a) of the Human Rights Code, 1981…for that Section dealt with the right of the Commission *NOT* to deal with a complaint! The letter was accompanied by a "Case Analysis" by none other than the previously noted Gilles Lepalme, and in his 'analysis' Mr. Lepalme made the startling observation that Ms. Martel could have dealt with her problems under the Ontario Labour Relations Act. This despite the fact that under the Contract Agreement between OECTA and the Board there was no provision for grieving any discrimination based upon health.

Then, as if to emphasize their rather strange conclusion, and in the face of all the evidence that Ms. Martel's human rights had been sorely abused by the Sudbury Separate School Board, a repeat of the same letter (this time dated January 26, 1995) was again sent to Ms. Martel!

Just what was going on here? And, perhaps more to the point, why was it going on? Here is a case where an employee is handicapped by a disease…admittedly an ill-understood disease …and yet this sick employee is denied her employer's legislated assistance , and who when she turns to the Human Rights Commission for the assistance the legislation was designed to provide, she is told over a year later that she should have been seeking help under other legislation altogether!

If the Human Rights Commission knew this over a year before, why had they not told Ms. Martel at the outset…grieve your treatment under the Labour Relations Act?

And if the Board knew this over a year before, why not, at the outset say to the Human Rights Commission… this complaint should be grieved under the terms of the Collective Agreement?

Instead, both parties participate in a fraudulent charade playing a mean-spirited game with an employee who is ill. And under the terms of their charade they come up with a one-sided accommodation which the employer then begins almost at once, to short-cut and circumvent. And, finally when the complainant goes back to the Human Rights Commission, their intake person at this late point (January, 1995) does a so-called 'Case Analysis' and suggests : "scrub the past two years of agony and abuse and start off all over again under other legislation!"

Human rights?

Then something happened which made it all clear… it turned out that there had been an informal, off-the-cuff agreement after Ms. Martel had reactivated her complaint to the Human Rights Commission which showed that Mr. Gilles Lapalme of the Human Rights Commission and Mr. Simon Ouellet of the Sudbury Separate School Board had agreed upon a course of action *before* Mr. Lapalme's "Case Analysis" dated December 5, 1994! Upon a careful review of the files I came upon a letter dated *November 22, 1994*…two weeks before the case analysis…from Mr. Ouellet to Mr. Lapalme. Here is what he wrote:

"*Re: Diane Martel.*
*As **discussed with you recently** (emphasis added), this will confirm that the Sudbury District RCSS Board, pursuant to Section 34(1)(a) of the Code, respectfully requests that the Commission not proceed with this matter. As you no doubt recall, this matter has been dealt with through the various means of the Collective Agreement…*"
Oh!

"Discussed recently…"? Who was at the meeting? Was the complainant notified or invited? Was the union representative notified or invited? Are private meetings conducted which deal with a human right of an individual without that individual even knowing about it?

One of the important qualities required in the administration of justice at any level is due process. That is, no party to a judicial process can surreptitiously approach any officer of the system and privately 'discuss' another party's rights or evidence or any other aspect of the "Case" without proper notification, record keeping, application of rules of evidence, and proper standards of testimony verification. Yet here there is evidence that one of the parties had discussed "Diane Martel" with the person charged with making a Case Analysis.

What was said? Was it true? Who were the witnesses? Were they sworn?

Who knows?

Then Mr. Ouellet writes: "…this matter has been dealt with through the various means of the Collective Agreement."

What?

Who 'dealt' with it? Under which Collective Agreement? Was the grievance settled? When? Under what terms? Was there an appeal to an arbitrator? If so, who was he, and when was the hearing?

Again, who knows?

Whatever the answers are to the above questions, we do know that two weeks later Mr. Lapalme was inspired to recommend a course of action to the Human Rights Commission which , to no one's great surprise, accepted Mr. Simon Ouellet's argument in its entirety.

At this point it is necessary to consider just what Mr. Lapalme in his Case Analysis declares to be fact and to compare this with the appropriate contracts, Acts, etc.

On page two of his Analysis Mr. Lapalme writes that the "above Act contains a grievance procedure which allows an employee to complain about any difference arising out of the interpretation, application, administration or alleged violation of the (collective) agreement (between the employer and the union) and the said Act.

This observation was totally irrelevant to Ms. Martel's situation, since the Collective Agreement under which she was employed provided for a 'Grievance Procedure' with a 'grievance' being defined as "any difference" in respect to "this agreement" and *there is nothing in that agreement about discrimination against an employee who is handicapped*. Since there were no grounds under the agreement for grieving, there was no violation of the agreement and no difference between the agreement and the Act.

Thus, since the Collective Agreement was silent upon the subject, and since the union and the employees looked to the Board to treat its employees in a manner which was respectful of their dignity as human beings, when that level of human rights was not observed the only recourse was through the Human Rights Commission.

There were other equally specious arguments in the Case Analysis that do not merit review. It is sufficient to state that Mr. Lapalme does not indicate anywhere in his presentation to the Commission that he has asked for or received any kind of witnessed report upon how the Board had fulfilled their original lock-step accommodation of Ms. Martel. There is nothing about the rude and harassing directions to be 'in the classroom tomorrow morning' or to 'report to Mr. Hammond's office at 8:30 Monday ' or requests to 'skip Step Three".

All Mr. Lapalme seemed able to come up with was a course of action suggested to him in a private and off-the-record conversation with the respondent.

The recommendation of Mr. Lapalme was accepted by the Commission which, over the signature of "Rosemary Brown", and dated "April 12, 1995" decided not to deal with the case. Ms. Brown, who had been appointed to her office by the New Democratic Party Government, appears to have looked no further than Mr. Lapalme's superficial and inaccurate assessment of Ms. Martel's situation and the manner in which she, as an ill and handicapped employee, had been treated by her employee.

It is perhaps appropriate to note at this point that the said New Democratic Party had long touted the fact that it stood for (among other things) human rights, labour rights, women's rights, prisoners' rights, etc.

It should also be noted that no where in Mr. Lapalme's Analysis is there mention of the fact that at the very time the Board was telling Ms. Martel that she could not work a fifty percent day on fifty percent pay, while getting a half day's pay from her insurance carrier, there were two employees of the same Board currently receiving that accommodation.

When the Commission sent Ms. Martel their ruling, they advised her that she had 15 days to make an application for reconsideration. Such a narrow time frame seems ironic in view of the fact that it had taken the Ontario Human Rights Commission almost 26 months to tell a sick employee that she should begin all over again under other legislation.

Within her window of opportunity, Ms. Martel wrote to the Commission on May 2, 1995 and formally requested a reconsideration of her case. At the time she did so she took the occasion to ask Mr. Lapalme why, if she should have made her case under the provisions cited he had not told her so at the outset. He replied that it had just been "within the past year" that the Human Rights Commission had been advised by some policy maker that they were to turn back as many cases as possible to the union-management grievance route as possible.

In other words, when the game is about half way along, it is time to change the rules!

On August 7, 1995 Ms. Martel was informed that the Commission had reconsidered her case and that the original decision not to deal with it would stand. When Diane persisted in her efforts she received another letter dated November 10, 1995 which stated flatly: "This decision is final and can not be further appealed."

So much for the way one handicapped employee was treated by a Human Rights Commission...one of whose officers felt it appropriate to 'discuss' a complainant with the respondent without the knowledge of that complainant. What did they talk about? Was it, perhaps, her illness, chronic fatigue syndrome? We don't know because the meeting was a private *tête-à-tête*. No one mentioned the nature of Diane Martel's illness... at least not on paper and not up to this point...but that was to change...when the Provincial Office of the Ontario English Catholic Teachers' Federation came into the case.

There Are Too Many Cases Of Chronic Fatigue
Robert Kirwan

Robert (Bob) Kirwan is a dedicated professional teacher. Not only is he committed to the best he can achieve in his classroom, he is also dedicated to the view that, as teachers, his colleagues are professional people who warrant respect from the school boards who hire them on behalf of the parents whose children are being taught. Because of his high professional standards which he believes can be achieved only by a partnership between the teachers and the board, Mr. Kirwan has for several years accepted election to various union offices so that he can make sure that the teachers receive the kind of professional representation that the board must recognize and work with. Mr. Kirwan is enough of a student of the history of teaching in Ontario to know that far too often boards of education have been dominated by persons who see themselves as 'bosses' and the teachers as 'workers'.

This master-servant attitude if allowed to manifest itself without any checks and balances reflects a lack of respect by many board members for the teachers which soon becomes internalized by the teachers themselves. And too often teachers promoted through the system to positions of authority are those who accept the boards' attitude and utilize it themselves in their dealings with their teaching col-

leagues. Thus, rather than being seen by their administration and boards as respected professionals who are to be consulted and honoured, the teachers are seen and treated as pawns to be moved as, when and where the 'boss' determines. Bob Kirwan is determined that such an attitude will not have its unchallenged way within the jurisdiction where he teaches.

Robert Kirwan was the elected President of the Sudbury OECTA Elementary Unit when Ms. Martel began experiencing the first symptoms of chronic fatigue syndrome. As with many other persons at the time he knew very little about the disease. All he needed to know was that a fellow professional whom he represented was ill and that this fellow professional was not being treated by the employing Sudbury District Roman Catholic Separate School Board with the dignity a human being warrants. When Diane brought her situation to him he agreed to assist her in any way that he could. As it was to turn out, he was the only professional in this whole affair who afforded Ms. Martel the respect a sick and handicapped professional deserves.

There were times over the four years of struggle that Ms. Martel and Mr. Kirwan had their differences. Such was to be expected for two reasons. First, almost without exception, everyone with whom Ms. Martel came in contact during her ordeal used her in a mean and disrespectful way. We have seen how Hammond and Ouellet treated her. And we have examined what happened when the professional 'defenders' of human rights took her case. We haven't yet noted how many others responded to her when she said "I am ill with chronic fatigue." There was , for example, a doctor to whom she was referred. After his initial examination he said to her that essentially, it was " all in your head"...whatever that means...She protested to him that she was ill; that she could not get through an ordinary day's work.

He remained adamant, but Diane persisted. Finally, at her expense, he ordered a variety of tests which it turned out revealed no abnormalities in her blood or tissue that would account for her condition. It was to be several months later that I was to learn why such negative results occur in such traditional tests; but, like me, the doctor didn't know what was evading him, and he said to her with a tightly controlled anger in his voice," For all the trouble you put our lab to I'm going to charge you $75 to $100."

Such an attitude, I came to know, was not the exception, it was generally the rule.

Another reason that led to a certain level of stress between Ms. Martel and Mr. Kirwan was the fact that although Bob responded to Diane in a humane and supportive way, he had little or no support from the central offices of OECTA. All he could do was give her his help at the local level. He knew from his contacts with the central office that little or no official union sympathy went out to victims of CFIDS. Thus, Ms. Martel was left to pay for extra medical file reports and for any legal advice she sought.

Finally, Diane told Bob that she would personally approach the central office and insist that they give her more help. Bob Kirwan yielded to his frustration, for not only had he been working very hard for her, he had at the same time been trying to cope with the Board which at one point on another matter set out to sue him for a variety of real or imagined reasons. He gave her OECTA's Toronto phone number and said "Good luck." It was only a few days later that each of these professional people came independently to the conclusion that they had been understandably impatient with the other and they exchanged apologies. But Diane's struggle with the brass at OECTA was just beginning.

Diane Martel usually tried to keep an accurate record of her experiences, and when she decided to deal directly with OECTA in Toronto, she kept notes of what followed. These notes capture the essence of events better than any comment I could compose from them, so they are set out in full below.

NOTES
As kept by Diane Martel

April ?/95 I got upset with Bob (Kirwan) regarding his negative attitude towards my case and he said that if I wasn't happy with the help or service he had given me that I should deal directly with Toronto OECTA.

I thought about what he had said and decided (after also consulting with my lawyer, Steve Horton) to call OECTA in Toronto.

I asked to speak to Claire Ross, the president. I told him of my desperate situation and he suggested that I call OECTA back and ask for 'Pat'. When I called back Pat was off sick and I explained the situation (somewhat) to his secretary. She said that Pat could be off for a time and that she would have Ed Alexander call me.

Ed called me and told me to courier everything down to his office. He said that he would be talking to union lawyers regarding my case, on Friday, May 5/95 & that I should call him back (to try all day if I had difficulty reaching him.)

Ed told me that he's extremely busy also that unless there's a 50-50 chance of winning my case, he wouldn't be able to convince the provincial executive to fight for me, legally.

We have 2 issues:
  1) disability case
  2) discrimination case.

I called Clare (sic) Ross president OECTA for the 2nd time after talking to Ed—the same day I think.

I told him that I wasn't pleased with the way Ed seem to be handling my case and that his attitude seemed negative & not helpful. I told him that I was upset that the meeting date of May 5/95 between Ed & the union lawyers was moved up to Monday, May 1/95 and that Ed said he wanted to get everything wrapped up when he would come to Sudbury on May 31/95. (Ed had said that he had 3 people to meet that day)

I told Clare Ross that Ed said the most the union may be able to offer me would be career counselling…

My lawyer Steve Horton suggested I take a nice break, go down to Toronto, see theatre & have dinner, and arrange to be present when Ed would meet with the union lawyer. Comment (I don't know where Steve thought I would get the money to do all this.)

I have a friend who was willing to drive me down to Toronto for this meeting.

I left a message with Ed's secretary, Janet, requesting to be present at the meeting between Ed & OECTA lawyers on Friday/May 5/95.

Ed called on Thursday April 27/95 at 2:32 & left a message on my machine.

This is verbatim:
"Diane, it's Ed Alexander returning your call. I will be talking to our lawyers now on Monday May 1/95 and I will get back to you after I meet with the lawyers. We need to do some preliminaries before we can take any other consideration for meetings & that kind of thing. So I'll get back to you after the meeting on Monday."

I told Clare Ross, that was not what I was looking for, "what I want is…*Fair Union Representation.*" I re-iterated my desperate financial situation.

Mr. Ross said that he would go to Mr. Alexander's office immediately to discuss my situation & that he would call me back.

Clare Ross called me back & said that Ed had my whole file and that I should go ahead and meet with him on May 31/95 and that I should call him & tell him this. He also said that a very competent young person was replacing Ed, in June, upon Ed's retirement.

Summary
Meeting With Ed Alexander & Bob Kirwan
May 31/ 95 2:30 p.m.
OECTA Barrydowne office (Sudbury)

Ed: I have a quite a big file on you. I haven't read it over lately. So tell me Diane, what's happening with you at this time?

Diane: Bob, haven't you told Ed about the job offer from Ritari Travel, as we discussed last week?

Bob: Yes I just briefly went over what was happening to you.

Diane: Well, Ed, I'm facing starvation & bankruptcy, and have therefore, been put in the position of having to take this job. {1}

Bob: (to Ed) What would you like in your coffee?

Ed: I want it straight, just like I drink my rye straight.

Diane: I explained my job offer to Ed & situation I was in.

Ed: Talked on about how there were too many cases of chronic fatigue and that the problem with having CFIDS accepted by insurance companies was due to the lack of objective medical evidence, in the medical world as to the causes of CFIDS, and referred to a particular doctor (I can't remember his name) who claims that CFIDS is a mental disorder. He said this physician is used by a lot of insurance companies to refute such claims as mine. He went on to say that in order for CFIDS to be accepted, the Atlanta Control Centre for Disease , guidelines had to apply.

Comment: Ed had obviously not read the medical report from Dr. McFarthing, which definitely referred to the Atlanta Guidelines.

Diane: I have read some material on chronic fatigue and the articles indicate that chronic fatigue or fibromyalgia are caused by a virus. Often, a traumatic event or surgery can trigger the onset of these diseases. My body has not been well especially so, after having the angiogram on my heart.

Ed: There is NO use in bringing your case before provincial executive. Your case isn't strong enough. I consulted our lawyer and he felt that, seeing as though you already had a lawyer fighting for the appeal, another lawyer would not bring about an acceptance of your claim. Your appeal will once again be denied, so there is no use appealing again.

(See letter from Ed Alexander dated May 4/95, telling me to contact Bob Kirwan to begin the appeal. I called Bob and he said that we would have to wait until May 31/95 until Ed came up to Sudbury and that we would all sit down together and talk about *Disability & Human Rights Case.*

Ed, obviously changed his mind about the appeal between May 4/95 - May 31/95.

I waited for an entire month and then- to be told there's really nothing we can do for you- you should take this new job offer.

Diane: Ed, I insist that the union appeal my disability claim with Great-West Life. I sent all the photocopied material, + all the lawyers letters to Great-West Life & the responses, the Human Rights Correspondence, the doctor's reports, and I just paid $60.00 to Dr. Franklyn for my entire medical file, as requested by Great West Life in their last letter of correspondence. I want the union to submit this additional medical information, along with my latest medical report from Dr. McFarthing & Dr. Lafreniere. The least the union can do is to submit an appeal on my behalf.

Ed: O.K. Bob, you can submit the additional information (reports) from your office. But I have to make it clear, we (union) will not be providing you with our lawyer.

Bob: Wouldn't it be better ,Ed, if it was submitted from the provincial office? It might have more clout.

Ed: Alright, we can draft a letter, with OECTA letterhead & basically just submit the additional information requested by Great West Life.

Note: I met with Bob, about 1 week before meeting with Bob & Ed, & brought in photocopies of pertinent information, updated medical reports from Dr. Lafreniere & Dr. McFarthing, plus the most recent copy of the letter from Great-West Life (as a result of my personal letter of appeal).

Ed obviously had not been faxed or made aware by Bob before our meeting this additional information re: my personal letter of appeal, the response & the recent medical reports

Ed: talked on about how teaching had changed and that a person needed to be quote "STRONG" to remain in the teaching profession today. He said that I returned to a job that I was basically not suited for.

Diane: I taught for the Board for 5 years prior to working at Air Canada and I was a successful teacher. What has made it difficult to succeed in this career now, was the Board's unfair treatment.

Ed: Went on to talk about how teaching was so demanding and didn't involve teaching but dealing with opposing parents etc. (sic). A person had to be strong to handle everything.

He talked about his wife, being out of teaching for a long period of time, while she was raising their children, and that she then, returned to do supply teaching. He said she would come home wiped after 1 day of supply teaching, looking like many teachers who have the June (end of year) exhausted.

To Ed and Bob: I apologize for my severe reactions at times, throughout this mess. I have felt as though the union weren't representing me, at times, and I came to the point of not trusting in you (both) helping me out. I need to trust that you are on my side, because there's no one else to represent me.

Bob: We understand it's difficult and we're not walking in your shoes.

Ed: We're used to taking flack from the members. It goes with the job.

Diane (to Ed) When Ed said that my appeal was not accepted due to the lack of objective medical evidence, I pointed out to him that GW Life's refusal was based more on the fact, that I was on a rehabilation (sic)program with the school board and that GW Life claims that I was performing 60% of my original duties, and therefore was not considered disabled. *Showing Again*...he hadn't read over the documentation thoroughly.

Ed: He went on to say that GW Life's interpretation of a teacher's duties could be quite broad, as outlined in Education Act. Being that I was in the school 100% time they could interpret that all my duties related to being a teacher.

Conclusion

-Ed Alexander agreed to bring the additional medical information , back to Toronto, and to submit it on Wednesday June 7/95 (date) when he would be returning to his office.

-that I was presently on a leave of absence without pay, and that I could start the job on June 5. When my appeal (decision) came through ...if it was not accepted...(as he once again said that he did not ex-

pect that a positive decision would be rendered), at that time , Bob would apply for a leave of absence for a period of one year, giving me a one year leeway, just in case I wanted to go back to teaching. He said: "You probably won't want to return, but just as an added protection, we should apply for the leave.

Re: Human Rights Case Meeting with Ed Alexander, Bob, Myself —31 May/ 95

Ed: As far as the Human Rights case goes, the story goes on. It's not a case of sexual or racial discrimination; it's not as clear cut, although there's a certain amount ? ? (can't remember what he said) Whether or not the union should give you representation on this one- was debatable.

Diane: I have had several well-educated, professional people read over my case, and they all feel it is a clear cut case of discrimination. I will definitely ask for the union to represent me with their lawyer, in this instance.

Ed: Went on to explain the Human Rights & Grievance Procedure—often Human Rights put it back to the union.

Bob: But we don't have a discrimination clause in our contract.

Ed: recommended that Bob himself respond to the letter from Human Rights Commission (regarding my request for reconsideration) before the 15 day period was up.

End of Ms. Martel's notes

It was about this time that Diane Martel phoned me, and we arranged to meet on June 10, 1995 as I have already summarized.

When I finished my reading, re-reading, and telephone calls to Bob Kirwan and one or two to OECTA in Toronto, I drafted and sent the letters I have cited to the Sudbury Board and got their brush-off reply. I also sent a letter to the Human Rights Commission citing the further inconsistencies also cited above. Again I received the pro-forma brush-off.

It was clear that Diane Martel had been bullied and abused by her employer and they didn't much care how their actions looked to me. It was also clear that the officer for the Human Rights Commission who was charged with the task of interviewing Ms. Martel and taking appropriate action had at the very least, been superficial and, from the correspondence between him and the respondent in the case, it appeared that he had connived to limit Ms. Martel's request for help under the Code.

On my third review of the case I focussed on the role of the union (OECTA) and sought to match that role against the claims made by her employer about her being represented at all times by her union, and the decision of Mr. Lapalme to accept this argument as grounds for *NOT* hearing her complaint.

As I again leafed through the files I felt fatigued and frustrated. With the exception of Bob Kirwan, no one in a professional capacity (encountered to this point) had treated Ms. Martel as a sick and handicapped employee. Why was that? Answers to this question began to show forth in the statements made by Ed Alexander. He could make such statements on the record because he was "on her side!" He could preface them by saying things like: "Well, people say" or "Well, the insurance companies feel". He, of course, didn't harbour such abusive thoughts himself! But the actions he took or failed to take, suggested that Ms. Martel's union had basically abandoned her when she came down with chronic fatigue syndrome.

It is appropriate at this point to examine some of those actions.

"...unless there's a 50-50 chance of winning my case, he wouldn't be able to convince the provincial executive to fight for me, legally."

Such a statement raises the question: does one launch an action for justice in a case of discrimination because one has a chance to win, or does one launch such a suit because one has been discriminated against?

"I will be talking to our lawyer now on Monday, May 1/95..."

When this change was made, it was after Ms. Martel had made arrangements to get a ride to Toronto so that she could participate in her own case. The change was not explained by Mr. Alexander, and one can only wonder whether it was made in order to keep Ms. Martel from the discussion? Certainly, Mr. Ouellet and Mr. Lapalme had apparently found it convenient to discuss her case without any chance for her to participate.

"I have quite a big file on you. I haven't read it over lately. So, tell me, Diane, what's happening with you at this time."

What a superficial way to commence a meeting with a sick employee whom you and your organization (OECTA) are supposed to be representing!

"...there are too many cases of chronic fatigue."

Can anyone imagine a professional person saying "There are too many accidents on the job, so we are giving up on trying to solve the problems that cause them"?

If there are "too may cases of chronic fatigue" then there must be an epidemic...and when there is an epidemic it is the responsibility of everyone in a civilized society to do his upmost to stop that epidemic...not to wash one's hands of any role he might play.

"...a person needed to be *strong* to remain in teaching."

How *strong* was a *sick employee* expected to be?

"The union will not pay for your lawyer".

How can this be rationalized with Mr. Lapalme's December 5, 1994 claim that Ms. Martel was " always well represented by a union agent"?

My next letter was to the Ontario English Catholic Teachers' Federation, and the final results are still pending. However, before I reviewed the outcome of these and related actions, I had felt the need to study this illness called chronic fatigue syndrome, and try to understand why its victims were to such a great extent, bullied, harassed, intimidated, and often ridiculed.

I was to find that this type of treatment was not a random or isolated response. It was the response most victim's received. And, I was to learn, it was an attitude carefully devised and propagated by significant groups whose best interests were better served by silence or lies than by telling the terrible truth about chronic fatigue syndrome. My novitiate had just begun.

Summary

Diane Martel came to me in early 1995. She needed help from someone because although she was sick and disabled from doing her job as a teacher, she was being bullied and harassed by her employer; treated superficially by the Human Rights Commission and largely ignored by her union, OECTA. My review of her heavy files bore out her claim of being discriminated against and of being unfairly dismissed by agencies that should help her.

But the way she had been used right across the board raised another general question of great significance: Why were people, ill with chronic fatigue syndrome, treated as if they were malingerers and unworthy of the help that is normally afforded to ill persons? What I was to learn made it essential that I tell Diane's story, not just for her sake, but for the hundreds of thousands of other victims of CFIDS, and of other victims about whom I had no inkling when I began my research.

FOOTNOTES

{1} Ms. Martel had no desire to avoid work. Her concern was that she was a trained professional who was not being treated in a humane and sensitive manner by an employer. The job offer at the travel agency gave her parttime work on flexible hours with an understanding employer. Although she needed the money, she did not want to compromise her perceived justified right to proper treatment from her employer and her union.

ENDNOTES

[1] Letter of March 8, 1993, in author's files.
[2] "Human Rights Complaint", a summary prepared by the Complainant, Ms. Martel and given to the author. p.5
[3] *Ibid*, p.5
[4] "The Examiner" Frank Scott in *Poems Worth Knowing*, Eds. Claude E. Lewis and John Bennett (Toronto: The Copp Clark Publishing Co. Ltd. 1958) p.114
[5] Ms. Martel's Summary, *supra* 10

CHAPTER TWO

OSLER'S WEB

"But a handful of more senior medical investigators, whose expertise bound them together in what amounted to a kind of secret fraternity, were amply aware of previous outbreaks of illnesses that seemed to presage the Lake Tahoe disease."
Hilary Johnson: *Osler's Web*, p. 196.

When I met Diane Martel and learned her story about a mystery illness with a protean range of symptoms and about the abuse she had to endure at the hands of her employer, her union, her insurance company, I had only a vague memory of the June, 1994 judgement that had been delivered by The Honourable Madam Justice B.J. Rawlins of the Alberta Court of Queen's Bench. [See Chapter Eight: "When I'm sick, call a historian."]

Justice Rawlins had determined that fibromyalgia did not exist as a physical condition but was a 'personality disorder'. Shades of Robert Hammond and Ed Alexander!

At the time that I had briefly noted the media reports of Madam Justice Rawlins' decision, I had no idea what fibromyalgia was and I had no idea that it is a variant of Diane Martel's chronic fatigue syndrome. However, a little over one year later, after several hours of interviews with Diane, and after reading her thick files, and after dealing with her employer, her union, her insurance company, I went back to Rawlins 'Reasons for Judgment'[1].

Rawlins 'Reasons' were supported by 'authorities' so I turned to them to see how the Justice could possibly conclude that fibromyalgia/ CFS did not exist. From this exercise I was to learn much about where Diane Martel's bullies and bureaucrats had come from. A trail was beginning to emerge in the under growth that could be traced back from Rawlins to a person named Edward Shorter of the University of Toronto, and from Shorter back to a doctor Stephen Straus of the National Institutes for Health in the United States. And, it was also becoming vaguely apparent that there were other trails that suggested where this 'mystery disease' and other equally mysterious diseases had their roots.

Justice Rawlins had based her decision that 'fibromyalgia does not exist' upon a book by the above mentioned Edward Shorter titled *From Paralysis to Fatigue*.[2] I bought the book and read it carefully. Shorter's theme was that chronic fatigue syndrome and fibromyalgia were not physical diseases but were imaginary diseases conjured up in the minds of those people (mostly women) who could not cope with the stress of modern life. Such a theme was dramatically at odds with the symptoms presented by Diane Martel and I arranged an interview with Dr. Shorter upon which we report in Chapter Eight.

It was about this point in time that I came upon a magnificent book by Hillary Johnson: *Osler's Web*.[3] I have since come to the conclusion that *Osler's Web* is one of the most important books ever written! This sounds like pure hyperbole, but I mean what I have said, and as we follow the ill-defined trails I have mentioned above, using Johnson's masterpiece as our guide, I trust that you will come to recognize the justice of my claim. In *Osler's Web* Johnson takes us, as her sub-title puts it, "Inside the Labyrinth of the Chronic Fatigue Syndrome Epidemic". A labyrinth marked by intrigue, double-dealing, secrecy, and misrepresentation. Elements that I had seen in the way Diane Martel had been treated and which are elements of Dr. Shorter's rant.

A hint of what *Osler's Web* reveals is to be found right from the beginning in Ms. Johnson's "Acknowledgments" where we learn that she received some funding from the Fund for Investigative Journalism in Washington, D.C. There is a clear distinction to be made between researching the source of a disease and investigating that disease. Ms. Johnson was well aware of that difference.

We also learn from her "Acknowledgments" that in the course of investigating her subject, she had to resort to the Freedom of Information Act, and that the Public Health Agencies, CDC and NIH were far from forthcoming in these efforts. What did these Agencies have to hide? Why did the Public Health Agencies resist responding to this new disease in an open and honest manner?

The significance of this resistance must be emphasized for the CDC and the NIH are agencies of government, yet by refusing to reveal evidence in their possession to affected citizens, they are attempting to circumvent the laws of the nation made by the representatives of the people of that nation.

Ms. Johnson was not asking for nuclear secrets protected in the interests of national security. She was asking for information about an emerging disease to which more and more citizens were succumbing. What was there about chronic fatigue syndrome that made several top government functionaries struggle so hard to keep hidden?

Ms. Johnson does not speculate as to what the reason for their resistance to public scrutiny might be. All she does in over 700 pages of carefully marshalled details is set out the history of CFS from 1984 to 1994 in 'prose of reportorial calm.'

The answer to the mystery of new and unusual diseases such as CFS and to the equally mysterious official government agency deceit was to emerge slowly for this writer over the years since that day in June, 1995, when Diane Martel phoned me. And the answer to the mystery of why employers, unions, insurance companies and others were so cruel to those afflicted by one of these new diseases was also to emerge.

A Decade Of Deceit: 1984 To 1994

Hillary Johnson begins her study of chronic fatigue syndrome with the year 1984, in San Francisco, California. In that city over the preceding eighteen months, Dr. Carol Jessop had treated fifteen patients with a similar array of symptoms that resemble those which Diane Martel described in 1995: fatigue, nausea, depression, myalgias, headaches.

In her review of these patients and their symptoms, Dr. Jessop saw hints that suggested lupus, rheumatism, multiple sclerosis, and even some signs that brought to mind another new mystery disease first officially diagnosed just three years before: acquired immunodeficiency syndrome…AIDS.

But, no one of these diseases could be totally diagnosed in any one patient. Each patient seemed to have his or her own particular spectrum of symptoms, and none seemed to demonstrate by the usual blood and tissue tests, a specific disease.

From San Francisco Johnson pans to places in Nevada, North Carolina, Florida and even Toulouse, France. In all of these places and others the same protean range of signs and symptoms was disabling previously healthy people. And other factors were already being spotted.

Among these factors was the 'psychobabble' theme which Diane Martel had found in William Hammond and Ed Alexander: it was a syndrome of 'neurotic women' who couldn't cope with stress!

Another factor kept coming up for consideration: AIDS. Jessop had consulted with early AIDS researcher, Jay Levy of the University of California's medical school. But Levy declined to help her…he was too busy with the AIDS cases that he was studying.

Then Johnson reports upon another high level researcher who dismissed the new mystery disease: Dr. Thomas Merigan of Stanford University Medical Center. Merigan, at the request of Dr. Herbert Tanney, had examined well-known motion picture director, Blake Edwards who was ill and who presented with the symptoms noted above. Merigan reported to Tanney that Edwards had mononucleosis.

But, I was later to learn, there was more to Thomas Merigan and his research than met the eye in 1984. It was later to be revealed that ten years before the outbreak of AIDS and its 'mirror image', CFIDS, Thomas C. Merigan with David A. Stevens had delivered a report for the American Association of Immunologists on April 15, 1971 titled "Viral infections in man associated with *A*cquired *I*mmunological *D*eficiency *S*tates.[4] [Emphasis added] The final four words of that title form the acronym *AIDS* used ten years before the first official case of that disease!

Adding to the mystery of such a coincidence is the fact that the work by Merigan and Stevens had been funded by none other than a Public Health Service Grant A1-05629. The very people who, as Johnson has revealed, later resisted responding to the new epidemic with a scientific and serious study.

Just what was going on here?

On the one hand there were the Public Health Agencies and their 'media asset' Dr. Edward Shorter, who were refusing to respond to the disease and who were mocking its victims; and, on the other hand there were the obviously disabled victims and Hillary Johnson's objective account of the nature of the disease.

In my own experience there was Diane Martel, a tragically ill lady whose symptoms matched those of the victims brought vividly to life by Johnson and whose treatment by her employer, her union, her insurance company, her lawyer and even some of her medical care givers reflected the NIH/CDC 'psychobabble' line and its major spokesman, Edward Shorter.

With the tragic reality of Diane Martel in mind, and while I worked with her to improve her personal situation, I did four things: first, I re-read *Osler's Web* and things that I had missed on my first reading emerged with dramatic significance on the second reading.

Then I did what my university training had taught me to do: I prepared and circulated a six-page survey to some fifty CFIDS/ FM victims. There is no scientific substitute for clear trust-worthy data in dealing with any new problem.

Third, I turned to my files and took out a document sent to me by a friend in the United States some three or more years before. It was titled " Department of Defense Appropriations for 1970; Hearings before a Subcommittee of the Committee on Appropriations–House of Representatives" and it was dated June 9, 1969. Its subject was the U.S. Department of Defense plans to develop two new biological weapons. One weapon would kill its victims by destroying their immune system, and one weapon would disable its victims. [Chapter Four, "June 9, 1969."]

The fourth thing I did was to ask the help of my son William (Bill) Scott to assist me in my research. He agreed and together for the past seven years we have struggled to find the truth about chronic fatigue syndrome [CFIDS] and acquired immunological deficiency states [AIDS] and (as it turned out) other medical mysteries such as fibromyalgia [FM], Gulf War Illnesses [GWI], multiple sclerosis [MS], amytrophic lateral sclerosis [ALS] and several other neuro/systemic degenerative diseases.

What follows is no longer an account of a one-man search for truth, it is a two-man search. Bill's first assignment was to read over my dog-eared and much under-lined copy of Osler's Web and then to study the June 9, 1969 Congressional Hearings.

With Johnson's wealth of detail about CFIDS and our own survey of CFIDS victims as our base, the Congressional Hearings took on a new and startling relevance. As Bill and I discussed the evidence it began to come clear! And one-by-one the mysteries were solved. We learned where CFIDS and AIDS had come from. We learned why Public Health Agencies had sought to disparage CFIDS and why President Ronald Reagan would declare that not one cent of public money would be spent on AIDS. We came to see why Dr. Edward Shorter would write a rant against the tragic victims of CFIDS and how that rant had come to affect Judge Rawlins in Al-

berta and the thinking of Diane Martel's employer in Sudbury.

And we learned why CDC Head, Dr. Brian Mahy, who had misspent and "lost" millions of dollars voted by Congress to investigate CFIDS, has still managed to stay on the government payroll: the government doesn't dare fire him; he knows too much!

YOU WON'T LEARN if YOU DON'T ASK

It was evident from a study of *Osler's Web* that Diane Martel was not alone. There were obviously hundreds of thousands of CFIDS victims in the United States and Canada…and as we were to learn in many other countries. Yet both Bill and I had been under the impression that numerically, Ms. Martel suffered from a relatively insignificant disease. Only when we began telling friends and family about our research were we to learn differently.

As already mentioned, we had the results of our six page survey of CFIDS/ME/FM victims. With the help of a local fibromyalgia support group (with whom Ms. Martel had put us in touch) the survey was sent to about 100 persons diagnosed with CFIDS or ME/FM. Fifty-three completed the survey and returned it to us. It was at this point that we became aware of how close to home CFIDS/ME/FM was.

Some months before, my son Bob had phoned to say that he had experienced chest pains and that the doctor had ordered him to the hospital for some tests. Later he had phoned to say that the doctor had diagnosed "stress" and had put him on tranquillizers. Only when we told him of our research into CFIDS/ME/FM did he say "That's what I have…fibromyalgia"!

About the same time, my daughter-in-law, Debbie, had phoned to give us the results of a visit she had made to her doctor. She, too, had been experiencing pain in her chest and at times her heart had palpitated at an alarming rate. When my wife got off the phone she gave me the report: "Debbie has chronic fatigue syndrome."

Bill and I turned to our fifty-three survey respondents.

Fifty-Three Victims of CFIDS

The first thing that struck us was the disproportionate number of female victims. Four of our respondents were male and forty-nine were female. This corresponded with some results quoted in *Osler's Web*. A survey by Ted Van Zelst[5] reported by Johnson showed a ratio of three females to every one male. Our survey revealed a ratio of twelve to one. The results could well vary due to the small number in our sample (here-after referred to as the 'Scott Survey'). However that may be, there was an obvious gender bias. We were later to discover the apparent basis for this bias[6]

In the Van Zelst survey, over forty percent were between thirty-five and forty-four years of age. In the Scott Survey, the average age of respondents was 48.97 and they had been sick for an average of 6.68 years. In other words, they had become ill on average at the age of 42. In the Van Zelst survey half had been ill less than five years. Of the respondents to the Scott survey, 65.3% reported that their symptoms had become worse with the passage of time, 23% felt that their symptoms had remained the same, while only 11.5% had experienced an easing of symptoms.

At the onset of their illness, 90% of the Scott survey had been working. None was a student, and 10% were at home. The majority, 65.5% were married at the time they became ill, 13.7% were single, 17.24 % divorced and 3% were widowed.

Eighty-eight of the Scott respondents were parents with an average of 2.3 children each.

Before they had become ill, most Scott respondents had regarded themselves as more active than most people their age. They had engaged in sports, danced often, belonged to social or other groups where they often played an active leadership role.

All the respondents to the Scott survey reported that fatigue, unrestored by sleep, was their major symptom. They ranked their other symptoms as follows:

Non-restorative sleep	89.6 %
Aching joints/ muscles	88.0
Forgetfulness	75.8
Mood swings	68.9
Balance problems	65.5
Vision problems	62.0
Numbness	62.0
Headaches	58.6
Light sensitive	55.2
Low grade fever	48.2
Cognitive problems [7]	48.2
Swollen glands	44.8
Disorientation	41.3

At the onset of their symptoms, sixty percent had sought medical help immediately, while the rest waited from three to six months 'hoping it would get better'. When medical advice was sought, over sixty percent of the doctors responded in what was seen to be a 'casual' manner, and many of these suggested that the illness was 'all in your head.' Less than forty percent seemed concerned and of these most ordered tests such as an X-ray or blood test. Only four ordered a magnetic resonance imaging [MRI] scan.

The diagnosis of 'depression' was the one most frequently given (52%) while Epstein-Barr was next with 20%. The other diagnoses ranged from encephalitis, neuromyasthenia, multiple sclerosis, and myalgic encephalomyelitis. Interestingly enough, in contrast with what we were later to read in Dr. Edward Shorter's book [Chapter Eight] not a single doctor diagnosed 'hysteria'.

Ninety-six percent of the respondents worked indoors, and ninety-eight percent recall the air being 'smelly', with a variety of solvents, floor cleaners, machine oil etc, noticeable most of the time. Fifty-nine percent of the victims in the Scott survey knew of someone else who had CFIDS, which is significantly higher than the figure in the Van Zelst sample where 'nearly half' of the respondents knew of someone else with the illness.

Sixty percent of the Scott survey reported that their spouse, family and friends were generally supportive, while their employer usually ranked as 'unsympathetic' or even as hostile.

Most of the people who had to leave work in the Scott survey were denied pension benefits that they would otherwise have received if their diagnosis had been cancer or an obvious injury. Many attributed their denial of benefits to unsympathetic letters from physicians. As a result of the poor response from employers and insurance companies forty-one percent of the victims had suffered a deteriorated financial situation, while in twenty-four percent of the cases the deterioration was 'serious' or 'catastrophic'.

When members of the Scott survey had received a diagnosis of 'fibromyalgia' or of 'chronic fatigue syndrome', most felt relieved to have a name put onto their condition. So many had been told by their initial doctors that "I can't find anything wrong with you" that they had begun to doubt their sanity. However, given that slight margin of relief at being diagnosed at last, sixty-two percent continued to fell depressed because after being diagnosed, they were usually told by their medical care-giver "We can make you more comfortable, but we don't have a cure." Thirty-five percent felt angry at no one in particular, but found it hard to be cheerful in their previous social circles. One fifth of the victims felt 'embarrassed' when asked about their illness. "Chronic fatigue sounded like I was always loafing" was a common complaint.

Nearly one fifth had considered suicide.

Although most of the Scott respondents had never associated their illness with the possible government testing of biological weapons, eighty-five percent had heard that such tests had been or were still being conducted, and that 95% of the human guinea pigs were not volunteers or even knew that they were the objects of a test. The respondents had never thought just who might be the victims of such tests, and none had ever thought that they might have been the targets.

Ninety-eight percent of the Scott survey believed that it was quite possible that such biological testing had resulted in accidents, none could recall any specific incidents.

Unfortunately, only 13.7% had read Osler's Web. However, of those who had read the book, all believed that Dr. Stephen Straus of the National Institutes of Health [NIH] had misused government research funds, had sabotaged private CFIDS research, and was aware of the U.S. Department of Defense testing biological weapons. The respondents also believed that Straus and some of his cohorts had worked to cover-up the real source of their disease, and that he had given leadership in efforts to discredit the victims.

Ninety-eight percent of the Scott respondents want Dr. Stephen Straus charged with fraud and medical malpractice.

Finally, ninety-seven percent of the respondents to the Scott survey want a Royal Commission along the line of the Commission appointed by the Government of Canada to study the safety of the blood supply. [The Krever Commission] Of this group, one hundred percent believe that knowing the truth about the disease and its source will help achieve a cure. The same group expressed shock when advised that the Government of Canada had in 1953 given the U.S. Government permission to spray the City of Winnipeg, Manitoba, in a test of a carcinogenic chemical.

The Scott survey demonstrated for us that Diane Martel was not alone in her tragic illness. Her symptoms and the response to her illness were similar to the way mounting numbers of people, mostly women, were suffering and were being badly abused.

We were on the right track with our quest.

SUMMARY

Except for a variety of relatively minor 'mystery' diseases that had occurred in many places both before and after World War Two, it was not until 1984 that major epidemics of what was dismissively called 'chronic fatigue' hit a variety of communities in the United States and Canada. As the community-centered epidemic stage seemed to wane, the scattered incidence grew, and soon there was hardly a community in North America that didn't have several victims of 'CFS' or 'CFIDS'. The response to these mystery outbreaks and then to the growing incidence of illness by the Public Health Agencies in both the United States and Canada, was at the least casual, and at the worst, criminal. As an apparently well-planned strategy, the public health agencies not only failed to respond to a great and growing health crisis, but even encouraged certain media assets to misrepresent the disease to the public. It seemed evident that someone had something to hide.

ENDNOTES

[1]. Action No. 9201-12776. In the Court of Queen's Bench of Alberta Judicial District of Calgary. Between Yvonne Mackie and Ronald Mackie Plaintiffs -and- Patrick Wolfe Defendant, June 10, 1994.

[2]. Edward Shorter; *From Paralysis to Fatigue* (Toronto; Maxwell Macmillan Canada, 1992)

[3]. Hillary Johnson: *Osler's Web* (New York: Crown Publishers, Inc. 1996)

[4]. Thomas C. Merigan and David A. Stevens; Viral Infections in man associated with acquired immunological deficiency states." *Federation Proceedings,* Vol. 30, No. 6. November-December, 1971. pp.1858 to 1864

[5]. Johnson, *op cite*, p.566

[6]. Our later research strongly suggests that the disease agent involved in CFIDS/ME/FM is a bacterial DNA particle called the 'mycoplasma.' It appears that the mycoplasma presents with symptoms under particular conditions of concen-

tration, body temperature, barometric pressure and blood pH. When the level of pathogenic concentration reaches a certain point and the victim experiences a trauma of some sort, the mycoplasma begins a disease-inducing process of up-taking pre-formed sterols in certain host cells that it has accessed. See Chapter Fourteen: "The Mycoplasma Hypothesis" for further details.

[7]. It was interesting to note that several of the respondents when asked about their cognitive problems told how when they would attempt to add figures they would actually subtract: ie."seven and two is five". Another strange problem was their inability to draw a pencil sketch of the human figure. Even with a person standing right in front of them, they would for example make a drawing with the arms coming from the hips, rather than from the shoulders.

CHAPTER THREE

"I think the CDC is doing a cover-up job"

One gets the impression while reading Hillary Johnson's "Acknowledgments" in the opening pages of *Osler's Web* that the U.S. Federal Government has something to hide. When Johnson expresses her thanks to attorney Quinlan J. Shea Jr., for his help in getting the release of documents from the National Institutes of Health (NIH) after 'long hours' of negotiations, a thoughtful reader's interest is piqued. Why would a government health agency created to serve the citizens of a country, resist the sharing of research with a professional reporter and well-regarded writer?

The initial impression that some secret is being rigorously protected and kept from public view is re-enforced as one studies the careful record presented by Johnson in the 700 pages of her important book. It also becomes evident that, although Ms. Johnson states that the Centers for Disease Control (CDC) were 'generally responsive to FOIA requests' this Agency ,too, has secrets it prefers to safeguard. The first clue to this is to be seen in the fact that the 're-sponsive' attitude of the CDC had only become apparent after the FOIA had to be utilized.[1] In other words, little of what either the NIH or the CDC was finally prepared to divulge was shared willingly!

The question is, 'Why?'

Both the NIH and the CDC are agencies of the U.S. Federal Government, under the umbrella of the Public Health Service. There are separate areas of responsibility assigned to each of the NIH and the CDC, but at times there are subtle 'turf wars' as to where the line between them is to be drawn. In broad general terms the NIH is responsible for programs designed to improve the health of the U.S. population [2] while the CDC is intended to be a more activist disease fighter, primarily engaged in monitoring and containing cholera, dengue, lyme disease and other epidemics including, since October, 2001, anthrax, in the United States and its territories.

On occasion the CDC has been called upon by the World Health Organization and by some national governments to assist in containing infectious diseases such as the 1976 outbreak of Ebola in Zaire.[3] The 'help' of the CDC in such international humanitarian efforts has not always been seen

in a positive light by the afflicted recipients of their ministrations; the CDC 1966 war on smallpox in fourteen sub-Saharan countries, in fact, was viewed with justifiable suspicion by many political leaders in those countries,[4] while the purported role of the NIH in the development of the AIDS virus, a role publicized in September, 1986, when a report was distributed at the Harare, Zimbabwe, summit of nonaligned nations, caused many participating nations to view the NIH with great concern.[5]

The report in question had been prepared by East German scientists, Jacob and Lilli Segal, and it sought to prove that the AIDS virus had been created in Fort Detrick, Maryland, by the U.S. Department of Defense [6] and had been introduced into the world as a consequence of a laboratory accident and faulty test procedures. The Segal scenario was publicized in Europe and Africa, as well as in certain other Third World countries, but was largely ignored by American media.

The suspicion with which the CDC and the NIH were viewed outside of the U.S. was, to a lesser extent, shared by many in America...especially by Black Americans, who recalled the role of the CDC's predecessor in the infamous Tuskegee experiments.[7] In the latter program several hundred Black men with syphilis were left untreated (while being led to believe that they were being treated) so that the Public Health 'scientists' could monitor the progress of the disease as it ravaged the bodies of its unsuspecting victims.

Thus, readers and researchers who are familiar with the murky past and the unexamined rumours of an even murkier current role in the development and spread of AIDS, are alerted by Johnson's references to her struggle to obtain documents under the Freedom of Information Act from both the NIH and the CDC. What, one again feels compelled to ask, needed to be kept hidden from the American public?

His Limbs Were Encased In Lead

Marc Iverson[8] 'awoke one morning in 1979 with the disconcerting sensation that his limbs were encased in lead.' Although he didn't know it at the time, he was just one of several persons throughout the United States in the mid-seventies and early eighties who had become ill with a mysterious malady. A malady whose most characteristic symptom was a deep-set fatigue which was not ameliorated by rest. There were several other symptoms which accompanied the fatigue but not all patients shared the same constellation of such. These symptoms included low-grade fevers, sore throat, swollen lymph nodes, headaches, sore muscles, and strangely enough in view of the common quality of fatigue…insomnia. What sleep the bone-weary victims did manage to get was generally non-restorative.

Over the next eight to nine years this mysterious 'syndrome'[9] was sufficiently common that in 1984-85 three research articles were published: one in the *Southern Medical Journal* and two in the *Annals of Internal Medicine*. The former was written by Richard DuBois, an infectious disease specialist from Atlanta, with the help of eight co-authors. The articles in the *Annals* were by Stephen Straus of Bethesda, and pediatrician James Jones of Denver. It is probably coincidental that Atlanta, the city where DuBois, et al had encountered the syndrome, was the principal site of the Centers for Disease Control, while Bethesda , where Straus did his research, was the site of the campus of the National Institute of Health devoted to Allergy and Infectious Diseases.

Because some of the patients of Dr. DuBois and his colleagues had developed the syndrome after a bout of what had been diagnosed as mononucleosis, the authors agreed to call the malady 'chronic mononucleosis syndrome'. However, regardless of what it was called, the DuBois group, James Jones and Stephen Straus had all discovered a 'preponderance of high Epstein-Barr virus antibodies among patients,'[10] leading Straus and Jones to propose Epstein-Barr virus as a potential cause of the syndrome.

Significantly, Straus and Jones concurred upon another important possibility. '(B)oth researchers postulated that the chronic malady might in fact be a form of *immune dysfunction*' (emphasis added).[11] Straus suggested a possible immune impairment of an *'entirely distinct cause'* while Jones drew attention to the fact that the victims of this mystery illness had something in common with AIDS victims…the latter also suffered from persistent or chronic Epstein-Barr virus infection! Both Jones and Straus noted that the disease exacted a heavy toll in their subjects' lives…many of whom had lost their jobs.

Their financial status had deteriorated, often their friends and even their families had abandoned them. But both Straus and Jones seemed to be clear on the point that these tragic consequences and the depression that often resulted, had followed the onset of this unusual disease which had so many significant yet variable and elusive symptoms and etiology.

Apparently Stephen Straus was later to experience a profound change of opinion, or at least of emphasis, for he emerged shortly after with a view that the syndrome was more psychosomatic than physical and that it 'reflects an excessive risk for educated adult white women' who have 'histories of unachievable ambition, poor coping skills, and somatic complaints.' [12] Since he offered no supporting data for his comments which were as Hillary Johnson was to observe 'jarringly antithetical to the spirit of scientific inquiry',one could not engage in a meaningful dialogue with him about his claims. All one could do was to watch in wonder as the National Institutes of Health 'scientist' coped with the emerging disease by blaming it on its victims.

The record of the NIH under Straus in its response to the syndrome was to be a record of dishonesty, misrepresentation, and sarcasm. Hardly what one would expect of a senior scientist in a government agency whose mandate, broadly speaking, was to improve the health of Americans. What had happened to effect Stephen Straus' switch from his early mix of scientific evaluation and psychosocial problems of patients with '…evidence of Epstein-Barr infection' to his single-minded emphasis upon mal-adjusted middle-aged women? And why was it that it was the female victims who had the 'unachievable ambition, poor coping skills, and somatic complaints' while the male victims were apparently free of such character deficiencies?

And where did his initial speculation about an 'immune impairment of an entirely distinct cause' disappear to? Is it possible that he was at that point covering all the bases in case someone, somewhere, later came up with clear evidence that the victims of this new disease had a demonstrable etiology that involved a new virus which did, in fact, attack the immune system? If such were to happen, he would always be able to point to his first written views and say "See, I suggested as much right at the outset." While if a firm, physical base for the myriad of symptoms never did come to light, he could let his earlier, open-minded, speculation fade away, leaving only his 'somatic' thesis intact.

As we read and discussed *Osler's Web*, we realized that Diane Martel had been responded to as if she were one of Straus' mal-adjusted middle-aged, under-achieving women with a shortage of coping skills! Where had Superintendent Hammond and union representative Ed Alexander picked up on that theme?

If it were simply a case of Stephen Straus positioning himself to make sure that his professional reputation did not suffer from premature and scientifically unfounded speculation, no great harm would have resulted. However, much more was at stake, for Stephen Straus was to be the individual who, more than any other, would control and direct federal government research funds in the years ahead. How he used that power is set out by Hillary Johnson and it raises further questions as to who was giving Stephen Straus his marching orders and whether these people really wanted the world to know what this new syndrome was and where it had come from.

This Sounded...well...strange, Not Urgent

While Stephen Straus was doing his thing in the National Institutes of Health, Larry Schonberger in the Centers for Disease Control was developing that agency's response to the dramatic increase in the mystery malady characterized by profound fatigue and a long and varied list of other symptoms. A new syndrome that more and more seemed to be a 'mirror image of AIDS'; another scourge that had broken upon the world at about the same time and one which, like its mystery fatigue-marked syndrome, was characterized by a dysfunctioning immune system.

Larry Schonberger was the chief of the CDC's Epidemiology Office within the Division of Viral and Rickettsial Diseases. He had joined the CDC in 1971. This, as we will come to see, was a significant year in matters of human health, for in that year President Nixon and his National Security advisor, Henry Kissinger, had appropriated over $125 million for 'population control'... An undertaking about which both Nixon and Kissinger were to later be completely silent in their self-serving accounts of that time.[13]

It was Schonberger's job to monitor any biological weapons testing by the U.S. Department of Defense when the latter tried out any new 'strategic' weapons designed to meet the population threat as perceived by Kissinger and his mentor, Nelson Rockefeller.

Schonberger also directed the CDC research into the outbreak of any new disease or the re-appearance in epidemic proportions of any well-known or well-established disease. Since Schonberger was a scientist with disease as the focus of his enquiring mind, one would anticipate that his efforts in respect to the mystery malady of 1975 would be careful, thorough, and objective. However, as the record was to show, his response can best be characterized as lackadaisical; although the disease had been simmering in various places throughout the U.S. for over ten years, it was not to be until 1985 that Schonberger would deploy two of his 'medical detectives' to the scene of a particularly dramatic outbreak which occurred in Incline Village, Nevada.

Explaining his strangely unimaginative and lethargic response to thousands of people across the country coming down with a mysterious illness, Schonberger was to say:

"We get these calls all the time...If someone had said 'I've got an acute case of paralysis here-it may be polio,' you respond immediately. You go out there-because that's a public health crisis. This sounded...well...strange, not urgent."[14]

The Epidemic Intelligence Service officers dispatched to Incline Village were Jon Kaplan and Gary Holmes.

Jon Kaplan was the senior of the two EIS officers, and his experience included a visit to Hawaii a few years earlier to investigate the outbreak of a paralytic disorder called Guillain-Barre syndrome. As it turned out, this latter outbreak was the consequence of a CDC snafu directed by David Sencer who had previously presided over the Tuskegee syphilis experiments. Sencer had personally persuaded President Gerald Ford to undertake a mass swine flu vaccination program in 1976. Unfortunately the shots caused over 500 cases of the paralytic syndrome [15] and more people died from the vaccine than from the flu itself.[16] We will have occasion to consider Sencer's contribution to America's health when we discuss his role as New York City Health Commissioner in early 1982 where the CDC had tested a Hepatitis "B" vaccine on the gay male population.[17] Unfortunately a very high percentage of the co-operating gay men who took the new vaccine were to come down over the next few years with AIDS. After walking in David Sencer's footsteps at least as far as Hawaii, Incline Village should have been a cake-walk for Jon Kaplan. It didn't turn out that way.

The second member of the two man team was Gary Holmes who was on his first field trip for

CDC and who was pre-disposed to believe that the syndrome was linked to the Epstein-Barr Virus. He would obviously be influenced by Jon Kaplan's more experienced disease sleuthing.

SOMEONE ABOVE THEM WAS CALLING THE SHOTS

The detective work by Kaplan and Holmes who were dispatched to Incline Village, Nevada, appears to have been greatly influenced by the attitude of their lackadaisical superior, Larry Schonberger. When one considers that the two 'foot soldiers' of the CDC were going to a small community where over 200 citizens manifested the symptoms of a mysterious syndrome, it comes as something of a surprise to learn that between the two researchers they only examined *ten* patients. At one point Holmes was later to claim that they had seen *sixteen* patients, but he soon dropped this number and went back to the ten. It also comes as a surprise to learn that senior researcher, Jon Kaplan, decided after just one week, to return to Atlanta, leaving his neophyte assistant to search for answers about this new medical mystery.

"He seemed to have already made up his mind about us," said one victim after a cursory examination by Holmes.[18]

Another puzzling aspect of the CDC investigation was the fact that Kaplan and Holmes seemed " vastly more interested in studying patient charts than patients."[19] Almost as if they knew before they ever got to Incline Village what it was that they would find in the victims... but what they didn't know was just how extensive the illness was, and that it was this which they needed to determine. They seemed to be quantifying consequences rather than seeking causes!

Such 'bookkeeping' could be done by Gary Holmes, so he had to linger a little longer, while, as we noted Jon Kaplan wound up his 'intensive' disease sleuthing in a week!

And it was to be upon this 'Mutt and Jeff' investigation that the Centers for Disease Control would base its response to the "mystery" disease even up to the present.

Thus, ten years after the syndrome with its long list of symptoms had begun to show itself, and after a lackadaisical Larry Schonberger of the CDC had finally sent a lethargic two-man team to Incline Village to 'investigate' one of several cluster outbreaks the official agency of disease control in America was about to issue its findings. But even here there was a long and unexplained delay: it was not until May 30,1986 that the *Morbidity and Mortality Weekly Report* was to present the Kaplan-Holmes research in a *seven paragraph* monograph. And the report stands today as the first official U.S. Government view of the disease that has wrecked the health and destroyed the lives of hundreds of thousands of people. A disease which has cut short promising careers and hopes of accomplishment in the arts, science, sports and other walks of life; which has reduced many victims to poverty and has driven others to suicide.

And what was the essence of the Schonberger-Kaplan-Holmes' efforts? The essence was paraphrased by a strangely accepting media, one example of which was the story based upon the monograph that appeared in the *Atlanta Journal* which informed its readers that "there is no conclusive scientific evidence that Chronic Epstein-Barr Virus actually exists" ![20] A theme that was to echo down over the years when people such as Madam Justice Rawlins in Alberta, Canada, was to rule in a Canadian court case that "fibromyalgia does not exist." [Chapter Eight] Much as, later on, the American and Canadian Departments of Defense health officers were to declare that "Gulf War Syndrome does not exist."

In other words the Centers for Disease Control corner stone for their position on this epidemic was to be 'denial', heavily laden with ridicule for the victims.

When Dr. Paul Cheney of Incline Village saw this strange and dishonest document he generously excused the team of Kaplan and Holmes: "...someone above them was calling the shots...I get the feeling they were told to ...publish this view." [21]

If Dr. Cheney's surmise is accurate, the question naturally arises: Who would need to deny the existence of a tragic and spreading disease, and why would they feel that need? And, five years later, who would need to deny the existence of Gulf War Syndrome, and why would they feel that need?[22] The starting point in the quest to find answers to all these questions can be found in the testimony of a Department of Defense researcher to a group of U.S. Congressmen on June 9, 1969...but that is getting ahead of ourselves.

LIKE WHY WAS GALLO INTERESTED?

Some time before Monday, May 11,1987, at least one and according to some reports, possibly two, persons visited Pierce Wright in the *London Times* office where he wrote major stories for that prestigious newspaper.[23] The visitor (or visitors) had some information for him about the growing crisis of AIDS in Africa. The story had actually been around since September, 1986, when as we noted above, it had surfaced in Harare, Zimbabwe. According to Jacob and Lilli Segal, the AIDS virus had been invented in Fort Detrick, Maryland.

The story passed to Pierce Wright was essentially the same, but there were some added details. When the virus that came to be known as Human Immunodeficiency Virus [HIV] had been developed, it was used, claimed Wright's source(s) by the World Health Organization and certain elements of the U.S. government in a project to reduce the population of Africa. The killer virus was to be disseminated under the guise of providing a program of smallpox vaccinations.

Most people when they first encounter this story are inclined to disbelief. It is altogether too horrible to think that educated, adult persons would use their skills in a plot which ranks with or even far beyond the Nazi holocaust as an example of evil incarnate.

However, when such sceptics reflect upon the process by which a story like this gets onto the front page of one of the world's most prestigious newspapers, they are compelled to suspend their tendency to disbelief and to look for further evidence about the subject. After all, an experienced writer (such as Mr. Wright must have been to hold the position he did) does not accept stories without requiring substantial proof that they are firmly rooted in provable facts. Then, if his sources can convince him, he must then convince his editor. Editors, generally speaking, do not hold such positions unless they are able to ask tougher questions about sources and evidence than their best writers ask. Whoever it was that brought evidence to Pierce Wright, must have been able to produce substantial credentials, for the story was run on the front page of the *London Times* on Monday, May 11,1987.

We will have occasion to return to the question of whether AIDS was invented, but at this point the subject has to be broached because a particular researcher into AIDS had been fingered by those who were circulating the story as the principal villain in the whole Satanic enterprise. That person was Dr. Robert Gallo, the researcher who was later to be credited, under murky circumstances, with the discovery of HIV, which is touted as the purported

cause of AIDS. And, as has been noted, the emerging 'mirror image' of AIDS, CFIDS, the mystery malady which debilitated its victims but did not (apparently) kill them, was also characterized by human immune dysfunction.

There were other parallels between Acquired Immunodeficiency Syndrome and the as yet officially unnamed Chronic Epstein-Barr Syndrome CE-BS. Both syndromes had emerged in the mid-seventies in isolated instances. Both then seemed to erupt in epidemic proportions in the early eighties. Both displayed a high incidence of Epstein-Barr antibodies. And the initial response to both had been official denial and a put-down of the victims. There was, however, soon to be a major difference: since AIDS killed its victims and since it was obviously very contagious, denial was not an option, and the syndrome soon had its own well-funded Agency within the National Institutes of Health.

Conversely, since CE-BS did not kill its victims… in fact many of those afflicted looked the very picture of health…and since there was no demonstrable evidence that it was highly contagious, the best that an official agency of the U.S. Government could come up with was a Mutt and Jeff visit to the site of one cluster of the disease. A visit followed by a seven paragraph monograph that dismissed the very great tragedy that had entered the lives of two hundred Incline Village citizens, and was soon to number its victims in the thousands.

Against this bewildering background of denial, dishonesty, misrepresentation, and evil rumours, it was to be expected that, when Dr. Paul Cheney of the Incline Village patient group learned from a researcher with the Wistar Institute that none other than the Dr. Robert Gallo wanted some blood samples from Cheney's patients that Dr. Cheney, according to Hillary Johnson's account, felt compelled to ask "…like why was Gallo interested?"[24]

Despite his initial misgivings about acceding to Gallo's request, Cheney agreed to allow the use of his patients' blood samples. Cheney believed that Gallo was probably looking for a retrovirus but actually the researchers were following another trail. They were looking for a new class of herpes virus, and were amazed to find that nearly every sample sent to them from Incline Village tested positive for the antibodies that seemed to signal the presence of that virus.

The confusion was mind boggling. There were over 200 victims of a strange new malady in Incline

Village, Nevada. Yet the disease detectives for one government agency, the CDC, had just declared that in effect, there was no disease. Another agency, the National Institute of Allergy and Infectious Diseases, presided over by Dr. Stephen Straus, had arrived at the conclusion that the disease, if it existed at all, was a psychosomatic condition of overly ambitious but under-achieving women with poor coping skills. And now there was another agency of government, the National Cancer Institute under Dr. Robert Gallo which had no apparent official role in respect to the syndrome, had found that the under-achieving women with a non-existent disease, had blood which carried evidence of a new version of herpes virus!

Few researchers and even fewer medical care givers had any idea that for much of the previous two decades, Robert Gallo had been busily engaged in an enterprise called 'The Special Virus Cancer Program' which had, in turn grown from an earlier military /CIA program called 'MK-SVLP'. And few if any knew that among Gallo's research partners in MK-SVLP there were people such as Dharam Ablashi, a doctor of *veterinarian medicine,* and Paul Levine. These and others who had been in the murky shadows of MK-SVLP were to emerge in the 1980's as experts on the two mystery diseases: AIDS and CFIDS!

Could such confusion arise naturally among honest researchers looking for answers about some new illness that had sprung into being almost over-night? Or is it possible that, as Dr. Cheney had speculated, that someone, somewhere, for reasons not available to the doctors and their patients, was giving the researchers their marching orders which were to be followed regardless of the evidence that was emerging? Could it have anything to do with the secret military/ CIA MK-SVLP program? We consider more about this possibility in Chapter's Twelve and Fourteen.

The mystery of both the disabling disease of Incline Village and the official government response to it was to deepen over the years, as both the NIH and the CDC maintained their policies of cover-up, misrepresentation, patient put-down, and actual fraud. Some of these qualities can be seen in the following paragraph from Osler's Web. It is just one such example of many.

> *"When he was asked…in 1988…Stephen Straus (of the NIH) refused to discuss either the nature of the tests performed on Peterson's patients or the results; he refused, too, to release any documents related to these investigations when they were sought under a Freedom of Information Act request, a petition originally made in early 1989…after the agency failed to comply fully with the original request. In violation of the federal Freedom of Information Act, Straus's superiors at the agency did not force him to comply with either request even when…James Mason, then the assistant secretary for Health and Human Services, instructed them to do so."(Emphasis added)[25]*

This amazing paragraph raises all manner of questions.

Why, if the disease was just in the minds of a bunch of neurotic women, would Straus require extensive testing of some of the victims and then refuse to say what it was his researchers were looking for and what, if anything, they had found?

How is it that Straus was allowed, not only to *defy* the law, but was also left in his job when he defied assistant secretary James Mason, his titular boss?

What was there about the test results that just could not be made public?

And finally, just who was in charge here anyway?

WHAT'S IN A NAME

The bewildering range of symptoms that characterized the syndrome whose dominant feature was 'bone crushing' fatigue, made it a difficult entity to label. And, as it was to turn out, such a difficulty created an opportunity for the CDC to trivialize the disease and to reduce public sympathy for its victims. The CDC had stalled as long as it could before it officially chose the name 'chronic fatigue syndrome', for after all, if a patient or a doctor cannot say what the victim has, the question lingers, does he really have anything? This latter possibility had apparently occurred to Stephen Straus of the NIH who didn't want a name and 'diagnostic criteria (published) anywhere.'"If it was published," he warned," clinicians might use it as a tool to diagnose patients"![26] This lack of a name would of course mean there would be no ready way to report the incidence of the disease. Just one more example of the denial that permeated the NIH and its sister agency, the CDC.

However, by 1987 there was little choice left for the CDC and that agency officially launched the label of 'chronic fatigue syndrome'.

This label opened the door for further labels…all of which picked up on the CDC lead and vied to find catchy ways to convey the view that CFIDS was a trendy label for upwardly mobile people who found their careers stalled and who were taking shelter behind a make-believe illness. *Time* magazine won the prize in the 'bad mouthing' sweepstakes when they coined the term "yuppie flu."

Score another one for the CDC, not in the realm of disease detective work which one might hope would be their principal objective, but in the realm of cover-up, for what's in a name? Well, if the name is 'chronic fatigue syndrome' there are ideas conjured up of malingerers, psychosomatics, and frustrated middle-age women. Re-enter Robert Hammond of the Sudbury Separate School Board and Ed Alexander of the Ontario English Catholic Teachers' Federation.

To the terrible tragedy of a debilitating disease is added a heavy burden of guilt and embarrassment for victims like Diane Martel. And, when the victims visit a run-of-the-mill doctor who is limited in imagination and concern for his patients' well-being, and who takes his direction from the published 'findings' of the researchers at CDC and/or NIH, such patients are told 'it's all in your head' or 'buck up and get more exercise'.

The Need To Soft-pedal The Disease

Meanwhile, back at the NIH ranch, Stephen Straus was continuing his insidious and invidious ways. When he wasn't busy telling jokes about CFIDS victims,[27] he was engaged in some experiments with a cluster of patients, one of whom was a psychotherapist, Susan Simon.

The latter experiment involved the use of acyclovir, a drug developed by a British firm which had been used successfully against herpes viruses. An important warning given to researchers who had decided to try the drug against illnesses characterized by immune system dysfunction was that patients during their treatment regime were to receive large quantities of fluids to protect their kidneys. Dr. Straus, it appears, neglected to observe sufficient precautions by failing to tell the patients and their care-givers about this important warning. As a consequence his treatment caused temporary kidney failure in some of his subjects.

Another of Dr. Straus' experiments necessitated, he claimed, a muscle biopsy of a twenty-two year old CFIDS victim, Sally Bentson (a pseudonym).

To make the test as valid as possible the doctor required that three slices of muscle be pared from her arm without the use of an anaesthetic. The patient endured the excruciating pain of the procedure, but was never to receive any results from Dr. Straus. She had been put to the long trip from Yerington, Nevada to Bethesda, Maryland; put through four days of testing, including several sessions with psychiatrists who were intent, it seems, upon getting her to realize that it was all 'in your head'; and finally the brutal biopsy, only to be told that the researchers at NIH had no report to offer about what they had found.

Such acyclovir treatments which damaged the patient's kidneys, or the anaesthetic-free paring away of live muscle was almost enough to make some of Dr. Straus' patients feel that maybe the disease was better than being treated. Especially when the pain they were put to did not produce results of any benefit to them. In fact, not only was there often no apparent purpose nor results to Dr. Straus' ministrations, some patients believed that he was guilty of medical malpractice. One patient, the above-mentioned psychotherapist Susan Simon, began to discuss charging the head of the medical virology section of the National Institute of Allergy and Infectious Diseases, Dr. Stephen Straus, with malpractice.

Unfortunately, before she could proceed with her suit which in the courts could well have resulted in much of what was going on at the NIH being held up to public scrutiny, a large truck in New York City hit Ms. Simon on her motor scooter and killed her instantly.[28]

The experience of Susan Simon and Sally Bentson were apparently not exceptions to the rule at Dr. Stephen Straus' NIH laboratories. The NIH record was so wide spread that by 1991, Barry Sleight, a volunteer advocacy activist for CFIDS victims was to declare (among other things) that:
 – Straus was biassed against women
 – NIH performed needless invasive, often high-risk, and frequently painful procedures on victims
 – research grants were unduly controlled by Straus to the disadvantage of independent research
 – Straus misled Congress.[29]

The evidence was clear that at NIH there was indeed, a deliberate effort to deny the very existence of the disease. Was their denial based upon the possibility that they, too, had something to hide?

Summary

When a mysterious malady began to appear throughout the United States, and to a lesser extent in Canada, New Zealand, Australia and Britain, in the mid-seventies, it did not generate wide-spread public concern. Its victims often appeared to be in robust good health and hence were easily tagged with the label of 'malingerer'. In 1984 there was a dramatic increase of the disease in several, relatively remote areas which affected not single patients, but clusters of them. Generally, the clusters centered on a single building such as a school or a hospital.

By 1985 the disease was of sufficient extent to merit the appearance of reports in professional journals, and also to be reported in the public media. The official government response to these clusters was very unusual. Instead of the Centers for Disease Control and the National Institutes of Health devoting their time and expertise to the study of the disease, these government agencies embarked upon a program of misrepresentation, dishonesty, put-down of patients, denial of research money and expertise. It seemed to many concerned doctors and lay-persons that there was a massive official effort to deny the existence of the disease and to down-play the extent of the epidemic.

In the face of such official government neglect, thousands of victims were relegated to the ranks of under-achieving "yuppies" whose careers were failing. Such victims, denied proper acceptance as genuine victims of a terrible disease, lost friends, family, careers and financial stability. Furthermore, to a very noticeable extent, elements of the major media went along with the official line that the disease (finally labelled 'chronic fatigue syndrome') was just a cover for mal-adjusted middle-aged persons. The victims were made the butt of black humour and were denied insurance, worker's compensation, pensions and other benefits they would have received if they were able to show an obvious physical or mental disability.

That was where Diane Martel was when she gave me a telephone call [DWS] and I gave my son, Bill, a call for help. Bill's double Honours degree in History and Political Science were to add a valuable dimension to our study.

Endnotes

[1].Johnson, *Ibid*, xi

[2]."National Institutes of Health", *The New American Encyclopaedia*. Philadelphia: The Publishers Agency, Inc., p.5218

[3]. Arno Karlen, *Man and Microbes* (New York: Simon and Schuster, 1995) p.166-7

[4].Pascal James Imperato, *Medical Detective* (New York: Richard Marek Publishers, 1979) p.28

[5].Mirko D. Grmek, *History of Aids* (Princeton, New Jersey: Princeton University Press, 1990) p.151

[6].It may be significant that although the report caused many Third World politicians great concern, it was largely ignored by the American media.

[7].Randy Shilts. *And the Band Played On* (New York: St. Martin's Press, 1987) p.532

[8].Hillary Johnson, *Osler's Web*, Most of the cases referred to in this chapter are based upon the reporting by Ms. Johnson. In order to avoid unnecessary endnotes only those cases derived from other sources will be identified from this point on.

[9].A 'syndrome' is a constellation of symptoms and physical signs manifested in an ill person, but which lack the specificity of a 'disease'.

[10]. Johnson, *Ibid*, p.21

[11]. Johnson, *Ibid*, pp. 21-2

[12]. Johnson, *Ibid*, pp. 268-9

[13]. You may search in vain through: Richard Nixon, RN; *The Memoirs of Richard Nixon* (New York: Grosset & Dunlap, 1978) and the two Volumes of Henry Kissinger, *White House Years* and *Years of Upheaval* (Boston-Toronto: Little, Brown and Company, 1979)and 1982. respectively for any mention about how $125 million was to be spent to 'control population' in several third world countries identified by Kissinger in his" National Security Study Memorandum 200" to Nixon. In the latter Memorandum, Kissinger develops the theme first given executive reality by Robert McNamara in 1966 under President Johnson. The essence of the theme was that the burgeoning population in the named countries posed a greater strategic threat to the U.S. than a nuclear bomb attack. McNamara was to note that some way would have to be found to 'increase the death rate' in these countries.

[14].Johnson, *Ibid*, p.32

[15].Karlen, Arno, *Ibid* ,p.8

[16].Shilts, Randy, *Ibid*, p.532

[17].Shilts, Randy, *Ibid*, p.67

[18].Johnson, *Ibid*, p.49

[19].Johnson, *Ibid*, p.49

[20].Johnson, *Ibid*, p.136

[21].Johnson, *Ibid*, p.137

[22]."Pentagon finds no 'Gulf War disease'" Delaware State News. August 2, 1995

[23].Strecker, (Dr.) Robert. Monograph published by (Dr. William Campbell Douglass, M.D.P.O. Box 1568, Clayton, Ga., 30525) p.4

[24]. We qualify Cheney's questioning of Gallo's interest because as will be developed later, Cheney's role in the whole mystery of chronic fatigue syndrome raises many problems.

[25]. Johnson, *Ibid*, p.171

[26]. Johnson, *Ibid*, p.217

[27].It is necessary to point out that at several points in her careful and low-key report in *Osler's Web,* Johnson notes the hilarity with which many doctors greeted accounts of the suffering of CFIDS victims. Every few pages one reads of incidents such as the speech to the Institute of Underwriters held in Toronto, where the guest speaker, Dr. Irving Salit of the University of Toronto, presented "a *Saturday Night Live* stand-up comedy routine with CFIDS patients as the brunt of the joke". One can only imagine the outrage that would have resulted if Dr. Salit had taken his Seinfeld routine laced with jokes about blind people falling down elevator shafts to a meeting of the Canadian National Institute of the Blind. The whole tragic pattern of mocking the victims of this terrible disease is so pervasive as outlined through *Osler's Web* that one comes to suspect that it is part of the strategy designed to deal with the disease. If nothing else, such 'jokes' encourage many people to view the disease with something less than the seriousness with which it should be accepted.

[28].Ms. Simon's death has a suggestive similarity to several other deaths in recent American history which involve a witness who has evidence to offer about questionable activities by government or government agency persons. In a number of such cases the witnesses have been accidently killed before their evidence was placed upon the record. Rose Cheramie of Dallas, Texas was one such accident victim. Ms. Cheramie had heard two employees of Jack Ruby discussing the impending murder of President Kennedy two days before the crime was committed. She was hit by a car on Stemmons Freeway a few days before she was to be interviewed by the House Committee on Assassinations. Another witness was Lee Bowers, also of Dallas. Mr. Bowers was a railroad employee whose quick action led to the arrest of E. Howard Hunt moments after the assassination of the President. Although Hunt, who was later to turn up working for President Nixon, was taken into the front door of the Dallas Police Station and let out the back door with no record of any questioning about what he was doing dressed as a tramp on the overpass approaches , was not charged, he must have felt relieved when he heard that key-witness Bowers had died in a suspicious auto accident. Then there was former J. Edgar Hoover deputy William Sullivan who had just been fired from the FBI. Mr. Sullivan approached John Dean with an offer for President Nixon: Sullivan would tell all about some seedy FBI misdeeds in return for protection and a job. A few days later, before Nixon could put him on the White House payroll, Sullivan was killed by a rifle bullet while he was standing on the patio behind his Maryland home. It seems that the son of the local sheriff was out hunting and took Sullivan for a deer. The bullet between Sullivan's eyes killed him instantly and he never was able to 'tell all'. There are at least twenty other cases that could be cited, but the point is clear: if you are contemplating sharing evidence that might threaten an official in a key government agency, take extra precautions about your safety.

[29].Adapted from Johnson, *Ibid*, p.456

THE DENIAL OF TRUTH about the INFECTIOUS
causes of Myalgic Encephalomyelitis
(aka Chronic Fatigue Syndrome)

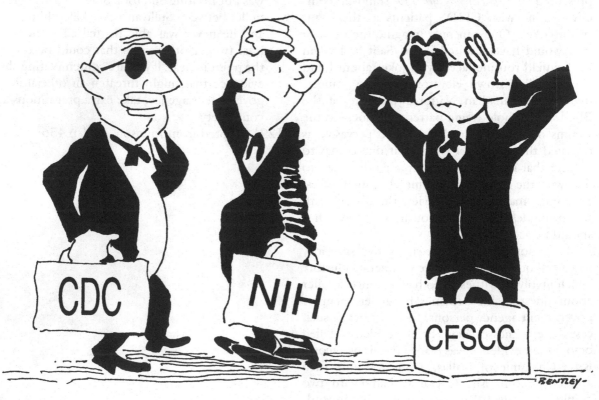

CHAPTER FOUR

JUNE 9, 1969

Certain dates stand out in human history. Some have a significance that is limited to a specific group...religious, ethnic, political...such as Mohammed's capture of Mecca in 628, or Genghis Khan's conquest of Persia in 1218, or Columbus' discovery of America in 1492.

Such dates have a mix of elements which can be seen as objective, but to varying degrees they also have an overlay of the subjective which often exceeds the significance of the former. There are very few dates which can be deemed to be of both a universal and objective significance. One such date might be August 6, 1945 when the Allies dropped the first nuclear bomb on Hiroshima for with that action warfare between nations or other social entities could no longer be waged without the specter of a nuclear catastrophe which would dramatically affect the well-being of all human kind.

Other dates can be suggested, but the chances of any such receiving more than a limited level of support as being of both a universal and an objective significance are scant. One possibility for such acceptance may well be June 9, 1969.

The significance of June 9, 1969 is unlikely to be recognized by even the best informed students of history. The year certainly had its share of dramatic events and some of these may occur to an informed reader. Richard Nixon was inaugurated as the 37th President of the United States... but that was in January. And James Earl Ray plead guilty to a crime he didn't commit (the assassination of the Rev. Martin Luther King, Jr.) and was sentenced to 99 years in prison, but that was on March 10.[1]

One reason that few if any historians will recognize the significance of June 9, 1969, is that the events that are the subject of this study took place in camera, away from the prying eyes of journalists or others not directly involved. Another reason is that, although a written record of proceedings was kept, it, too, was kept secret until under Freedom of Information provisions, it was brought into public view by the late Theodore Strecker.[2]

There is, however, another very powerful yet subtle reason why very few will recognize the date, and that reason is based upon the need of many Americans to deny the extent of the evil that would have to be acknowledged if they were to consider in an objective and fair-minded way what had transpired on that date.[3]

A final reason, and one which will be developed more fully later is the extent to which the American media is the hand-maiden to the powers which give rise to the kind of meeting we must consider. As Charles A. Reich has written:

"...corporate giants, especially those already in control of other forms of mass communications such as newspapers, gathered the lion's share of the licenses, often controlling multiple stations. In addition, the major networks and stations have been given over exclusively to commercial use, so that they are dominated by large corporate advertisers...It means that corporate America completely dominates the public airways, and nothing that is disapproved of by corporate America is likely to be heard by the public."[4]

And, as will be developed in this chapter, the discussions which took place in Washington, D.C. on June 9, 1969, gave rise to a social and human catastrophe which has already cost billions of dollars in medical expenses and lost production. Those discussions also gave rise to human suffering unequalled before in history. And, if the truth is finally acknowledged and justice is done then millions of sufferers in all parts of the world will be entitled to reparations for the crimes committed against them. Crimes which were placed on a written record on June 9, 1969, and then kept hidden until now.

And, if the truth is finally told, then perhaps those who wield their great but hidden powers will be dragged 'kicking and screaming' into the broad sun-light so that acts of evil cannot be committed without accountability for them, and the reason for the CDC/NIH coverup of CFIDS and AIDS will become obvious.

The proposals made and the decisions taken on this day in history explain why Diane Martel is sick with CFIDS and why Ed (Boyd) Graves is sick with AIDS.[See Chapter Six]

Monday, June 9, 1969

The meeting that convened on Monday, June 9, 1969 was that of a Subcommittee of the Committee on Appropriations of the House of Representatives who gathered to receive a report from scientists and officers of the United States Department of Defense. The report on this particular day dealt with 'Chemical and Biological Warfare' and was under the Chairmanship of George H. Mahon of Texas..." the Big Daddy of all appropriations."[5] The members of this Subcommittee are listed on the cover page of their *Hearings* but there is no indication whether all were present.[6] From the record it is clear that the following participated for they engage in conversation during the meeting: (besides George Mahon) Robert Sikes of Florida; Mr. Daniel J. Flood of Pennsylvania; Mr. William E. Minshall of Ohio; Mr. Joseph P. Addabbo of New York; Mr. George W. Andrews of Alabama; Mr. Frank E. Evans of Colorado.

These Representatives met with Dr. Donald M. MacArthur, who was the Deputy Director (Research and Technology) of the Department of Defense. He was accompanied by his Deputy Assistant Director, Dr. B. Harris, and his Acting Deputy Assistant Secretary of the Army, Dr. K.C.Emerson.

Two senior Army officers also accompanied Dr. MacArthur: Brig. Gen. W.S. Stone, Jr., and Col. J.J. Osick.

As indicated above, this group of men were gathered together to talk about what the Department of Defense was doing in the realm of chemical and biological warfare, both for purposes of defense against an 'enemy' and for purposes of being able to utilize the latest technology in any offense that might have to be undertaken. The particular areas of concern for this Subcommittee were developed over the next few hours of secret discussions.

Before those discussions are examined, it may be pertinent to consider just who the Representatives were in terms of their political and ideological bent.

The Chairman, George Mahon of Texas, was nominally a 'Democrat' but with this important qualifier...he was a 'Southern' Democrat. To give some idea of his position on the political spectrum of the time, we have a testimonial from Richard Nixon:

"Throughout my presidency my strongest and most dependable support in foreign affairs came from conservatives in both parties."[7]

He then cites George Mahon among others. If Nixon's assessment of Mahon is correct, then one can reasonably assume that when Henry Kissinger presented Nixon with National Security Study Memorandum 200, Mahon would know of it and would approve. As we shall note in a later chapter, NSSM 200 was a top secret document on why the United States should take action to reduce the rate at which the population of the world was growing.

George Mahon was also one of the few people, another being Robert Sikes of Florida, who had control of a huge secret fund of money which, on occasion, he used to meet certain Nixon requests. As Gulley and Reese put it:

"There was (besides Mahon and Sikes...Ed) only one guy in the Chesapeake Division, a commander who was assigned to them but responsible to the White House Military Office, who was aware of the actual purpose, amount and, more important, the actual destination of money from the Secret Fund."[8]

In 1969, George Mahon was recognized as one of the strongest 'hawks' in Congress...'Mahon supported the Nixon-Ford Vietnam policy to the end.'[9] The significance of this characteristic will be seen when the subject of the June 9, 1969 meeting is examined.

Representative Jamie L. Whitten was another Southern Democrat and a well-known hawk. Of significance is the fact that :

"Whitten also favoured a strong defence establishment and supported every major controversial weapons system proposed by the Administration"[10]

Among the Republicans were those who were equally as hawkish as the Southern Democrats, including John J. Rhodes of Arizona who '...favoured a strong defense, endorsed the (Nixon-Ford) Administration's Vietnam policy and backed foreign military aid.[11] He also had the distinction of sticking with Richard Nixon after the Watergate scandal broke for longer than almost any other Republican.

On a more general level it is important to make the observation that the Representatives who were involved in the activities of June 9, 1969 were disproportionately Southern in their geographic origins and most tended to support any weapons system that held out hope for the defeat of the 'enemy'...more specifically of the Soviet Union...in the war which many of them felt was bound to come. And, among such weapons systems were included the development of biological agents which would kill or disable. Weapons which would later be provided to Iraq by the Reagan Administration for use against Iran, and would come back to disable thousands of Gulf War service men and women.

Dr. Donald M. MacArthur

The person the Representatives had come to meet was 38 year old Donald M. MacArthur, who had taken most of his university at St. Andrews in Scotland. Shortly after completing his Ph.D. he found work at Westinghouse in the United States where he soon became manager of the Chemistry and Life Sciences Research Center. One of his areas of interest within a large number of defense programs was 'biology'...the science of 'living matter.'

However, the question arises as to what particular slant on 'life sciences' were MacArthur and Westinghouse interested in? After all, a person is often judged by the Company that keeps him...and Westinghouse has a spotty record as to whether their interest was in preserving life or in finding ways to terminate it at a profit.

In the early 1950's Westinghouse had helped develop the F3H jet fighter. In test flights, eleven of the planes had crashed, causing the deaths of several pilots. When Congressional committees considered scrapping the plane it was strongly defended by Admiral Lloyd Harrison so the huge contracts to Westinghouse/McDonnell Aircraft were continued. When Admiral Harrison retired in September, 1955, he was lucky enough to land a job with Westinghouse partner, McDonnell Aircraft as a vice-president.[12]

It is also significant to note that Westinghouse had a long and at times morally questionable[13] relationship with John J. McCloy who had served several years on its board of directors. Thus, the Company can easily qualify as a member of what President Eisenhower had called the military/industrial complex when he warned the American people to keep alert to the dangers of allowing too much power to pass to that shadowy group.

In 1966 Dr. MacArthur, in a move that was a reversal of normal transfers, went from Westinghouse to the Department of Defense, where among other things, he was responsible for research in 'medical and life sciences' which can reasonably be translated to 'diseases and death sciences.'

The Introductory Remarks

When the meeting of June 9, 1969, gets under way Representative Mahon observes that Congress had, over a period of years, supported a program of 'considerable significance' in chemical and biological warfare, and he wonders out loud whether the testimony about to be received should be put into the record.

Dr. MacArthur is, of course, alert to the sensitivity of the subjects that he will be raising and suggests that he will indicate as he goes along, the 'level of classification' the topics should receive.

In this exchange certain points should be carefully examined. In the first place, the idea that research and development in 'biological' warfare had been going on for a 'period of years' would probably have caught most Americans by surprise. The general public was well aware of the fact that military hardware was being developed and tested all the time... but did they suspect that someone somewhere in the military establishment was using knowledge gained in the 'study of life' to develop better ways to wage war and to terminate life?

It is also significant that if the research has been going on, then at some point the results of that research would have to be tested. If such testing had indeed been done, upon what or whom were the tests performed and with what consequences?

At this point it may be useful to review the experiences of 'David' as reported by W.H. Bowart and consider these experiences with some of Dr. MacArthur's testimony to the Congressmen. First to Dr. MacArthur [14]

On page 114 of the Hearings, Dr. MacArthur reports upon 'Agent BZ'. It is, says the doctor, an agent which will cause 'complete mental disorientation as well as sedation which induces sleep...The individual is completely confused as to what he is doing or what he is supposed to do.'

With this frame of reference we can now read of the experience of 'David'{1}

"Through the gray waters of amnesia he drifted, coming back from blind coma... For several hours he lay that way, perfectly still...then his eyes opened...'I couldn't remember anything. I couldn't remember how I'd gotten there or why I was in the hospital'...He asked nurses...why he was there. They told him he'd have to ask his doctor..."[15]

As it turns out, David had been the guinea pig for

military experiments with a mind-altering drug. Had it been Dr. MacArthur's 'Agent BZ'?

If, as Dr. MacArthur indicates, agent BZ were tested upon someone, had that someone given his consent? Certainly, Dr. Frank Olson hadn't given his consent when he was given LSD in a military experiment and had then 'died when he fell, jumped, or somehow exited from a twelfth-floor hotel window in New York'[16]

With the introductory statements out of the way, Dr. MacArthur then reads the "U.S. Position With Regard to Chemical and Biological Warfare" into the record.

Again, there are points worthy of particular emphasis. First it is important to note that Dr. MacArthur states that a program of research and development in the area of chemical-biological offensive capability will *continue*. In other words, with or without the Congressmen knowing about it, someone has been and still was working in this area. The significance of this is that an 'offensive' weapon does harm to the 'enemy'; it is not something that simply protects Americans. And, if it is to be tested, someone has to be subjected to it. If the tested agent is lethal, how will the military find volunteer guinea pigs?

Dr. MacArthur then touches a sensitive nerve in people like Mahon, Whitten and the others whose support for innovative weaponry was well known. He tells them that the U.S. is sorely lacking in some areas of biological warfare and that the "United States could not launch an immediate, massive retaliatory chemical or biological attack."

On page 108 of the Hearings it is revealed that $31 million has been authorized for expenditure in 1969 for *offensive* research and development. Only later do we learn that he would like another $10 million for some really dramatic biological weapons.

There is of course, danger when one plays around with chemical and biological agents, but Dr. MacArthur assures the Congressmen that there is no chance any American weapon will ever get out of control or produce toxic effects for any significant time period.

To illustrate the latter point he tells his listeners that 'agent orange' that was presently being sprayed all over the hapless state of Vietnam, showed 'no evidence of substantial permanent or irreparable damage.' Small comfort can be drawn from his words today when it is a well known fact that many pregnancies in Vietnam still terminate in miscarriages and many babies who happen to be carried to term are born with gross physical and mental deformities.

There was, however, that 'extremely unfortunate Skull Valley incident' of which more later.

By page 114 something entirely new is introduced into the equation with a chilling question by Mr. Flood:

"Mr. Flood. Wouldn't it be more effective to disable than to kill troops? Wouldn't it cause the enemy more trouble to disable him than to kill him."(sic)
"Dr. MacArthur. Yes, it imposes a greater logistical burden on the enemy when he has to look after the disabled people."

This will not be the last time that we will hear about incapacitating agents that disable their victim. But at this point it is sufficient to note that the idea is part of the military's thinking and we can rest assured that the idea will recur, as it does on page 117 when Dr. MacArthur moves one step further by telling the Congressmen that "In addition to chemical incapacitants you can have *biological* incapacitants." That is to say, the Research and Development experts in the U.S. Department of Defense can utilize biology...the science of life...to disable a target group of human beings. This in addition to being able to use the life sciences to kill.

It is at this point that Dr. MacArthur lets something slip. Bearing in mind that he is telling the Congressmen what they might be able to develop, he suddenly reveals:

"We have had some of the top scientists in the country working for years on how to get more effective incapacitating agents. It is not easy." (p.117)

Significantly, none of his listeners picks up on the point. None asks whether these new incapacitants work. None asks where and how the agents to incapacitate have been tested. Is this because they already knew, or just missed the point, or were well aware that there were many things going on that they, the nominal bosses were just not advised of?

By page 120 of the Hearings 'biological weapons' have taken center stage, and several chilling points are made.

First, Dr. MacArthur advises that biological agents would probably have to be delivered 'as a primary aerosol and infect people inhaling it.' Then he reveals that once one person was so infected, the agent could be carried from 'me to you' by an insect vector- a mosquito, for example.

For this reason, Dr. MacArthur is apprehensive:

"Dr. MacArthur. A contagious disease would not be effective as a biological warfare agent, although it might have devastating effects. It lacks the es-

sential element of control which I alluded to earlier since there would be no way to predict or control the course of the epidemic that might result."

On the next page he is still concerned about an agent that might get away from the scientists and which might then create:

"...a worldwide scourge or black death type disease that will envelop the world or major geographic areas if some of these materials were to accidentally escape."

Then he goes back to that mysterious incident in Skull Valley where, it would appear, something got out of hand, and just as he had consoled the Congressmen that agent orange would have no permanent or irreparable effects, he now assures them:

"That could not possibly happen with the biological agents that we have."

At this point there is another statement which, as later history would reveal, has a significance far beyond that given to it at the time by the Congressmen. Dr. MacArthur admits:

"However, to keep the record straight, we have done a small amount of research on a few agents that do not satisfy this constraint"

In other words, his researchers, without Congressional approval, had been working on 'a few agents' that might cause a worldwide scourge or black death. Could this be the AIDS epidemic that he is referring to? As we shall learn this was indeed the case.

Then there is another chilling comment which, at the time, did not have the significance it now has. Dr. MacArthur states that "...for most of these agents there is natural *Immunity.*" So, by inference, there are agents being developed that the human victim will not be able to cope with because he has no natural immunity. Dr. MacArthur foreshadows the development of synthetic biological agents that the human immune system is not naturally equipt to handle, agents which can either kill or disable their victim. And on page 129 there is the revelation that renders this June 9, 1969 date more significant than the August 6, 1945 date when the first nuclear weapon took over 100,000 lives.

On June 9, 1969, Dr. MacArthur was to ask for and to get Congressional approval to continue with plans to develop the AIDS pathogen!

Acquired Immune Deficiency

On page 129 of the record of the June 9, 1969 meeting Dr. MacArthur of the United States Department of Defense makes a statement to the assembled Congressmen that every human being should read carefully and think about deliberately.

The statement is of significance to every man, woman and child wherever they are in the world, for it deals with the survival of humanity as a species. On a more immediate level the statement is significant to all those persons whose lives have been destroyed or the quality of whose lives has been radically altered by the onset of AIDS or of chronic fatigue syndrome (CFIDS) in themselves or in someone they love.

Plain and simply put, Dr. Donald M. MacArthur says that his scientists have done enough unauthorized work to convince them that they can invent a new class of diseases based upon the destruction of the human immune system. That is, if they are given $10 million and 5 to 10 years the scientists in the Department of Defense laboratories will invent AIDS and its 'mirror image' which we have already noted in *Osler's Web:* chronic fatigue syndrome.

Here is the critical dialogue between Dr. MacArthur and Mr. Robert L.F. Sikes of Florida:

"Dr. MacArthur...eminent biologists believe that within a period of 5 to 10 years it would be possible to produce a synthetic biological agent, an agent that does not naturally exist and for which **no natural immunity could have been acquired.**

Mr. Sikes. *Are we doing any work in that field?*

Dr. MacArthur. *We are not.*

Mr. Sikes. *Why not? Lack of money or lack of interest?*

Dr. MacArthur. **Certainly not lack of interest.**

The reference to 'eminent biologists' is important because it means that according to Dr. MacArthur's expert opinion, the persons who believe that a synthetic agent that attacks the human immune system could be invented are not idle theorists puttering away in a basement laboratory. These are research biologists working in significant research settings. Another point to make is that MacArthur speaks of these 'eminent' researchers in the plural. That is to say, there are several persons with the necessary expertise who, if given enough money and time, will produce a brand new biological agent.

Note the time frame: 5 to 10 years. Thus, if these eminent biologists get the money they need...and don't forget that Mahon and Sikes in particular can authorize all of that given their role on the powerful Appropriations' Committee...then, sometime between 1975 and 1980 the scientists will produce a 'technological surprise' for America's enemies and they will be looking for a place to test the new agents on unsuspecting human guinea pigs, under the supervision of the Centers for Disease Control and of the National Institutes of Health.

As we shall see, Congress was to accept Dr. MacArthur's proposals and was to vote him the money. Almost immediately a defence contract was awarded to Dr. Leonard Hayflick of Stanford University. The contract was to permit Hayflick to acquire, store, inventory and disperse to selected scientists a disease agent named the mycoplasma.[17]

In 1972 there were two unusual scientific/ medical papers published under the auspices of the World Health Organization. One of these papers by Allison, et. al.[18] suggested that, just as Dr. MacArthur had indicated was possible, synthetic viruses could be developed to attack or impair the human immune system. Another scientific paper by Amos. et.al.[19] suggested that one way to test such new agents would be to introduce them into selected vaccination programs.

And, as we have already noted, in 1987 there was another unusual article published. This time it was in the *Times of London* [20] under the by-line of writer Pierce Wright.

It then turned out that when, in the late 1970's, WHO teams had visited Kenya, Uganda and other African nations, they had offered free vaccination against smallpox to anyone who volunteered. Thousands of otherwise healthy people lined up to accept this gift. Then, three years later an unusual illness began to show itself over the whole vaccinated area. The spread of this mystery disease was phenomenal and unlike the victims of CFIDS, the victims of this new disease faced the prospect of almost certain death.

By 1992 the poor medical records of the affected areas established that at least eight million people were HIV positive.[21]

It is useful to recapitulate these dates:

1969...Dr. MacArthur promises to invent an AIDS-like synthetic virus

1972...WHO publication suggests that the testing of an AIDS virus could be achieved in a vaccination program

1972...WHO, financed primarily by the U.S. and manned by CDC personnel, begins widespread smallpox vaccination program in Africa

1981...AIDS epidemic begins to sweep areas vaccinated against smallpox

1987...*Times of London* article says that the AIDS epidemic was created in a western nation laboratory and was introduced into Africa under the guise of vaccinating the population against smallpox.[22]

Returning to the record of the conversation between certain U.S. Congressmen and key researchers from the *Biological Warfare* Branch of the Department of Defense. When Robert Sikes hears about a new weapon that will be a 'technological surprise' and which will be a synthetic agent that does not naturally occur and which will be refractory to the human immune system he is immediately interested... 'Are we doing any work in that field?' When he learns that no work is being done, he wonders why and Dr. MacArthur tells the guy with his hands on the purse strings that although his researchers are interested in developing this agent, they don't have the money needed.

At this point in the record there is some additional information provided later by Dr. MacArthur and two more key points are made in item '4'. First, it is revealed that tentative plans had been made two years *before* to develop this deadly new synthetic agent, and that *"...there are many who believe such research should not be undertaken lest it lead to yet another method of massive killings of large populations."*

It is only towards the end of this momentous day's Hearings that Dr. MacArthur gets back to that "extremely unfortunate Skull Valley incident." On page 142 he explains what happened on March 13, 1968 near the Army's Dugway Proving Ground in Utah. It turns out that on that day a plane had flown over the testing grounds and had sprayed out a deadly nerve agent VX. After the test flight the pilot had shut down the spray system...but the release valve malfunctioned and the deadly agent continued to spray beyond where it was supposed to be. Then another unforeseen development: the "meteorology changed". This is MacArthur's colourful way of saying that as it is often wont to do, the direction of the wind changed and the nerve gas was made available to all living organisms down wind...and "range sheep began sickening and some{2} died later."

Thus the 'extremely unfortunate Skull Valley incident.'

Now, in the great order of things, and especially in view of all the evil things that have been done by certain people with power to those, witting or unwitting, who lack power, the loss of the sheep does not loom very large on any crisis scale. However, the point is very clear :No matter how certain one is that he has everything under control, there is always something that might possibly go wrong. On March 13, 1968 a fouled-up test killed some sheep.

Is it possible that fouled-up tests of Dr. MacArthur's deadly new diseases are creating a 'Skull Valley' of our whole world? Is that what CFIDS and AIDS represents? The evidence suggests it is.

Or, even more horrifying to consider: was the AIDS virus introduced into Africa in a deliberate attempt to reduce the population of that most unhappy continent?

Harare, Zimbabwe—The Skeletal young man with jerking, sweat-drenched limbs waited four hours for care in emergency.

He finally made it to a ward with other AIDS sufferers, where he spent a few days before being sent home to die. With him went a leaflet on basic AIDS care for those unable to afford medication with tips such as sucking overripe tomatoes to soothe mouth lesions.

Zimbabwe's state hospitals and clinics offer little else for victims of "mukondombera"–which means "the big kill" in the local Shona language. AIDS has spread so far and fast in the southern African country that government resources and medical care cannot keep up.

No one is exempt-soldiers, scholars, politicians, babies in the womb…[23]

Summary

On June 9, 1969, several United States Congressmen met in a secret session to learn the latest news from the Biological Warfare experts of the U.S. Department of Defense. At this meeting they learned that the scientists in their employ could create a synthetic biological agent which would attack the human immune system and leave the victim dead (AIDS) or disabled (CFIDS). They were warned that in the testing of such new synthetic agents an error or some unforeseen developments might release a black plague like disease which would sweep vast geographic areas and kill or disable millions of innocent victims. The Congressmen were also promised that they could get this new agent for $10 million, but it would take 5 to 10 years time. Ten years later, in 1981, the first case of AIDS was diagnosed and was attributed to some highly unusual activities involving a Canadian airline steward, a black woman who had been bit by a green monkey, and the homosexual population of New York City, San Francisco and Los Angeles.

Footnotes

{1} "David" is a pseudonym for an American serviceman who joined the U.S. Air Force in 1969. He told his story to W.H.Bowart on condition that his identity would be protected. The full account can be found in: W.H.Bowart *Operation Mind Control* (New York: Dell Publishing Co.,1978) pp.27-41

{2} MacArthur's use of "some" helped hide the extent of the disaster. Over 4,000 and by some accounts up to 8,000 sheep died within 24 hours. One can only wonder what would have happened if the plane had flown over a school yard!

Endnotes

[1].The best source on the framing of James Earl Ray is the 1995 book by William F. Pepper: *Orders to Kill* (New York, Carroll & Graf).Another important source is Frame-Up by the Dean of investigative researchers, Harold Weisberg. The book is available from the author, Route 8, Frederick, Maryland.

[2]. Leonard Horowitz: *Emerging Viruses: Aids and Ebola*. Massachusetts; Tetrahedron Publishing Group. (1997) p.86. It is important to note that Mr. Ted Strecker died under suspicious circumstances a few months after achieving the historic release of Congressional documents revealing US Military plans to develop the AIDS pathogen.

[3].Professor Peter Dale Scott develops the theme of 'denial' in his book Deep Politics and the Death of JFK .This book is required reading for anyone who has ever wondered how it is that a popular president of a nation such as the United States can be executed in broad daylight before hundreds of people and yet have the crime go uninvestigated in an honest, objective manner. As Professor Scott convincingly demonstrates,it is not just the extent to which great power is exercised by persons beyond the public view, but it is also the extent to which so many Americans will go to deny the reality of this power distribution. The book is published by the University of California Press.

[4].Charles A. Reich *Opposing the System* (New York: Crown Publishers, Inc.1995) pp.43-44

[5].Bill Gulley with Mary Ellen Reese *Breaking Cover* (New York: Warner Books, 1980) p.178

[6].Hearings (i)

[7].Richard M. Nixon RN (New York: Grosset & Dunlap, 1978) p.351

[8].Gulley and Reese, *Ibid*, p.44

[9].Eleanora W. Schoenebaum *Profiles of an Era* (New York: Harcourt Brace Jovanovich, 1979) p.417

[10].*Ibid*, p.667

[11].*Ibid*, p.521

[12].Fred J. Cook *The Warfare State* (New York: The Macmillan Company, 1962) pp.190-1

[13].See, among other sources, Kai Bird *The Chairman* (New York etc.:Simon & Schuster, 1992) p.640

[14].To be found in the Hearings, on page 114 of that document.

[15].W.H.Bowart, *Operation Mind Control* (New York, Dell Publishing Co., 1978) p.27

[16].*Ibid*, p.88

[17].*Special Virus Cancer Program*, Progress Report Number Eight, Page 255: Contract: Stanford University,(NIH- 69-2053)

[18].Allison, *et.al. Bulletin*, WHO (1972) VOL. 47, pp.257-263

[19].Amos, *et.al.* WHO Federation Proceedings (1972) Vol. 31, p.1087

[20].Pierce Wright, *Times of London* May 11,198.

[21].*The Cambridge Factfinder* (New York: Cambridge University Press, 1993) p.124

[22]. This brief summary does not give the full complicated picture of the various vaccination programs that were being foisted upon unsuspecting citizens of various African countries by the United States, France, Belgium and other nations. For a comprehensive and scholarly study of the subject the reader is referred to Edward Hooper's: *The River*: (Little , Brown and Company, Boston, New York, London, 1999)

[23].Angus Shaw, *Sudbury Star,* May 2,1996

Chapter Five

Legionnaires' Disease

Thirty-two year old Chris Guthrie, a married mother of one child and anxious to have another, knew something was going seriously wrong.[1] A former teacher who had left that job to become a meter reader for Sierra Power in Kings Beach, California, Ms. Guthrie walked twenty miles a day, five days a week. She enjoyed the independence and the fresh air as she paced through the community, and had an excellent attendance record. However, near the middle of 1984 she began to experience a series of nagging illnesses…strep throat, low grade fever, and a persistent, agonizing fatigue. Finally, on December 30,1984 [2], she was unable to complete her route:

"I called my boss and told him,'I can't make it in, I can't finish,'Guthrie recalled … three years later. Her husband left his workplace in Reno to collect her; found his wife collapsed on the road shoulder outside Kings Beach." [3]

It was the beginning of a long and tragic ordeal which defied definitive diagnosis. Guthrie was to be hospitalized several times with pneumonia, dehydration, or dangerously high fever:

*"At various stages of her illness, she would appear to have **Legionnaires' Disease**, multiple sclerosis, and lymphoma; she would never again be able to work."* [4]

To her doctor, Paul Cheney, the most dramatic abnormality to emerge from the many tests he performed, was *low or nonexistent antibodies to Epstein-Barr nuclear antigen*, a symptom previously observed only in patients *whose immune systems had been depressed by some radical event such as AIDS…*

This early, tenuous link to AIDS, was to be a harbinger of things to come, but at the time Dr. Cheney did not make a connection. What he did recognize was that, amidst the plethora of possible diagnoses was one of Legionnaires' Disease…another mysterious plague that had struck an American Legion Convention in Philadelphia in 1976 and had claimed several lives. But this diagnosis, like so many others, was tantalizing in its elusiveness. At one point the *Legionella pneumophila* bacterium seemed to be there, but at a later point it had disappeared. Dr. Cheney knew that something awfully unusual was going on, but he had no idea what it might be.

Ms. Guthrie's experience in 1984 was not unique, but Dr. Cheney's attention was. To an amazing extent the medical profession of the United States and to a lesser extent the rest of the world, took their lead from the United States Centers for Disease Control which right from the start had refused to accept victims of this mysterious malady with the kind of caring attention they merited as sick people. It is a pattern that persists to the present day and which warrants the special attention given to it in Chapter Six of this work.

But there was more about Ms. Guthrie's situation than just the care with which Paul Cheney responded to her illness. There was the unusual combination of something that was affecting her immune system and the hints of Legionnaire's Disease that blood tests revealed. A combination made all the more significant when one places it in its time frame as related to the meeting on June 9, 1969 when Dr. Donald MacArthur of the Biological Warfare Branch of the United States Department of Defense had promised a cluster of United States Congressmen a *new* agent which would (a) attack the human immune system and (b) either kill its victims or incapacitate them. Both AIDS and CFIDS are diseases which reflect an impaired or destroyed immune system as Dr. MacArthur suggested was possible, and one of these was certainly more fatal than most known diseases, while the other was characterized by Ms. Guthrie's 'bone crushing' fatigue.

Thus, if in 1970 Dr. MacArthur and his scientists continued their work which had already begun[5] with an additional $10 million then in approximately 1976 they would be looking both for ways to test their handiwork and for human guinea pigs who, wittingly or unwittingly, would provide the testing grounds for the modified bacterial and viral agents …their bodies. Bacterial agents which would withstand the conditions necessary to introduce them by aerosol projection into the atmosphere and viral agents which would attack the human immune system.[6]

Such a bacterium would resemble that which mysteriously appeared in 1976 in Philadelphia and which was able to remain lethal even though it had to endure the chill of a hotel's central air-conditioning system. Such a virus (AIDS) suddenly appeared in the same year but was to remain undiagnosed until 1981. And characteristics of both were to hint at their presence in Ms. Chris Guthrie in 1984!

In addition to the general biological warfare challenges that Dr. MacArthur developed with the Congressmen, there were more site specific problems dealt with by other people interested in the subject. For example in a meeting between Richard Helms' CIA operatives and the Fort Detrick 'Special Operations Division' the question as to whether an agent could 'be produced to knock out everyone in a building?'[7] was examined. The discussion apparently was a part of a top secret operation code-named 'MK-NAOMI' that came to light during the Church Committee's hearings in September, 1975.[8] Unfortunately the records (which we were later to learn, were collectively known as "The Special Virus Cancer Program" under numbered 'Progress Reports') were ordered destroyed by the person who helped launch the whole evil enterprise in 1953...Richard Helms. The answer to the question about knocking out a whole building might well have been provided by the experience of the American Legionnaires who had gathered in Philadelphia for their Convention. After all, when one invents a new way to kill one's enemies, one must find a way to test it to make sure that it works.

Germ Warfare....the Problem Of Testing

In his hauntingly beautiful account of hell on earth, William Allister tells the story of his nearly four years as a prisoner of the Japanese during World War Two.[9] At one point Allister and forty-nine other prisoners-of-war were ordered to prepare to be moved from the shipyards where they had worked for over two years:

"Where were we to be sent? There was no information and the void was filled by morbid speculation and rumour. Repatriation? Oh sure. We'd been there too often. Germ experiments? That was too horrible. We'd heard vague, half-formed hints of a camp in Manchuria where prisoners were used for experimentation. No one knew where this had come from- could be from Shinagawa, the Tokyo hospital, where someone may have picked up some gossip from top doctors..." [10]

But it was not just gossip...the fact was that in 1923 the Japanese, despite being signatories to the Geneva Protocol on chemical and biological warfare (but never ratifying it) had initiated studies of chemical warfare. Over the years they expanded into the study of biological weapons, and soon after their occupation of Manchuria in 1931 they established the first of several test sites where they employed prisoners-of-war as human guinea pigs. Most were Chinese prisoners, but rumours persist that these were later joined by American, British and Australian POWs. The truth, however, will probably never be known for, like Richard Helms and his records of MK-NAOMI, when the war ended the Japanese high command destroyed all records and executed any surviving eye-witnesses.[11]

Then an extraordinary bargain was made between the occupying American Army and the former commanders of the Japanese germ warfare experiments. The Americans:

"...offered immunity from prosecution if, in exchange, the Japanese would hand over details of their experiments..." [12]

The Japanese, happy to escape with their lives, shared their evil secrets, and the American Army kept the deal hidden for over thirty years. And, in their interrogation of the man in charge, General Ishii Shiro, they accepted his explanation that the research had indeed been conducted, but purely as a means of defense against possible enemy attack. It is interesting to observe that Dr. Donald MacArthur, the 1969 American counterpart to General Ishii Shiro, used exactly the same rationale in explaining his experiments to the Congressmen on June 9, 1969:

"...(W)e have done a small amount of research on a few agents that do not satisfy this constraint- the reason for this is that a potential enemy might use them against us and we have to be prepared to defend ourselves." [13]

Thus, the Japanese were discovered to have been using prisoners-of-war in tests to determine the efficacy of the biological weapons they had developed, and the United States became accomplices after the fact when they purchased the lessons learned at the cost of secretly sparing the criminals involved.

However, with no prisoners to use as guinea pigs, the United States biological warfare researchers had to look around for other test victims, and they found them in three principal places: the armed services, prisons and hospitals. In some cases the persons used in their tests had actually volunteered, with a more or less honest explanation of what was being fed to them, injected into them or breathed by them. In other cases, advantage was taken of the defenceless quality of their relationship to those in charge. One way or another, biological weapons had to be tested on living human beings to see if the planned effects could actually be achieved. There is also evidence that some agents were tested in other countries on the armed forces, prison populations or hospital patients. Canada seems to have been an especially willing host for such programs.

An example of Canadian complicity is to be found in the activities of Dr. Ewen Cameron of McGill University in the 1950's. Dr. Cameron, in what must be seen as his professions' lack of perception as to whom among them was fit to treat patients and who was himself certifiably insane, had been elected as the first president of the World Psychiatric Association.[14] At McGill University where he was the Director of the Psychiatric Hospital he employed funds provided by the CIA to subject helpless patients to weird and cruel treatments. He injected them with LSD and watched the often horrifying results. On another occasion he put them into a drug-induced , thirty day sleep...during which time he had tapes played to them over and over again to see if he could 're-program their brain'. One colleague, Donald Hebb, described Cameron's efforts this way:

> "If you actually look at what he was doing and wrote what he wrote, it would make you laugh. If I had a graduate student who talked like that, I'd throw him out." [15]

Such actions by Dr. Cameron may have been enough to make Dr. Hebb 'laugh', but the damage to the unsuspecting patients was anything but laughable. It is also a commentary upon the life-attitudes of people engaged in what is termed the 'intelligence services'. They are evidently drawn to the covert world because they have learned from experience that if they shared some of their inspired efforts to defend their nation from some real or imagined 'enemy' with the public at large they would be seen to be luminously insane.

Furthermore, if the insanity that allows for distinguished scientists to meet with right-wing politicians to discuss ways and means to utilize biological science to destroy or disable other human beings were simply an exercise in lunatic speculation, it would do no harm. However, the politicians who met with Dr. MacArthur on June 9, 1969, had the power to vote vast sums to permit him to realize his research goals. All they needed were enough people like Dr. Ewen

Cameron who would abuse his obligation to his patients by subjecting them to whatever new biological agents Dr. MacArthur came up with.

The experiments at McGill came to light only after an astute American researcher employing the Freedom of Information legislation of the United States was able to gain access to the documentation. However, this was just one case and there were hundreds of other biological agents developed and tested the details of which are yet to be revealed . In 1977 the CIA admitted that there had been 149 sub-projects involving forty-four colleges and universities, fifteen research foundations, twelve hospitals or clinics and three penal institutions. Just what was developed and upon whom were the developed agents tested?

Was one of the tests conducted at Philadelphia in 1976 when hundreds of American Legionnaires gathered from across the nation for their Convention?

Before one leaps to judgement consider the words of Fritz Haber, a pioneer in the development of gas warfare, when he accepted the Nobel Prize for Chemistry in 1919:

> "In no future war will the military be able to ignore poison gas. It is a higher form of killing." [16]

Or, even more chilling, consider the 'Most Secret' minute from Prime Minister Winston Churchill to the British Chiefs of Staff on July 6, 1944:

> "It may be several weeks or even months before I shall ask you to drench Germany with poison gas, and if we do it, let us do it one hundred percent. In the meanwhile, I want the matter studied in cold blood by sensible people and not by that particular set of psalm-singing uniformed defeatists which one runs across now here now there." [17]

The fact of the matter is that evil weapons have been contemplated and actions taken to develop and use them by all manner of sensible men ranging from Churchill through Dr. MacArthur and Congressmen such as Sikes, Mahon, Rhodes and others, to lunatics such as Allen Dulles, Richard Helms and Fritz Haber. And the whole operation requires that at some point their evil products are put to the test.

LEGIONNAIRES' DISEASE
Motive, Means and Opportunity?

When Dr. MacArthur met secretly on June 9, 1969 with a group of largely right-wing, hawkish United

States Congressmen, he concluded his presentation with a summary of the priorities of the Biological Warfare branch of the Department of Defense. One of these priorities is especially worthy of note:

"Questions such as efficiency of dissemination, whether viruses and bacteria can be mutated to new forms resistant to vaccines, the longevity of microbes in aerosols, and others must be quantitated so that we can accurately assess our vulnerability and develop effective defense." [18]

If one is to 'quantitate' (by which term we presume Dr. MacArthur means 'quantify') any results of a scientific test it is necessary to have a sufficiently large sample to achieve anything statistically meaningful. For example, if one were seeking some pathogenic agent which would achieve Richard Helms' objective of knocking out 'everyone in a building', one could not test it on mice or dogs. That would be a start, but when it came right down to quantifying how many human beings in a targeted building would succumb to a newly created pathogen introduced by an aerosol agent one would have to have several hundred human beings in a building for the necessary test period during which the pathogen is released. Then, after the release of the agent, one would have to have some control over the activities of the exposed victims. To just release an agent into a building where everyone exposed was free to head for all parts of the city or state and to consult hundreds of doctors in a wide range of hospitals, clinics and medical offices would never be subject to effective quantification. Everyone exposed might have become sick, or none of those exposed might have suffered any adverse reaction.

The need to 'quantitate' must, therefore, be emphasized.

A further goal that Dr. MacArthur set for his researchers was to determine the 'efficiency of dissemination'. This, of course relates to the need to quantify results, but to have more than one test site so that different disseminating techniques can be compared to each other. One could never test two methods at the same time since there would be no way to establish which method achieved which part of the end result.

These two criteria are normal for any scientific testing of a hypothesis or method. It is the question 'whether viruses and bacteria can be mutated to new forms resistant to vaccines?' that is cause for the greatest concern. Dr. MacArthur is referring to the 'synthetic biological agents' that he had introduced

on page 129, when he talked for the first time about an agent for which no natural immunity could have been acquired…i.e. AIDS.

The final question in the sixth point of the priorities enunciated by Dr. MacArthur was to determine the longevity of microbes in aerosols.

Before we examine the outbreak of a mysterious illness among the Legionnaires gathered in Philadelphia in 1976 for their annual Convention, considering as we do so the challenge Dr. MacArthur would face in testing the new 'virus/bacteria' agent he was working on, it is important to remind ourselves that his Branch of the Department of Defense had already been doing such research since 1947 when they recruited the Japanese murderers into their research and since 1952 when they entered into their secret agreement with the CIA to develop biological weapons for 'covert' operations.

Even twenty years ago the Bellevue Stratford Hotel in Philadelphia was an ancient dowager among hotels of that city. However, it still attracted good convention business because it was large and economical. All manner of middle income travellers could afford a few days at the Bellevue Stratford, and that is why the Oddfellows fraternal group selected it for their Convention in 1974…just five years and one month after Dr. MacArthur had met with the Congressmen, and *two years before the Legionnaires were to gather in the same hotel!*

The Convention started off well enough, but after two days the celebrants were beginning to suffer from a mix of symptoms that defied immediate diagnosis: some felt sick at the stomach, others developed a mild headache. Still others experienced rapidly rising fever and nonproductive coughs. Although several had symptoms, only 20 sought medical care and of this number two died. No doctor who was consulted by the ill victims was able to identify the pathogen and the outbreak faded out of view. [19]

Two years later, almost to the day, another group of Convention-goers checked into the Bellevue Stratford Hotel in Philadelphia. Like the Oddfellows of two years earlier, they were basically middle-aged and middle-income Americans. And, like the Oddfellows before them, in two or three days the Legionnaires began to manifest the symptoms seen two years earlier: headaches, rapidly rising fever, myalgias, nonproductive coughs. Before many days several Legionnaires were ill and of those, 182 sought medical attention. And, where ten percent of the Oddfellows had died, nearly sixteen percent of the

Legionnaires died. In addition, there were another 39 cases among persons who were not attending the Convention. Some were hotel employees, some were around the hotel on family or other business, and of this group five died. Unlike the Oddfellows whose tragic get together had largely faded from the public mind, the plight of the Legionnaires became headline news across the country, and they gave the disease its distinctive name: Legionnaires' Disease.[20]

The higher profile of the Legionnaires' epidemic motivated certain researchers to look back over the recent past for traces of similar outbreaks. They identified two that seemed to fit the template...one outbreak in 1965 in St. Elizabeth's Hospital, a large psychiatric facility in Washington, D.C. There had been 81 cases and 14 fatalities...approximately 17 percent, and another outbreak in Pontiac, Michigan, in 1968 where 144 employees of a health department building had become ill, but none had died.

Although all four outbreaks came to be labelled as "Legionnaires' Disease" and all did indeed share several characteristics, there were significant differences between them. The most important of these was the fatality rate...from no deaths in Pontiac, through ten percent among the Oddfellows, sixteen percent among the Legionnaires and over seventeen percent among the patients of the psychiatric hospital.

These statistics based upon the varying fatality rates in the four cases under review calls to mind Dr. MacArthur's concern that "before an agent can be classified as an incapacitant we feel that the mortality must be very low...Now this is a very difficult job. *We have had some of the top scientists in the country working for years on how to get more effective incapacitating agents. It is not easy.*" [21] The question arises, how do these top scientists tell just how lethal their new agents are unless they test them on statistically significant samples?

Another problem faced the researchers...by what medium had the pathogen made its way to the victims? In the Bellevue Stratford Hotel the blame was fixed upon the central, water-cooled air-conditioning system, while at St. Elizabeth's Hospital blame was placed upon dust stirred up by construction work in the parking lot. In Pontiac researchers could not finger a specific medium. This in turn again takes us to Dr. MacArthur's questions...how to determine the efficiency of dissemination. Is there any significance in the fact that in one case of Legionnaires' Disease the agent was dust while in another it was water?

Several important characteristics , however, were shared by all four sites. In each case all victims occupied a large building for a significant number of days. They were not in and out of a mall, or seated for two hours in a movie theatre. Furthermore, the victims were relatively easy to track. The Bellevue Stratford guests had all registered, while the patients at St. Elizabeth were on record as were the employees of the Health Department Building.

Such factors would help anyone minded to do it to 'quantitate' the effects of each outbreak, with a somewhat reduced capacity in respect to the Oddfellows group. The co-incidence of two outbreaks in the same venue would also help anybody trying to measure some factor that they might be aware of, but which would not be apparent to the uninitiated.

A very important characteristic of the Legionnaires and the patients in the Hospital was the fact that in both cases, researchers would have ready access to medical histories which would be helpful in analysing any anomalies.

The most important point that must be evaluated is Dr. MacArthur's suggestion that his scientists were going to try to mutate viruses and bacteria to create new forms that would be resistant to vaccines. When the virologists and other specialists turned to the blood samples of the victims of Legionnaires' Disease they found that they could not trace the pathogen to any known virus or bacteria. Whatever it was, it was 'unresponsive to penicillins, cephalosporins, and aminoglycosides.' Furthermore, according to Don J. Brenner, *et al,* "It is unlikely that the LDB (Legionnaires' Disease Bacterium) is related to any well-described pathogen." [22] In other words, seven years after the Biological Warfare specialists suggested that a new agent could be created which would have to be tested for a range of qualities including dissemination, longevity of microbes and resistance to vaccines, a major outbreak of a new infectious agent among a group of Legionnaires apparently introduced into the atmosphere by aerosol technique took 34 lives. If anyone was monitoring the results he could have 'quantitated' them by comparing them with what happened in three other cases.

In conclusion, it must be noted that although Dr. MacArthur and the Congressmen never mention the possibility that tests will be performed upon unsuspecting human beings, the " researchers were nevertheless able to base much of their work upon a compendium of case studies which supposedly did not exist." [23]

Summary

At the conclusion of World War Two the United States military spared the lives of the Japanese researchers who had used allied prisoners of war as biological warfare guinea pigs in return for the results of their evil experiments. In 1952 the U.S. move towards the development of biological weapons was advanced when the CIA entered into a secret agreement to continue the activity for 'covert' operations against the 'enemies' of the U.S. Over 149 tests were conducted under the latter agreement, including tests on unwitting persons in prisons, psychiatric hospitals and the armed services. These tests even extended into Canada, Britain, New Zealand and Australia. In the period from 1965 to 1976 a new pathogenic agent made its presence known on four separate occasions, taking approximately fifty lives. This new disease named after its Legionnaire victims has an almost perfect fit with the template of criteria identified by Dr. Donald MacArthur when he met with several U.S. Congressmen on Monday, June 9, 1969.

Endnotes

[1].The details of Chris Guthrie's experiences are drawn from Hillary Johnson's remarkable book, *Osler's Web* (New York: Crown Publishers, Inc.,1996) For anyone interested in chronic fatigue syndrome, acquired immune deficiency and biological warfare experiments, Ms. Johnson's book is essential background reading.

[2].It is important at the outset to emphasize the year...1984...As this study reveals, something very significant was initiated in that year.

[3].Hillary Johnson, *Osler's Web* p.24

[4].Johnson, *Ibid*, p. 25

[5].Although on June 9, 1969, Dr. MacArthur was asking for research money, the evidence is clear from the conversations during the meeting that, with or without Congressional approval, the development of biological weapons was already well under way. Not only does Chairman George Mahon state at the outset of the Meeting that 'This subcommittee and the Congress has, over a period of years, supported the appropriation of funds for chemical and biological warfare', but there had been such developments carried on by the CIA and the Fort Detrick biological warfare experts from as early as 1953 when the then Director of Plans, Richard Helms, asked for and received the approval needed from Allen Dulles to establish a 'program for the covert use of biological and chemical materials.' This quote appears in Robert Harris and Jeremy Paxman's significant study *A Higher Form of Killing* (New York: Hill and Wang, 1982), p.205

[6].*Ibid*, p.129

[7].Harris and Paxman, *Ibid*, p.212

[8].Referred to in Endnote 30 on page 262 of Harris and Paxman. MK-NAOMI is still a very closely guarded 'black' project which some careful researchers believe was given the job of developing the chronic fatigue retrovirus.

[9].William Allister *Where Life and Death Hold Hands* (Toronto: Stoddard Publishing Co.,1989)

[10].Allister, *Ibid*, p.174

[11].Harris and Paxman, *Ibid*, p.79

[12].Harris and Paxman, *Ibid*, p.152

[13].Hearings, p.144

[14].Celina Bledowska and Jonathan Bloch, *KGB/CIA* (London: Bison Books Ltd.,1987) p.164

[15].Bledowska and Bloch, *Ibid*, pp.164-5

[16].Quoted in Harris and Paxman, p. xiii

[17].Harris and Paxman, *Ibid*, p.107

[18].Appendix (i), p.144

[19].Gilda L. Jones and G. Ann Hebert *Legionnaires'* (Atlanta, Ga.,:U.S. Dept. of Health, Education, and Welfare, 1978) p.5

[20].Jones and Hebert, *Ibid*, p.5

[21].Hearings, p.117

[22].Quoted in Jones and Hebert, *Ibid*

[23].Harris and Paxman, *Ibid*, p.152

CHAPTER SIX

ACQUIRED IMMUNE DEFICIENCY

Nelson Aldrich Rockefeller

Nelson Rockefeller was never a member of the United States Central Intelligence Agency...or at any rate not in any publicly acknowledged capacity...yet, on page 62 of what is almost a semi-official 'photographic history' of that Agency is a picture of Nelson Rockefeller and his brother, Laurance.[1] Beneath the picture is this important statement:

"Rockefeller ran his own secret operations in Latin America as a private businessman..." [2]

This masterful understatement just alludes in passing to the role of Nelson Rockefeller in the world of covert activities, and it masks the fact that he and his brother, David, had inherited the Rockefeller family bent for exercising the power of the family wealth and control of banking, oil, and a multitude of other financial institutions in support of what was (and probably still is) effectively an alternate government, not just of the United States, but of many other nominally independent nations.

This concept of an alternate government has been developed by a number of writers, ranging from those who believe it is just a loose cluster of powerful people who happen to share a range of political/economic beliefs, to those who believe that there is a far more structured and coherent power cluster which exercises its collective will through key figures in government, finance, journalism, and other significant areas of influence.

In the former category is Charles A. Reich who has written about 'The System' which he sees as being run by a managerial elite..."formed on the basis of shared knowledge and assumptions...Like other significant features of the System, this shared knowledge has no name, is never directly taught, is not written down, and prefers invisibility." [3]

At the other end of the scale is L. Fletcher Prouty who wrote in reference to the assassination of President John F. Kennedy:

"That assassination has demonstrated that most of the major events of world significance are masterfully planned and orchestrated by an elite coterie of enormously powerful people who are not of one nation, one ethnic grouping, or one overridingly

important business group. They are a power unto themselves for whom these others work. Neither is this power elite of recent origin. Its roots go deep into the past." [4]

Historian Arthur M. Schlesinger, Jr., identifies the power base as 'The American Establishment' and is more specific than Reich or Prouty:

"Its household deities were Henry L. Stimson and Elihu Root; its present leaders, Robert A. Lovett and John J. McCloy; its front organizations, the Rockefeller, Ford, and Carnegie foundations and the Council on Foreign Relations; its organs, the New York Times and Foreign Affairs.[5]

Prof. Peter Dale Scott in his meticulously researched study of the assassination of John F. Kennedy, states in his Epilogue:

"We still talk of an America of constitutional government. But in crisis after crisis the real power centers turn out to be institutions like the CIA, or the National Security Council, which the Constitution never contemplated and arguably cannot survive." [6]

Whether one identifies with Reich's 'loose managerial elite', Prouty's 'coterie of enormously powerful people', Schlesinger's 'American Establishment' or Scott's 'real power centers' one will find within his choice from among the options, the power of the Rockefeller interests being exercised in support of a private agenda and, during the period from 1931, when he went to work in the family enterprises, until his death in 1979, one will especially discover hints of the covert activities of Nelson Rockefeller. When one explores these activities more closely he will find that contrary to the public persona conveyed by a largely captive media, a persona characterized by liberal ideas, progressive racial attitudes, a love of art and a happy smile, the Nelson Rockefeller that lurks in the shadows is one of baleful influence.

Two years after Nelson Rockefeller joined the family enterprises, one of their most important holdings was Standard Oil, which, in 1933 and 1934, through various members of its Board of Directors, supported the American Liberty League, a group of America's wealthiest families and most powerful corporations determined to recruit retired Marine

Corps Major General Smedley Darlington Butler to lead a *coup d'état* and depose President Franklin Delano Roosevelt.[7] We have no way of knowing how much Nelson Rockefeller knew of the planned *coup*. Only closely guarded and possibly well-sanitized Standard Oil Board Minutes or the top secret Rockefeller archives could tell us that. However, it is unlikely that Nelson Rockefeller was 'out of the loop' in any Standard Oil role, given the fact that he of all the 'brothers' was most informed about that company's seedy history and 'the power and grandeur' as he termed it of John D. Rockefeller's founding role.[8]

Not only are most American history texts, out of an apparent deference for the sensitivities of the Rockefellers and other establishment figures, deficient in their reporting of the 1933-4 efforts by Standard Oil and others to stage a *coup d'état*, (and at the same time help the American public avoid having to face up to such fascist elements in their history) the same texts also pay scant attention to another Rockefeller family concern: population control.

In 1904 a significant amount of Rockefeller money, together with major contributions from the Morgan, Vanderbilt, and Carnegie families, went towards the creation of the "Station for Experimental Evolution" in Cold Spring Harbor, New York. Part of the Station was the Cold Spring Harbor Laboratory (which went on to become a major center of molecular biological research headed by James Watson, the co-discoverer of DNA). In 1910 the Harriman family made their contribution to the study of "eugenics" and population control by endowing the Eugenics Record Office, where, in the interests of developing a more perfect humanity, studies would be made of families whose mating was monitored and whose off-spring were followed through the early years of their lives. The sponsors preferred to think of it as 'social Darwinism' and they were intent on making sure that the fittest,(ie themselves) gave nature a helping hand.

By 1932, when Nelson Rockefeller, already well imbued with John D. Rockfeller Senior's population control philosophy, began to play an active role in the family business, the Third International Conference on Eugenics was convened. The wealthy Eastern elite was well represented by Mrs. H.B. Dupont, Mrs. Averell Harriman (mother of the Democratic Party luminary) Mr. and Mrs. Cleveland H. Dodge, and J.P. Morgan nephew, Henry Fairchild Osborn and again the Standard Oil Board was well represent-

ed by Mrs. John T. Pratt and Mrs. Walter Jennings. Again we have no record of Nelson Rockefeller's response to the event; however, his later efforts in 1952, when he played a part in the establishment of the Eisenhower Administration, suggest that he was aware of the philosophy and over-all direction of the population control movement. This philosophy and direction can be inferred from the fact that the Third International Conference on Eugenics unanimously elected Dr. Ernst Rudin as President of the International Federation of Eugenics Organizations. Rudin went on to develop Hitler's 'racial hygiene' policies and trained the medical personnel who conducted the Nazi's first extermination program, killing 40,000 mental patients. Final evidence that Nelson Rockefeller was at least a silent partner in moves to counter the threat some saw in the growth of the world's population can be seen in the fact that his brother John D. Rockefeller lll, in that same year (1952) established the Population Council with initial funding of $250,000.[9]

The consequences of five decades of Rockefeller support for the concept of population control will be seen later as the philosophy melds with other concepts of resource development, the protection of 'free enterprise' and the need to husband the world's threatened environment.

Besides being inclined to control what went on in areas that he deemed worthy of his attention through covert agencies such as his 'private intelligence apparat' in Central and South America, and his knowledge of and evident support for any effort to limit the unfettered growth of the world's population, Nelson also had an interest in business, but not in the same routine way that his brothers had. The latter approach was too staid and unimaginative for him, and in May of 1945 he united his business acumen with his love of the covert by participating in the creation of the British American Canadian Corporation S.A.(re-named the World Commerce Corporation in April, 1947, and referred to in this work hereafter as WCC).

The WCC possessed a number of qualities that make it worthy of careful attention. First of all, it was established largely by former intelligence officers from the United States, Britain and Canada.[10] Second, the organization had, according to Frank T. Ryan who had succeeded John Arthur Pepper as WCC president, "financial resources available" that "were substantial." [11] Third, the incorporation was registered in Panama, which put its financial transactions beyond the scrutiny of any of the governments of the founding members. Fourth, it had significant links with James Forrestal who was one of the controllers of a secret cache of Nazi gold seized during World War II and hidden from America's allies and from public scrutiny and which was used to finance a covert campaign against communism.

The WCC, with Nelson Rockefeller participation, engaged in a mix of legal and illegal activities for several years, the latter including the deliberate murder of several Social Democratic leaders in Italy on May Day, 1947.[12] But probably its most significant role as far as this study is concerned is that it served as one of the instruments for recruiting former German and Japanese officers into the developing American intelligence apparat. These efforts brought in the likes of SS Sturmbannfuhrer Alois Brunner of Germany who is known to have been directly responsible "for the murder of 128,500 people," [13] and General Ishii Shiro of Japan who had directed the Japanese biological warfare research and testing and in the process murdered several allied prisoners of war. [14] This whole evil enterprise which seems to have been characterized by an absence of any moral standards at all and which betrayed the debt owed to millions of holocaust victims and thousands of allied soldiers was headed up by Nelson Rockefeller, John J. McCloy, William Stephensen (a man called 'Intrepid') William Donovan, Allan Dulles and others. However, it was the recruitment of General Ishii Shiro, which was to lead to the research alluded to by Dr. Donald MacArthur when he met as we have seen on June 9, 1969 with a group of cold war champions of the United States House of Representatives, and the creation of a 'synthetic agent' for which 'no natural immunity could have been acquired'.[15] It was also to be marked by an ironic personal tragedy for one of its principal architects, Nelson Aldrich Rockefeller, and the death of his son Michael.

General Ishii Shiro, having been spared prosecution as a war criminal in exchange for Japanese research results and having been put onto the payroll of the United States taxpayers, claimed to have had all the documents destroyed, was able to convey a great deal of information to his new friends. One piece of information was that the Japanese had established a biological test station in New Guinea in the Dutch East Indies.

Just what General Ishii Shiro's researchers were working on is still an official secret, but in a few years after the war in the western reaches of the territory on the Island of New Guinea (now called Irian Jaya) the Stone Age natives of the area began to succumb to a strange new disease which was characterized by "loss of coordination, tremors, paralysis, and dementia; wasting and death followed the first symptoms within a year." [16] By an unusual co-incidence an American virologist, D. Carleton Gajdusek, travelled to New Guinea to study the epidemic in the late 1950's. He discovered that the disease, which the Fore tribe referred to as kuru, the trembling sickness, was caused by a virus which attacked the brain and left it in spongy ruins! It was, apparently, the same disease which had appeared in flocks of sheep in Iceland in the eighteenth century and which, although it killed sheep "did not seem to pass from sheep to other species." [17] Something or someone appears to have been able to get the virus to 'jump species'.

Evidence has now emerged that the Japanese were, indeed, experimenting with what they have labelled "sheep serum" in tests upon both natives and Allied prisoners of war.

"Murphy testified that Hirano had told him the serum was made from sheep blood and was safe to use. Hirano denied this during interrogation, although he claimed he indeed had sheep for experimental use at department headquarters." [18]

Although at a loss to explain where the virus came from, Dr. Gajdusek was to hypothesize that it spread due to a Fore tribe tradition.(Note: in any discussion of infectious diseases, one must distinguish between the source of the pathogen and the vector by which it is transmitted). Apparently, when a body of a deceased tribe member was prepared for burial, the women performing the rites, removed the victim's brain and ate it. Then the head was ready for the next step of being shrunk to form a totem. This, said Dr. Gajdusek, accounted for the fact that most victims of kuru were women since it was they (and occasionally a child) who ate the diseased brains.

It is now relatively common knowledge that the 'brain rot' in sheep and 'another sheep infection, visna, which produces something like human multiple sclerosis,' [19] was the starting point for the research Dr. MacArthur was doing in the early 1960's in Fort Detrick and other research centers, and which he had initiated after the April, 1953 proposal to Allen Dulles from Richard Helms had led to the secret CIA-military agreement under the codename MK-NAOMI. Their research had proceeded far enough to give him the confidence to promise the Congressmen on June 9, 1969, that in 5 to 10 years his researchers could develop the new synthetic agent we now know induces the disease state AIDS.

Then, in December, 1954, President Eisenhower appointed Nelson Rockefeller as his Special Assistant for Cold War Strategy.[20] It is hard to imagine anything more contradictory than such a title with the avowed nature of his duties which were to give 'advice and assistance in the development of increased understanding and cooperation among all peoples'! However, the rhetoric was just for the public…Rockefeller's real job was that of Presidential Coordinator for the CIA. In this role, according to biographer Joseph E. Persico:

"He completed his petrification as a Cold Warrior(and)…he enjoyed an intimate knowledge of and developed a lasting taste for CIA covert operations." [21]

Thus, in December, 1954 when he was appointed by Eisenhower to conduct the 'cold war' it all came together under Nelson Rockefeller: the fifty year family commitment to population control, the background in covert scheming, the links with the WCC, the alliance with Allen Dulles and Richard Helms who not only had their secret agreement with the biological warfare researchers at Fort Detrick, but also had the links with the Japanese germ warfare researchers. The latter treasure trove of deadly knowledge, purchased by the lives of the prisoners of war used as guinea pigs, gave America a leg up on every other nation in the development of new and deadly biological agents, including the results of the Japanese research in New Guinea which may well have been linked to the 'brain rot' among the Fore tribe. Nelson Rockefeller also had his enduring ties with a relative by marriage, Tracy Barnes, who was one of the controllers for the Gehlen Nazis that had been recruited into the CIA, together with Frank Wisner whose principal claim to fame today is that he was the person who recruited the luminously insane E. Howard Hunt into the CIA.

The challenge facing today's researcher is to piece together what transpired in Fort Detrick and other laboratories under the control of the CIA-Biological Warfare scientists between the December, 1954, arrival of Nelson Rockefeller in a command position (which post he held for approximately a year and a half) and Monday, June 9, 1969 when Dr. Donald M. MacArthur revealed what he and his 'life science' experts had been up to over the fifteen year period. For several years those who were in a position to tell had not volunteered what they knew even had they

been so motivated, and the power of the military-industrial complex has been sufficient to keep them from being compelled to reveal their secrets. However, as we shall reveal later in this work, those hidden records were to come to light. In the meantime, the researcher was left to fit together such pieces as he could find into a reasonable hypothesis based upon available clues from a variety of disparate sources was able after details of the so-called Special Virus Cancer Program were discovered in 2001 to replace his hypothesis with the facts. However, just as those engaged in the spy-trades make it a cardinal rule not to leave a trail of evidence, [22] and depend upon the naivete of a trusting public to lead them to assume that in the absence of evidence, all things done by the covert operators were moral and appropriate early researchers had to count upon their intuition to fill in the gaps. As Peter Wright has put it:

"Espionage is a crime almost devoid of evidence, which is why intuition, for better or worse, always has a large part to play in its successful detection." [23]

Another important element to be watched for by the researcher when trying to arrive at the truth that others are determined to keep from public scrutiny, is a working hypothesis of Professor Peter Dale Scott which he has termed the 'negative template'. That is, one must look at what has been left out of any 'revelation' for a clue as to what is really important. For example, having noted that several FBI reports had omitted the names of certain persons involved in the 'investigation' of the assassination of President John F. Kennedy, Prof. Scott was to write:

"These missing names were recurringly so sensitive that I formed the testable hypothesis that the index itself, or more specifically the residue of names missing from it, provided a negative template or clue for further investigation." [24]

In Fort Detrick, under the general cover name of MK-NAOMI, the research given over to developing the synthetic agent promised to the Congressmen by MacArthur which would attack the human immune system and either kill its victims, or ,in a variation, disable them as CFIDS does was conducted. However, when the CIA came under scrutiny by the Senate's Church Committee in September, 1975, Director William Colby had to confess that the CIA had deemed it prudent to destroy all records of MK-NAOMI. As we have noted above, some of these records accidentally escaped being shredded and were to come into our hands in 2001. What we learned therein is revealed in the final chapter of this work. They had apparently learned about more than germ warfare secrets from the Japanese. However, it was during these hearings that among the challenges explored by the MK-NAOMI researchers was the question whether biological agents could be developed to 'knock out a whole building'...as had later happened in the Bellevue Stratford Hotel in Philadelphia when it was the venue for a convention of American Legionnaires. And, it was during this period that:

> "...researchers were being sent on expeditions to far flung corners of the globe to gather plant or animal samples which might be used in the manufacture of new weapons." [25]

The latter expeditions corresponded in time with Dr. Gajdusek's happily co-incident visit to that 'far flung corner' of the world, New Guinea, where by another fortuitous co-incidence, the Japanese had recently operated a biological warfare station for reasons never publicly disclosed but which were probably part of the information provided to the United States biological warfare researchers. It was also an area where the brains of deceased tribesmen who had succumbed to a mysterious illness were eaten by the women who were preparing the victims for burial, and where the women themselves then became fatally ill with a disease long associated with biological efforts to create a new weapon of war.

As a starting point in this effort to develop what happened between 1954 and 1969, it will be useful to take a second look at what Dr. MacArthur told the Congressmen in the latter year, and to try to formulate reasonable hypotheses based upon evidence from other reliable sources and, as Prof. Scott suggests, look at what Dr. MacArthur failed to reveal as a clue to what was going on.

However, before moving to that stage, it is necessary to pause and consider a tragic personal event in the life of Nelson Rockefeller which has several ironic relationships to the story out of New Guinea.

In 1961 Nelson Rockefeller's son, Michael, travelled to the home areas of the primitive Kurelu [26] tribesmen of New Guinea where he:

> "...photographed babies being born, warfare with other tribes, the death of wounded warriors, and the ceremony preparatory to the cremation that sent the dead to oblivion."

A few weeks later Michael disappeared off the coast of New Guinea and was never seen again. However:

> "For years travellers returning from the Asmat brought back lurid stories of having seen natives wearing Michael Rockefeller's broken glasses around their neck and of having been shown what was purported to be his shrunken skull." [27]

And, in another ironic twist, Watergate burglar E. Howard Hunt who had worked closely with Rockefeller relative, Tracy Barnes, seemed puzzled over the Michael Rockefeller disappearance. On one occasion, while talking to Kerry Thornley about other things, Hunt suddenly remarked apropos of nothing in the conversation:

> "Kerry, one of Nelson Rockefeller's sons went on an expedition in the jungles of New Guinea and vanished. I wonder what ever happened to him?" [28]

We shall have cause to return to this question later.

On Green Monkeys And Airline Stewards

The 'eminent biologists' who could, according to Dr. Donald M. MacArthur of the Biological Warfare branch of the U.S. Department of Defense, create a synthetic agent for which no natural immunity could have been acquired must have been doing something somewhere between the years of 1952 and 1981 when, in terms of the 'official' history of the disease, there were the 'first reports of AIDS'.[29] This chronological listing about the mysterious appearance of acquired immune deficiency in a standard reference work gives a hint of just how uncertain the accepted view of things can be, and explains why, when dealing with this subject which should be rigorously scientific and objective, it is necessary to devote a separate chapter to the 'official mythologies' of AIDS, CFIDS, and biological warfare.{1} However, at this point it is useful to take a second look at Dr. MacArthur's testimony to the United States Congressmen on Monday, June 9, 1969, and to refer certain details to other sources. Then the 'official' story of the disease as told by Randy Shilts [30] and others can be reviewed to discover whether there are any 'negative templates' evident, and to determine the significance of the testimony in its relationship to other things going on in the realm of cold war politics.

Dr. MacArthur tells the Congressmen that the United States Department of Defense has a total of 76 in-house laboratories. This number should be noted since it gives a very good clue as to the extent of the U.S. research. To warrant identification as a laboratory, a site would obviously require from 20 to 30 scientists suggesting a personnel total of between 2,000 and 2,500. This estimate seems to be confirmed by MacArthur's later revelation that $90 million was being spent annually and that sum would fund over 2,000 personnel at 1969 wage levels. In other words, the amount of work being done was significant.

George Mahon's comment that:

"This subcommittee has, over a period of years, supported the appropriation of funds for chemical and biological warfare"

leads to the question of how many years? The answer is probably since 1945 when the Japanese scientists were recruited into the American efforts. However, some clues have emerged from other sources to confirm a time frame of at least ten years. Thomas Powers in *The Man Who Kept the Secrets* [31] writes:

"In 1960, when Richard Bissell asked his science adviser, Sidney Gottlieb, to undertake research on assassination techniques, and when he discussed the possibility of killing Castro...the CIA was also trying to assassinate Patrice Lumumba in the Congo, was at the very least considering the assassination of General Kassem of Iraq, and was deeply involved with a small group of dissidents in the Dominican Republic who were planning to kill Trujillo..."

Gottlieb was later to tell the Church Committee that he picked out a biological agent at Fort Detrick, Maryland from a list of materials which would cause tularemia (rabbit fever), brucellosis (undulant fever), tuberculosis, anthrax, smallpox, and Venezuelan equine encephalitis (sleeping sickness).[32] Fort Detrick, of course, is the place where the CIA-U.S. Army 1952 experiments were carried out under the top secret MK-NAOMI project.

The evidence is compelling...The United States Department of Defense had spent hundreds of millions of dollars over several years to develop biological weapons.

On page 114 of the Hearings, Mr. Flood of Pennsylvania asked a key question and elicited a chilling answer from Dr. MacArthur:

"Mr. Flood. Wouldn't it be more effective to disable than to kill troops?

Dr. MacArthur. Yes, it imposes a greater logistic burden on the enemy when he has to look after disabled people..."

Then Dr. MacArthur tells the Congressmen:

"We have had some of the top scientists in the country working for years on how to get more effective incapacitating agents..."

Just which disabling agents the Biological Warfare researchers were working on *for years* will be examined in Chapter Seven. At this point it is enough to ask: just who were these 'top scientists' who had been working 'for years' and what did they come up with? Was it an agent which would produce chronic fatigue?

However, it was Dr. MacArthur's statement that he and his researchers could over a 5 to 10 year period and at a cost of $10 million develop a new infective microorganism that might be refractory to the immunological and therapeutic processes upon which humans depend to maintain relative freedom from disease that merits top consideration, for, plain and simply, Dr. MacArthur was promising to invent AIDS! He had, he tells his listeners, 'a small group of experts' who believed that somewhere between 1975 and 1979 the biological warfare researchers of the United States could develop a 'synthetic agent' which would be refractory to the human body's natural defence immune system. One for which no immunity could have been acquired. Such an agent, if developed according to Dr. MacArthur's informed estimate, would be ready for testing on someone in the year 1976 or earlier...and , if it worked as planned, then, in or around 1979 the 'volunteers' or more likely the unwitting guinea pigs who had been injected with this new synthetic agent would be coming down with a disease which would be refractory to the human immune system.

In 1979 Dr. Lucille Teasdale, the first woman surgeon to graduate in the Province of Quebec, and a recipient of the Order of Canada and the Order of Quebec, was operating upon a Ugandan patient who among other things, was suffering from some strange malady. She and her husband, an Italian pediatrician, had dedicated their lives to working with the poor of that emerging nation. During the operation Dr. Teasdale somehow received some of the patient's blood into an open cut. Three years later Dr. Teasdale found herself suffering from the same debilitating disease of her former patient. She died in 1996 of that disease...AIDS.

It is of interest to note that Uganda, like several other sub-Saharan nations, had a few years before been the lucky beneficiary of a World Health Organization's American-financed campaign to eradicate smallpox by a vaccination program. The advent of AIDS among the poor of several Third World nations was to bear a striking similarity to the experience of several hundred homosexuals in New York

City, Los Angeles, and San Francisco a few years later [33]. An experience to be told later by Randy Shilts in his 1987 best seller, *And The Band Played On* [34] when Shilts chronicled the appearance and spread of AIDS from Christmas Eve, 1976 when Danish doctor, Grethe Rask struggled with the strange symptoms in Kinshasa, Zaire, until May 31, 1987 when the Third International Conference on Acquired Immunodeficiency Syndrome convened in Washington, D.C. Shilts' chronicle must be considered in relation to the testimony of Dr. MacArthur eighteen years before, and in relation to some developments involving Nelson Rockefeller protege, Henry Kissinger, and Robert McNamara, McGeorge Bundy and others who were busy grappling with some concerns about the future of the human race. Only with these concerns clearly in mind can one appreciate what happened between June 9, 1969 and Christmas Eve, 1987. The dates when a new disease was projected that would be refractory to the human immune system and the International Conference convened because just such a disease had already claimed nearly 10 million victims. It was almost as if, by some tragic co-incidence, Dr. MacArthur's expressed fear 'that there will be a worldwide scourge, or a black death type disease that will envelop the world or major geographic areas if some of these materials were to accidentally escape' had come to pass.

There Is No Other Way

On October 2, 1979, World Bank President Robert McNamara told a group of international bankers:

> *"We can begin with the most critical problem of all, population growth…short of a nuclear war itself, it is the gravest issue that the world faces over the decades ahead…Either the current birth rates must come down more quickly, or the current death rates must go up. There is no other way."* [35]

In this concern McNamara was being consistent with an attitude he held in 1966, just three years before MacArthur's testimony to the Congressmen, when he had joined the Population Crisis Committee, together with Gen. Maxwell Taylor, and McGeorge Bundy. The Committee had been established by General William Draper, who had a long association with the idea that the world's population was getting out of hand. As far back as 1932 he had participated in the Third International Conference on Eugenics which had given the career of Hitler adviser, Dr.

Ernst Rudin, a boost by naming him President of the International Federation of Eugenics Organizations. Draper later turned up in 1958 when he was appointed by President Eisenhower as a member of a Committee which was to study U.S. military preparedness. General Draper and his colleagues, which included Rockefeller associate, John J. McCloy, Joseph M. Dodge (whose father and mother had participated with the Nazi brain-truster, Dr. Ernst Rudin back in the 1932 Eugenics Conference) came up with the startling conclusion that population control should be an integral part of any military preparedness program![36] The concept is of critical significance when considered in conjunction with Dr. MacArthur's plan to create his synthetic agent which would be refractory to the human immune system, for General Draper was looking at population control as an element to be factored in when planning for American defense! With this linkage established one can now appreciate the *full* significance of Dr. MacArthur's statement on page 121 of his testimony:

> *"(MacArthur) The biological agents are considered **strategic** rather than **tactical weapons** but there are many limitations which I pointed out earlier. When we talk about **strategic** applications, we think of large area coverage, but as I said you can only cover so much because of the germicidal effects of ultraviolet radiation."*

Such a concept had the effect of making population control a national security issue! This explains why people like McNamara, and Generals Taylor and Draper took such an interest in world population growth…it was part of America's strategic defense planning, and that planning included the necessity of reducing the world's population by an 'increase in death rates' that McNamara had said was the only possible way of achieving that result. It is impossible to exaggerate the consequences of such a position for it ranked the increasing birth rates of Africa, India, Thailand and so on as being as much of an enemy of American defense interests as was the Soviet Union. Which brings us back to Nelson Rockefeller and his protege, Henry Kissinger, and the latter's National Security Study Memorandum 200.[37]

Henry Kissinger had worked with Nelson Rockefeller back in 1955 when the latter had been summoned by President Eisenhower to help win the cold war. Rockefeller had:

> *"…called together a group of academics, among whom I was included, to draft a paper for the*

President on a fundamental diplomatic problem: how the United States could seize the initiative in international affairs and articulate its long-range (ie 'strategic') objectives." [38]

When, in 1968, Richard Nixon had summoned Kissinger to the White House as his National Security Adviser, the latter took a number of his earlier Rockefeller position papers and re-worked them as National Security Study Memoranda...each dealing with a long term consideration of a critical area in national affairs, which now included the population growth in certain 'LDC's'...lesser developed countries. Over two hundred such studies were produced, and most were later released for public scrutiny. All but NSSM 200, which dealt with the sensitive subject of 'population control'. Here one can see an example of Prof. Scott's 'negative template', for practically no study of Nixon or Kissinger discusses NSSM 200. As a Jew, Kissinger was very sensitive to the evil connotations any mention of 'eugenics' or 'population control' was bound to arouse. After all, Adolph Hitler gained much of his notoriety by taking the advice of Dr. Ernst Rudin, who had also served as mentor on the subject to the Rockefellers and the other members of the eastern banking elite. Richard Nixon, too, was sensitive to anything that smacked of anti-semitism. During most of his public life he had been challenged many times by accusations that he was prejudiced against Jews.[39] Even Kissinger hinted as much when he told a journalist:

"You can't believe how hard it is, especially for a Jew. You can't begin to imagine how much anti-Semitism there is at the top of this (ie Nixon's) government-and I mean at the top."[40]

The National Security Study Memorandum 200 was withheld from the public until 1990. A review of its contents suggests why...it is a thinly veiled suggestion that the interests of the United States, from a national security point- of-view will be best served by seeking ways to reduce the population growth of the world in general and of thirteen geographic areas in particular where the U.S. was seen to have a special interest. The thirteen areas listed are: India, Bangladesh, Pakistan, Nigeria, Mexico, Indonesia, Brazil, the Philippines, Thailand, Egypt, Turkey, Ethiopia and Colombia.

These areas are important, said Kissinger, because they are sources of supply for the United States, and, if their population increases there will be a demand in these nations to expropriate property owned by 'foreign interests'. This, of course, will constitute a long-term, strategic threat to U.S. interests and so will require 'greatly intensified population programs.'

What possible 'intensified population programs' could be initiated by the United States? We have already noted Robert McNamara's view that reduced birth rates were impractical to expect. That would leave only one possible alternative: an increased death rate from disease.

However, such a strategic goal for a wide area would, as Dr. MacArthur had suggested, also be impractical because all known disease agents were reasonably well-handled by the human immune system. That left just one possible alternative...the United States would have to develop a new agent, one which did not naturally exist, and for which no immunity could have been acquired. Such an agent would, also according to Dr. MacArthur, meet the U.S. strategic needs for 'national security'. Little did the LDC's realize it, but they were on America's hit list. And, since 1952 following Richard Helm's agreement with Allen Dulles, efforts were on-going to co-operate with the U.S. Army to create biological weapons to achieve these defense ends by 'covert' means.

That is, reduce the rate of population increase in India, Africa, Thailand and other countries where U.S. strategic interests were threatened.

However, how would one get several hundred thousand people in these target countries to submit to a lethal injection of such a synthetic agent?

The answer is appealingly simple: tell them that you are going to give them a vaccination that will prevent them from catching smallpox. Then, three to five years later, the new agent will manifest itself in a mystery disease, one which seems refractory to the human immune system, but which is deadly in its consequences.

It is interesting to note that of the thirteen target areas for Kissinger/ McNamara 'national security' concern, most are today struggling against a terrible epidemic of AIDS...acquired immune deficiency syndrome.

There is no reasonable doubt for the conclusion that from the point when General Draper and his colleagues placed the issue of world population growth as a threat to the national security of the United States the latter country was covertly at war with the lesser developed countries whose death rates, according to McNamara and others, had to increase with some method other than a nuclear war.

The 'strategic weapon' they needed was found in Dr. MacArthur's new synthetic agent for which no immunity could have been acquired.

However, before the Eisenhower-spawned defense establishment could act in a serious way to tackle this newly identified threat, an election intervened, and in 1960, John F. Kennedy became President for 1,000 days, until the military-industrial complex had him assassinated. And just one of their reasons among several that they felt it necessary to execute Mr. Kennedy was the fact that he totally rejected the Malthusian population control doctrines of the Rockefeller, Dulles, McCloy, Dillon, Draper, Lemnitzer, McNamara coterie.[41] It is also an interesting co-incidence that after Mr. Kennedy had been murdered, five out of this group of seven served on either the Warren or the Rockefeller Commissions investigating the crime. It is also of interest to note that when Gerald Ford appointed Rockefeller, Lemnitzer and Dillon to one of the Commissions, he was asked why he had so many 'conservative and defense-oriented' members on the commission and, according to Daniel Shorr:

> *"President Ford explained that he needed trustworthy citizens who would not stray from the narrow confines of their mission because they might come upon matters that could damage the national interest and blacken the reputation of every President since Truman.*
>
> *"'Like what?' asked the irrepressible Times managing editor, A. M. Rosenthal.*
>
> *"'Like assassinations!' President Ford shot back, quickly adding, 'That's off the record.'"* [42]

A rule of thumb: if you want to keep a crime under wraps, appoint the criminals to investigate it. We shall have occasion to return to this maxim in Chapter Nine when we examine the role of the Centers for Disease Control in its 'investigation' of where acquired immune deficiency and chronic fatigue syndrome came from.[43]

SUMMARY

The eastern elite, referred to as 'The Establishment' by Arthur Schlesinger, Jr.,began to worry in the early 1900's about the threat posed to their established position and power by world population growth. Such a concern manifested itself over the next six decades in the creation of various groups to study the problem. Then, in a dramatic Report to President Eisenhower in 1959, some of the most right-wing members of the Establishment urged that world population growth be treated as an aspect of United States National Security, with a goal of reducing the rate of population growth, especially in certain designated resource areas which included sub-Saharan Africa, India, Pakistan and Thailand.

Various defense-minded persons such as Robert McNamara, Nelson Rockefeller and Henry Kissinger saw only one way to contain the problem: The death rate in certain 'lesser developed countries' would have to increase. At the end of World War Two several Japanese scientists who had been developing biological warfare weapons were recruited into the service of the U.S. Military and by 1969 Dr. Donald M. MacArthur, head of the Biological Warfare Branch of the Department of Defense told U.S. Congressmen that given 5 to 10 years and $10 million his scientists could produce a synthetic biological agent which would be 'refractory' to the human immune system…much like the disease that sprang into being five years later…AIDS.

He also promised another synthetic agent which would not kill, but would disable…much as chronic fatigue syndrome has done to millions of people since 1984. If Dr. MacArthur was correct in his estimate of five to ten years, then some way would have to be discovered to test his new synthetic disease agents without triggering a new 'black death' over vast geographic areas…unless the powerful coterie envisioned by Col. L. Fletcher Prouty …decided to solve their national security problem in Africa, India etc. by introducing the disease among the world's poorest and most disadvantaged people. Perhaps by telling them that the United States was going to give as many of them as could be reached, a free shot of vaccine against smallpox.

Dr. Don Francis of the Centers for Disease Control had carried out a smallpox eradication program in Africa a few years before the AIDS outbreak. Then, by a startling co-incidence, shortly after he had carried out a hepatitis 'B' vaccination program among the homosexual males in New York, Los Angeles and San Francisco a very high percentage of his vaccine recipients came down with AIDS.

Footnotes

{1} See Chapter Seven below.

Endnotes

[1].John Patrick Quirk, *The Central Intelligence Agency* (Guilford, Conn.,Foreign Intelligence Press, 1986) p.62

[2].*Ibid*, p.62

[3].Charles A. Reich, *Opposing the System* (New York: Crown Publishers, Inc.,1995) p.47

[4].L. Fletcher Prouty, *JFK*, (New York: Birch Lane Press, 1992) p.334

[5].Arthur M. Schlesinger, Jr., *A Thousand Days* (Boston: Houghton Mifflin Company, 1965) p.128

[6].Peter Dale Scott, *Deep Politics and the Death of JFK* (Los Angeles: University of California Press, 1993) p.313

[7].Curt Gentry, *J. Edgar Hoover: The Man and the Secrets* (New York :The Penguin Group, 1991) pp.201-205. The story of plans by America's power elite to depose FDR is an example of the problem faced by students of American history… the problem of secrecy and media control by that elite. One searches Rockefeller biographies largely in vain if one is looking for certain facts. Peter Collier and David Horowitz in their study: The Rockefellers - An American Dynasty don't mention General Butler nor the planned coup. Neither does Ferdinand Lundberg (The Rockefeller Syndrome) nor Joseph E. Persico (The Imperial Rockefeller).

[8].Peter Collier and David Horowitz, *The Rockefellers: An American Dynasty* (New York: New American Library, 1976) pp.196-197

[9].WE are heavily indebted to the piece on the Internet by Mike Morrissey wherein he develops this chronology of population control efforts by the families Rockefeller, Morgan, Harriman etc. Message ID:<Pine.3.89.9407041 143.A10968-0100000@netcoml2> From: m.m orrisey@asco.ks.open.de (Mike Morrisey)Editor: sisskind@sas.upenn.edu

[10].For further details about WCC see: Anthony Cave Brown: *The Last Hero*. (New York: Vintage Books, 1984 edition) pp.795-803

[11].Anthony Cave Brown, *Ibid*, p.798

[12].Peter Dale Scott, *Ibid*, pp.177-8

[13].Christopher Simpson, *Blowback*. (New York: Weidenfeld & Nicolson, 1988) p.249

[14].Harris and Paxman, *Ibid*, pp.75-76

[15].Hearings, p.129

[16].Arno Karlen, *Man and Microbes*, (New York: A Touchstone Book, Simon and Schuster, 1995) p.197

[17].Arno Karlen, *Ibid* p.196

[18].Tanaka, Yuki: *Hidden Horrors*. (Boulder Colorado; Westview Press, 1998) p.154

[19].Arno Karlen, *Ibid*, p.197

[20].Collier & Horowitz, *Ibid*, p.271

[21].Joseph E. Persico, *The Imperial Rockefeller* (New York: Simon and Schuster, 1982) p.86

[22].Generally speaking, those engaged in covert work do not like to leave a trail, but there are exceptions. For example, when E. Howard Hunt, a friend and employee of Richard Nixon, broke into the offices of Daniel Ellsberg's psychiatrist, he paused in his labours long enough to take a photograph of fellow burglar, E.Gordon Liddy, posing by the doctor's sign.

[23].Peter Wright, *Spycatcher*. (Toronto, Stoddard Publishing Co.,1987) p.300

[24].Peter Dale Scott, *Ibid*, pp.60-61

[25].Harris and Paxman, *Ibid*, p.213

[26].There is not, to my knowledge, any relationship between the tribal name 'Kurelu' and the name for the trembling disease, kuru. However, the similarity is arresting.

[27].Collier & Horowitz, *Ibid*, p.533

[28].Kerry Thornley, *The Dreadlock Recollections* p.142. This important typescript manuscript has not yet found a publisher, but it really should for it is of interest to any student of the 'deep politics' of the United States. It gives some idea of just how insane some of the people who function in the so-called 'intelligence community' really are. With Kerry Thornley it is hard to tell where fact leaves off and fiction begins…but the essential lunatic reality of the people he worked with can be seen in his work.

[29].David Crystal (Ed.) *The Cambridge Factfinder* (Cambridge: Cambridge University Press, 1993) p.161

[30].Randy Shilts, *And the Band Played On* (New York: St. Martin's Press, 1987)

[31].Thomas Powers, *The Man Who Kept the Secrets*. (New York: Pocket Books, 1979) p.184

[32].Thomas Powers, *Ibid*, p.437

[33].It is interesting to note that the two outbreaks

of AIDS (in several sub-Saharan nations and among the homosexuals of the United States) had an unusual factor in common. Dr. Don Francis, of the American Centers for Disease Control, had headed up the humanitarian smallpox vaccination program in Africa, before turning his attention to a vaccination program in the United States to wipe out Hepatitis 'B'. By a tragic co-incidence, both disease eradication programs were followed three years later with an outbreak of AIDS.

[34].Shilts, *Ibid*

[35].Quoted from 'Michael Morrissey' *Supra*

[36].Peter Collier and David Horowitz, *Ibid*, p.288

[37].For a valuable summary of the issue of population control, see Donald Gibson, *Battling Wall Street* (New York: Sheridan Square Press, 1994) pp.87-98

[38].Henry Kissinger, *White House Years* (Boston: Little, Brown and Company, 1979.) P.4

[39].Herbert S. Parmet, *Richard Nixon and his America* (Boston: Little, Brown and Company, 1990) pp.199-200

[40].Stephen E. Ambrose, *Nixon*, Vol.2 (New York: Simon and Schuster, 1989) p.641

[41].Among other reasons that the military-industrial complex of Rockefeller, McCloy, C. Douglas Dillon, Allen Dulles and others decided they had to murder the President were: the Kennedy-Kruschev nuclear test ban agreement; the move by Kennedy to normalize relations with Cuba; the refusal of Kennedy to commit combat troops to Vietnam and his view that the way to population containment was by helping the rest of the world to develop their resources and hence improve their standard of living. It was Mr. Kennedy's view that when people enjoyed economic security they were inclined to limit their family size. Furthermore, his decision to issue Treasury greenbacks to eliminate a budget deficit alarmed the Federal Reserve Banks.

[42].Daniel Schorr, *Clearing the Air* (Boston: Houghton Mifflin Company, 1977) pp.143-4

[43].At the risk of sounding less than serious, I feel that a personal anecdote illustrates my point. In 1943 when I was briefly posted by the Royal Canadian Navy to Montreal, Quebec to co-ordinate certain aspects of frigate construction at Vickers Shipyards, I and a Petty Officer Joe Ryan used to carry our brown-bag lunch to our third-floor office on D'Youville Square. After eating we would occasionally fill the bags with water and drop them on the heads of passers-by who could not enter the Naval Establishment without security clearance. One day P.O. Ryan and I decided to drop a water-bomb onto a Naval Commander passing the building. When the bag was well on its way to its target we hurried from the office, ran down a flight of stairs and entered the offices of the Naval Police. There, collecting himself calmly, Ryan called 'Anyone for a game of crib?' Two shore patrol police said 'Sure' and we sat down and began to play. Just then the door flew open and a water soaked Commander shouted 'Everyone in here come with me'. We all jumped up and rushed to the hall where the Commander said to Ryan and three others...'Place yourselves at those stairs...Don't let anyone come down.' Then he turned to me and four others...'Come with me,'and led us up to the third floor. There he said, 'Go into every room. Look in every closet and under every desk. Anyone in any room, send them to the hall to speak with me.' Well, we rustled out some five or six puzzled office people who reeked with innocence and talked their way out of further investigation. When we came down the back stairs and learned that no one had attempted to flee there, our Commander said 'Where in the hell could he have gone?' A seasoned old salt said...'Did you check the fire escape, Sir?' After a quick check the decision was reached...whoever had water-bombed the Commander had obviously fled down the fire escape. We went back to our crib game and the crime remains unsolved. Somewhat like having Rockefeller, Dulles, Dillon, Lemnitzer, and McCloy investigating the murder of President John F. Kennedy.

CHAPTER SEVEN

Official Mythologies and Media Assets

This chapter is regarded by the authors as critical to this study. It deals with the media in a democracy which serve as the channels of communication between those who wield power and those who are affected by that power. Thus, the media can be seen as the intermediary between a victim such as Diane Martel, the subject of Chapter One, and the world at large.

Diane, and hundreds of thousands like her, become ill with a tragic disease which, although disabling, shows few if any signs to those around her. She looks well and healthy, but she cannot function as she once did. She and the other victims depend upon the media to explain their tragedy, and here they have been let down.

Much of what we set out below will be hard to accept because it draws into question several people and institutions upon which many citizens have built their world view. The authors urge you not to believe what we have found in our research. We much prefer you to ask yourselves whether it can possibly be true, and then to turn to the sources cited and see the facts for yourself.

Larry Speakes has been quoted as saying: *"What's history is history, be it fact or fiction"*.[1]

Being so philosophically flexible was probably a help to Mr. Speakes when he served as the press secretary to President Ronald Reagan. Given the frequently bemused ramblings of the President, the syntactically and morally muddled pronouncements of then Secretary of State, Alexander Haig, and the devious mumblings of CIA Director, William Casey, it was undoubtedly useful to have a press secretary who was not bound to the quaint view that history was the record of what had actually happened at some point in the past, but was simply a perception of the facts conjured up by the people in power and passed to the public by the media.

The point is that a citizen of a nation only knows what goes on beyond his own limited personal sphere by what he is told through the various media. Those media include stories he is told by his family, friends, employer, and fellow workers. There are also the stories he receives from his television set or newspaper. At another level, there are the books, magazines and movies he reads or views. There are the sermons he hears in church and the political speeches and debates he may attend. In other words, each individual, depending upon his intelligence and capacity to remember what he sees, hears, reads, or otherwise experiences, has a world view composed of all that he has met, even though many details of such experiences fade over time and only the dominant images, ideas, concepts and memories remain in any conscious sense.

If a certain perception of reality is repeated often enough, many persons who hear that perception will accept it without question and it will become part of the 'mythology' of the society. Over time, such official mythologies may be questioned, challenged, and in some cases gradually replaced by a new mythology.

The government of a state can only maintain a comfortable and secure hold upon power if the official mythologies it seeks to establish about itself fit well with the existing mythologies of the majority of its citizens. That is why presidents keep 'press secretaries': they need someone to put the proper 'spin' upon events so that the official version of events going out through the various media provides a comfortable fit with what is already out there. And what is already out there is represented as 'history'. If it is actually history, then it must be the truth. If it is not the truth it is an invention that purports to be the truth. That is what Larry Speakes had in mind...the inventions created over the years and passed off as fact. And, if these inventions are not challenged or closely examined or if evidence in support of them is hidden or disguised or otherwise controlled, the invention comes to be accepted as 'history'.

An example of this process can be found in the account of the over-flights of Soviet territory by U.S. U-2 spy planes in the 1950's. Certain top officials in the U.S. knew that such flights were going on because they, of course, were the ones doing the deed. There was also a significant group of pilots, mechanics, radar operators (including Lee Harvey Oswald at one point) and airport operators who knew what was going on.

The Soviet Union also knew that such violations were taking place, but they said nothing publicly because to do so would be to admit that they did not have the technical weapons or skills to bring high altitude aircraft out of the air.

When, on May 1, 1960, a U-2 disappeared on a flight over the Soviet Union, the powers that be were convinced that the fragile craft would be so badly broken up that the pilot would not survive and the parts of the plane would be spread over miles of tundra. With such a belief in mind, President Eisenhower launched the 'official mythology' (ie: he started the lies) of the vanished plane…It was a weather plane that had strayed a few miles into the Soviet airspace by mistake. He also expressed hope that the Communists had not shot down an unarmed, helpless weather craft.

The American media took up the myth with vigour and righteous indignation at the thought that the 'evil empire' might have done so mean a deed as to shoot down an innocent pilot who had made an honest error.

The Soviet Government fed out all the line the President wanted as he told his lies to the press. Then, to the great surprise of the American Government, the Soviets produced the pilot, Gary Powers, who had parachuted to safety 1,300 miles inside the Soviet Union.

The official myth fell totally apart and President Eisenhower stood before the world as a liar.

But there are myths within myths. For example, the Soviets claimed to have taken the plane out with a radar-guided missile. However, when Andrew Goodpaster reported the U-2 missing to Eisenhower, Goodpaster said "The pilot reported an engine flameout…" [2] If this were so, it would probably mean that the plane had been sabotaged…undoubtedly by the CIA who was running the program, in order to scuttle the Summit Meeting scheduled with the Soviet Union for the following week!

The people who knew what the pilot had reported had deemed it better to allow the Soviet Union to claim a shoot-down than to reveal the pilot's 'flameout' report since that would alert several thousand handlers and pilots in the U-2 program about the duplicity at the upper echelon of their operation.

Ironically, Eisenhower had told some aides a few weeks before the incident that he, President Dwight D. Eisenhower, would have an advantage at the Summit because of his 'reputation for honesty'. This reputation, too, was part of the official mythology.

There are hundreds of further examples of official myths that turn out to be lies. For example: Johnson's Gulf of Tonkin story, about a non-existent attack upon U.S. destroyers in neutral waters, was used to panic Congress into voting the President a free hand to drastically escalate U.S. involvement in Vietnam; [3] or, Richard Nixon who was publicly calling for a cease-fire throughout Southeast Asia while "his administration was secretly expanding the war inside hapless Cambodia." [4] Another example is that of President Reagan and his insidious Vice-President Bush who had maintained consistently in the eight years of the former's administration that they were honouring the congressionally ordered non-intervention in Nicaragua. Then, an American plane was shot down over Nicaragua and Eugene Hasenfus captured alive.[5]

Official mythologies are invented at the highest levels of the United States government and are then trumpeted by a pliant media, in the name of 'national security.'

THE FREE PRESS

If the citizens in a democracy are to cast their ballots in a meaningful way and to share in the benefits of their citizenship, they have to be fully and honestly informed about what is going on.

To a very significant extent, the major media in the United States not only carry the official mythologies of those in power, but in very many cases they actively engage in the cover-up of the truth. An example of such duplicity is well-reported by author Christopher Simpson:

"Actually the media falsified their reports to the public concerning the government's role in Radio Free Europe and Radio Liberation for years, actively promoting the myth- which most sophisticated editors knew perfectly well was false- that these projects were financed through nickel-and-dime contributions from concerned citizens." [6]

The official cover-up of the true nature of the assassination of President John F. Kennedy is quite likely the most significant, and to date, successful, effort in history to misinform and mislead public opinion. The extent of the media participation in the cover-up demonstrates how surely and completely certain significant editors and publishers were a part of the plot. It is for this reason that we here summarize that participation.

And If You Believe That,
I Have An Ocean-Front Lot In Arizona

The apparently final shot that hit President Kennedy threw him back and to his left. The spray of blood, flesh and bone from his shattered head also went back and to the left, hitting one policeman on his motorcycle so violently that he at first believed he had been hit.[7] In other words the bullet had come from the front and to the right. If this were so, then it would have been impossible for one man such as Lee Harvey Oswald to have fired shots from the Texas School Book Depository behind the President and another six seconds later to fire another shot from in front of the President.

Two bullets from two different places provide clear evidence that at least two people were shooting at the President. This fact further indicates that there was a *conspiracy* to murder President John F. Kennedy.

The violent thrust of Mr. Kennedy to the back and to his left was captured on film by several people, the best known of whom was Abraham Zapruder who filmed the President's car from the time it turned left from Houston Street in Dallas onto Elm Street, until it finally sped under the railroad underpass on its way to Parkland Hospital.

That film shows the effects of the final bullet on the President...he was clearly thrown back and to the left.

The world at large had, of course, no first hand, detailed knowledge of what had happened in Dealey Plaza. They had to depend upon what they were told by the media.

The first newsman to see the Zapruder film was Dan Rather of CBS. He viewed the film the next morning and then ran with his 'scoop' to the CBS studio. Within seconds of walking into the studio, he was on the air *purporting to describe* what the Zapruder film showed. He made what he calls an 'error': "I described the forward motion of his head. I failed to mention the violent, backward reaction." [8]

The 'forward' motion described by Mr. Rather, of course, totally misrepresented the reality. This 'error', wittingly or unwittingly, was to re-enforce the official myth that only one person was firing at the President from one place. That myth was a lie.

The Zapruder film had also caught another action by the President. Just before the limousine passed briefly behind a Stemmons Freeway sign, the President had raised his right hand in a wave to the crowd. [9] By frame # 225 the President is 'clearly shot according to lip readers' and by frame #234 (about one half a second later) Mr. Kennedy has brought both hands to his throat as if a bullet had hit him just below the Adam's apple.

This interpretation was substantiated by one of the first Parkland Hospital doctors to see the President. That doctor reported :"I also identified a small opening about the diameter of a pencil at the middle of his throat to be an entry bullet hole. There was no doubt in my mind about that wound. I had seen dozens of them in the emergency room." [10]

Again the clear evidence is that someone had been shooting at the President from the front. Yet, the official myth was that only one man behind the President had done all the shooting. How do the people charged with the task of misrepresenting the facts, handle this evidence? For the most direct evidence of dishonesty and misrepresentation we need to examine Life magazine. Here for all the world to see is the clear evidence that if Dan Rather of CBS had made an 'error', Life magazine blatantly lied to their millions of readers. Here is how Life magazine accounted for a wound of entry from the front, and another wound in the President's back...obviously from the rear:

"The description of the President's two wounds by a Dallas doctor who tried to save him have added to the rumours. The doctor said one bullet passed from back to front on the right side of the President's head. But the other, the doctor reported, entered the President's throat from the front and then lodged in his body.
Since by this time the limousine was 50 yards past Oswald and the President's back was turned almost directly to the sniper, it has been hard to understand how the bullet could enter the front of his throat. Hence the recurring guess that there was a second sniper somewhere else. But the 8mm film (Zapruder film) shows the President turning his body far around to the right as he waves to someone in the crowd. **His throat is exposed-towards the sniper's nest- just before he clutches it.***"(emphasis added-Ed) [11]*

At the time that *Life* magazine, probably the most influential magazine in the world in that decade, published this total lie they controlled the Zapruder film which they had purchased for several hundred thousand dollars. Their writers and editors knew the truth, but they hid that truth and lied to the world.

And the effect of such lying was to re-enforce the official myth that the President had been assassinated by a lone lunatic killer. By creating and presenting this myth to the world, the truth of who it was that had killed Mr. Kennedy was kept secret.

Thus, the hidden powers that could execute a popular President in broad daylight in the middle of a large city, could also control what the media told the world about the crime. The media obediently told the world the official myth that Lee Harvey Oswald, acting alone, had killed Mr. Kennedy with a cheap, mail-order rifle.

And, if you believe that...

LIES, DAMN LIES, AND THE WARREN REPORT

Immediately after a dramatic tragedy, the world will receive and largely accept the reports from the media. Whether reports are in 'error' such as Dan Rather's claim that Mr. Kennedy was thrown forward by the final shot, when actually he was thrown back, or whether the report is a blatant lie told by Life magazine.

However, as life settles back into place, the state has to bring its law-enforcement capabilities into action and bring anyone guilty of a crime into a court of law where evidence can be presented under oath and witnesses can be cross-examined. Such would have happened with the accused assassin, Lee Harvey Oswald, but for the further tragedy that Mr. Oswald was shot dead in the basement of the Dallas Police Station while surrounded by seventy policemen. The killer of Mr. Oswald was one Jack Ruby, a member of the Lansky branch of the Mafia and a friend of many Dallas policemen.

Mr. Ruby wanted to kill Mr. Oswald; however, he didn't want anyone else, including himself, to get hurt in the melee, so he phoned the Dallas police the night before and told them that he was going to kill Lee Harvey Oswald, but meant to do no harm to anyone else.[12]

Even with Lee Harvey Oswald silenced, the state still had to participate in some official activity which would, apparently, delve into the details of the crime and present a reasonable judgement to the public. The people who had the power to murder the President and to direct a pliant media to lie about the crime, also had the power to control the 'official' fact-finding exercise. The new President, Lyndon Johnson, had to make sure that those conduct-

ing the official investigation of the crime, could be counted upon not to reveal any damaging evidence which would contradict the official mythology. To achieve this end, the President appointed a seven person 'Commission on the Assassination of President Kennedy', with one Commissioner, Chief Justice Earl Warren as the Chairman.

The seven men were hailed as a 'blue-ribbon' panel of 'august gentlemen' who would leave no stone unturned in their search for the truth. The fact was that three of the Commissioners were about as insidious as one could find. All three: Allen Dulles, Gerald Ford and John J. McCloy had long and unsavoury ties with the covert world and the crimes committed by the operatives in that world. The other three, Senator Richard Russell, Senator John Cooper and Representative Hale Boggs had at least some dependency upon the Mafia family of Carlos Marcello of New Orleans. However, at least Hale Boggs and Richard Russell seem to have been very uncomfortable with the travesty of justice in which they were engaged.

The insidious trio of Dulles, McCloy and Ford, were supported by equally insidious staff members such as Arlen Spector and David Belin. The Report that this Commission produced is a tissue of lies. One example can be found in paragraph six of Chapter Three when the Report tells how an 'eye-witness', Howard L. Brennan, saw Oswald fire the final shot:

"Well, as it appeared to me he was standing up and resting against the left window sill, with gun shouldered to his right shoulder, holding the gun with his left hand and taking positive aim and fired his last shot. As I calculate a couple of seconds. He drew the gun back from the window as though he was drawing it back to his side and maybe paused for another second as though to assure himself that he hit his mark, and then he disappeared."[13]

This account, like *Life* magazine's account of the throat shot, is demonstrably and totally false. It is a lie, told to the American people by seven august gentlemen on a blue-ribbon commission, chaired by the highest legal officer in the nation!

The reader must note: the window at which Oswald was supposed to have stood, was 12 inches from the floor and it was open 15 inches. If Oswald was to stand in that window and fire a rifle through it without breaking the two panels of glass he would have to have been approximately 18 inches tall, but capable of firing a rifle two and a half times his height.

Mr. Brennan's testimony was just one lie out of literally hundreds that are scattered through the 700 pages of the Warren Report. Yet this Report was not a cheap throw away novel; it was presented to the world as an official document of the Government of the United States! For one of the most painstaking, honest, fair-minded critiques of this terrible patch work of lies, the reader is referred to the work of researcher Harold Weisberg.[14] This brief review of the murder of Mr. Kennedy, the media cover-up and the official government stamp of approval to the lies is only meant to demonstrate that the world view held by the average citizen is often a view invented by those who really run the major affairs of the world from the shadows. They will work through public figures such as Gerald Ford when necessary. They will utilize the Chief Justice of the Supreme Court if they have to. They will employ the major media as they require. But they will have their way as long as the public will accept the official mythology as fact and will refuse to go to the source of that mythology.

Only when one faces this reality of the power structure of the world, will one understand why it was that a lady such as Diane Martel could be afflicted with a tragic illness and find herself bullied by her employer, largely neglected by her union, double-dealt with by the Ontario Human Rights Commission, denied benefits by her insurance carrier and largely put down by those around her.

These people in her circle were treating her the way they did because they held a view of chronic fatigue syndrome that seemed to justify their actions.

There is a mythology about chronic fatigue syndrome that has been invented by agencies of the United States Government, published in professional journals, misrepresented in the media, and used by the insurance companies to hide a terrible reality...the reality that chronic fatigue syndrome was invented in a U.S. Government laboratory as a strategic biological weapon, tested in certain supposedly isolated places, and sold to Saddam Hussein for use against Iran.

The myth about the origins of CFIDS, and about the victims of this tragic disease can be traced by reviewing the literature that purports to tell the story.

We have already noted (see Chapter Three) how Stephen Straus published articles that were based upon very narrow samples, which distorted the facts,

and which concluded with seriously flawed theses. Dr. Straus was the NIH equivalent of the *Warren Report*. However, Dr. Straus' "put-down" inventions needed to be projected into the public media so that the reality of the seriousness and epidemic proportions of the disease could be hidden. To launch his theses along this route he turned to the *Journal of the American Medical Association* or *JAMA*. Such a professional sounding journal would lend an air of authority to the NIH fabrications and would influence thousands of doctors who were too busy to research the disease for themselves. If *JAMA* told them that the Straus line was valid, they would be pre-disposed to admonish their patients to seek psychiatric help or to develop a more positive approach to life. No wonder the victims of CFIDS were often the butt of black humour at medical meetings. And we have noted how the popular media such as *Time* magazine ("yuppie flu") did its part in this process of popularizing the myth.

Again, however, one must look behind the myth presented to the world by the NIH, the CDC, *JAMA* and the trivializing articles in Time and on CBS. To begin, one must consider the record of *JAMA* in the murky world of covert myth making.

Of all the professional journals available in the United States few have taken a more active role in advancing the official mythology on any subject than has *JAMA*. An excellent example of this slavish adherence to the official line can be seen in the articles published by *JAMA* in support of the Warren Commission 'lone assassin' theory. In 1992, when the Oliver Stone movie JFK had re-opened the whole question about who had murdered the President, George D. Lundberg, the Editor of *JAMA* decided to run an article on a series of interviews with the military doctors who had performed the grossly distorted autopsy of the President at Bethesda Naval Hospital. One has only to read David Lifton's meticulous research into that autopsy to understand how it had been used to try to match the President's wounds to the official myth of one shooter who was firing from behind his victim. [15] Now, nearly 30 years later this medical journal devoted several pages to the re-enforcement of the official myth. Lundberg tried to justify such a strange subject in the Journal by claiming that many doctors around the nation had asked *JAMA* how the President had been wounded. *JAMA*, of course, felt that the best authorities on the subject would be the people who had botched the job in the first place.

A little over a year later Lundberg followed up with a second article, this time by none other than John K. Lattimer of the College of Physicians and Surgeons, Columbia University. Dr. Lattimer was given the chance to provide additional data on the shooting of President Kennedy.[16] Dr. Lattimer regarded himself as something of an authority on the subject, having written an earlier piece in the May, 1972 issue of the Resident and Staff Physician and Medical Times, Port Washington, New York. The latter article was replete with several diagrams and a rather unusual photo of Dr. Lattimer on page 58. The photo purports to be Lattimer's re-creation of Oswald's purported shooting…a myth to re-create a myth one might say. However, it is in total disagreement with the *Warren Report* myth that an eye-witness had seen Oswald *standing* in the window of the book depository, with his shoulder against the left side of a window. In Dr. Lattimer's fanciful re-creation, the good doctor's assassin is seated, with one foot up on a ledge. His rifle is resting on another ledge on what appears to be a roof, not an open window. Lattimer apparently didn't feel up to re-creating an 18" tall Oswald firing a rifle without benefit of a rest position.

How is one to account for the spectacle of a senior doctor at a prestigious university presenting such a distorted picture of an already distorted picture presented by the Warren Commission? There is no logical answer and that doesn't trouble the people who are creating the official mythology for they do not depend upon logic, they depend upon authority.

The question naturally arises as to just who Dr. Lattimer is and where has he come from? And again we have to peer into the murky past to get any idea at all of the answers.

The first record the present authors can find of Dr. Lattimer is that he turned up at the Nuremberg Trials after World War Two, working with Col. Leon Jaworski, Chief of the War Crimes Trial Section of the U.S. Army in occupied Nazi Germany.[17] Besides the business of trying 'war criminals' it now turns out that the U.S. Army was also on a recruiting mission in Nuremberg. They were offering freedom from prosecution to selected German scientists who had expertise in the uses of drugs and hypnosis.[18] As Bob Dean and Steve Jones were to put it: "Apparently Dr. Lattimer and Dr. Lundberg are the vehicles for advancing many other deceptions about the JFK assassination." [19] If official deception in the mat-

ter of Mr. Kennedy's murder is possible, then who better to engage in official deception about the origin and nature of CFIDS?

In passing it is well to note the linkage between the recruitment of Japanese biological warfare criminals and the recruitment of Nazi chemical warfare criminals, and the testing that would have to be conducted to find out how effective their new pathogens were.

From Nuremberg, John Lattimer went on to his distinguished career in medicine, arriving at the position of Professor Emeritus at the Columbia University Medical School and the author of a highly imaginative rendering of Mr. Kennedy's fatal head wounds in a book titled *Kennedy & Lincoln: Medical and Ballistic Comparisons of Their Assassinations*. His article of May, 1972 demonstrates how loosely Dr. Lattimer can be with history and logic. For example he says at one point:

"The author (i.e. Lattimer) had been surprised to hear it stated so many times that it was an 'impossible shot' for Oswald to have accomplished, whereas it did not seem that difficult to him, once the author had visited Dallas and sat (Comment: Wait a moment! Sat? Didn't the only 'eye-witness' tell the Warren Commission that Oswald was standing?) in the actual window used by Oswald.(Comment: What, Dr. Lattimer? A window 12" from the floor, open just 15"…for a total of 27 inches. Even when sitting, as your photo shows, with the rifle resting on a support the rifle is over 36" from the floor. How is it that the window wasn't shattered?) The author and his two young sons thereafter undertook a series of lengthy, unhurried, careful experiments to determine whether the shooting was indeed feasible, as alleged by the Warren Commission.(Comment: 'Unhurried', Dr. Lattimer? Didn't the assassin get off at least three shots in 6.5 seconds? And didn't the House Committee on Assassinations determine that at least four shots had been fired?) These experiments have been reported in detail elsewhere, and indicated it should have been quite easy to accomplish." (Comment: '…easy to accomplish', Dr. Lattimer? In Sudbury, Canada, the Sudbury Police SWAT Team firing at a stopped target could not come anywhere near the shooting skills attributed to Lee Harvey Oswald.)[20]

The very dishonest report by Dr. Lattimer in this and his other writings about the murder of Mr. Kennedy are bad enough. However, two more comments are in order. Under the photo of Dr. Lattimer wherein he re-creates the shooting in his own warped way, is the following report: "Dr. Lattimer has probably fired more Oswald-type cartridges, in Oswald-type rifles, at Oswald-type mock-ups than any other person." The repetition of the name of Mr. Oswald is rhetorical, and the fact that there is no evidence that Mr. Oswald had ever fired the Mannlicher-Carcano rifle at anything, let alone the President, tells an obviously unintended truth. And finally, the authors of this work had the opportunity to see a video of Dr. Lattimer and his 'two young sons' re-creating the rifle firing attributed to Mr. Oswald. The video showed a human skull sitting on the top of a three foot step ladder. A 6.5 Mannlicher-Carcano rifle was fired at the obviously still skull, from about fifty feet away. The skull , when hit, moved away from the shooter and with just the friction from its weight on the ladder, actually tilted the ladder away from the shooter as well so that the front legs of the ladder were lifted about three to five inches off the ground. When the ladder sat back down on all four legs it threw the skull forward and Dr. Lattimer intoned on the sound track that the bullet had caused the skull to move towards the shooter. Hence, when Mr. Kennedy was pitched to the rear, reasoned the doctor, it was towards the direction from which he had been shot. It never seemed to occur to this Professor Emeritus, that had the skull been strapped to the ladder, both it *and* the ladder would have been thrown over to the rear. It was Newton's law of inertia to the effect that for every action there is an equal and opposite re-action, that Dr. Lattimer's strangely sophomoric film demonstrated. It was also unusual that no one had drawn to Dr. Lattimer's attention the fact that John F. Kennedy's skull was not balanced precariously on his neck and that it was, in fact, securely fastened thereto by bones, muscles and skin.

Such weird distortions of reality by a Professor Emeritus would be simply diverting and humourous if they were family films about shooting tin cans from fence posts. However, it is important to emphasize, that Dr. Lattimer is a figure of authority in a great university who is re-creating in a most distorted way, the murder of the elected President of the United States of America! What is such a person doing presenting such silly nonsense to the world? Anyone in his audience who stops to examine Dr. Lattimer's efforts can only conclude that he has another, and far deeper purpose in defending the

execution of the President by the powers that can compel such deeds with such very dishonest writings, speeches and 'films'. Could it be related to the fact that in his early career he was a part of the military hierarchy and associated with Leon Jaworski who came to act as paymaster for covert CIA activities, and who turned up in Dallas, Texas and with the Warren Commission 'investigating' the murder of the President.[21] Some idea of Mr. Jaworski's commitment to justice can be found in his claim that "In no period of history, in no other country , has a government conducted so thorough and scrupulous an investigation".[22] Jaworski also turned up in Washington, D.C. between November 5,1973 and October 25, 1974, as Watergate Special Prosecutor, and it was he and Gerald Ford who made it possible for Richard Nixon to escape prosecution for all crimes 'known and unknown' of which Nixon stood accused.[23] Or could Dr. Lattimer's interest in and efforts on behalf of revisionist history be accounted for by the fact that from December, 1952 until June, 1954, Columbia University had a contract to work with the Biological Warfare researchers in Fort Detrick, Maryland? [24] And, were some of the German war criminals recruited into the U.S. secret war effort part of the Fort Detrick research team? Nazis who were hired after the war when Dr. Lattimer and Col. Jaworski were busy meting out justice at Nuremberg while part of their occupying Army was offering freedom from prosecution to such criminals in exchange for Nazi secrets?

Only a proper, dispassionate, non-partisan investigation by some of the millions of honest, liberty loving, democratic Americans will ever get to the truth. As long as the powers that lurk behind the scenes can control and manipulate make-believe investigations by people who are themselves part of the 'system', then just so long will official myths take the place of the real story.

In Dr. Lattimer it appears that the system has managed to secure a doctor of medicine who will help write revisionist history. And, as we will examine below, in Canada a doctor of history has been found who will write revisionist medicine.

It is evident that a clear path connects the CDC-NIH myth-making to the *JAMA* article writers and editors, through to the mass media. Thus was the image of CFIDS victims as malingerers and frustrated middle-aged women invented and passed out to the world to influence public response to people who looked healthy but were actually being wracked by a terrible new disease. However, the myth makers were not finished yet. They needed something with the imprimatur of the scholar so that those who were bullying the victims of CFIDS didn't have to wave a sheaf of *Time* magazine clippings to rationalize their treatment of the sick. And as luck would have it, the myth makers were blessed to find just such a scholar in their midst.

Enter Dr. Edward Shorter

In 1992, eight years after the earliest American clusters of chronic fatigue had burst upon the scene in several places, which were hundreds of miles from each other and isolated geographically (except for a significant group of 'left-leaning' writers, actors, and other movie-industry personalities in Hollywood and Beverly Hills, California), a new book was released which summed up in one neat, polemical package, the official mythology of the tragic syndrome. According to the author of this contribution to medicine the victims of the new disease were poorly adjusted people, mostly single, middle-aged women, whose careers had stalled and who now sought a sheltering excuse for their lack of achievement in the 'trendy' disease called 'chronic fatigue syndrome.' It was , said Dr. Edward Shorter, a disease that had *'no physical cause.'* [25] And, of course, he should know because he is a doctor! However, this note of authority is set at nought when one learns that Dr. Shorter of the Faculty of Medicine, University of Toronto, has actually a doctorate degree in history, not medicine. The name of Dr. Shorter's book is *From Paralysis to Fatigue.*

The appearance of Dr. Shorter's book dealt a terrible blow to the victims of CFIDS and to the professional medical doctors who accepted these victims with dignity and respect. Such doctors said, in effect, 'I cannot find the organic or physical basis for your illness, but I will deal with you as a rational human being who is ill."

Dr. Shorter in his self-admitted snide style says of such doctors: "The saga of chronic fatigue syndrome represents a kind of cautionary tale for those doctors who lose sight of the scientific underpinning of medicine, and for those patients who lose their good sense in the media-spawned 'disease-of-the-month' clamour that poisons the doctor-patient relationship." [26] In such a superficial comment Dr. Shorter demonstrates an insidious capacity for ignoring

the major characteristic of those few doctors who accepted the suffering victims of CFIDS with respect. To balance Dr. Shorter's warped view, one is urged to read Hillary Johnson's *Osler's Web.*

Where was Dr. Shorter coming from, both academically and personally? The authors determined to place his polemic in perspective.

Academically, as Johnson points out: "Predictably, Shorter invoked the research of NIH scientist Stephen Straus" who was labled by Shorter as "a distinguished internist".[27] That was sufficient answer for the first part of our question. Dr. Shorter's cruel put-down of the victims of CFIDS and of the doctors who treated these victims with dignity and respect, was based upon the 'official mythology' emanating from the government agencies...the National Institutes for Health and the Centers for Disease Control. And Dr. Shorter's snide style was Time magazine writ large.

To answer the second part of our question... where, personally, was a person such as Dr. Edward Shorter coming from? We determined to ask for a personal interview. Dr. Shorter was quite agreeable to such when we phoned him, and he confirmed a one hour interview by letter.

Before our interview we looked into Dr. Shorter's history. It turns out that Edward Shorter had been born and raised in Illinois, the son of Joan and Lazar Shorter. He was obviously a bright student for he graduated from high school and university with little apparent trouble. Then, for us, the story gets interesting.

It turns out that Edward Shorter enrolled at Harvard University in 1968 to take his doctor of philosophy degree in history. The date and place caught our attention for Harvard was the University, and 1968 was the date when none other than Dr. Henry Kissinger, protege of population-control, eugenics-patron Nelson Rockefeller, was sharing his worldviews with graduate students in the Government Department of that University. It was also interesting to note that both Kissinger and Shorter had focussed most of their graduate studies and doctoral theses on nineteenth century Austria-German history and political philosophy. It was also interesting to note that McGeorge Bundy was the dean of the Government Department at the time, and that the latter had been a student and disciple of Richard M. Bissell, Jr., Allen Dulles' principal aide in the Bay of Pigs fiasco. There was, we were to learn, much more to McGeorge Bundy that we develop in Chapter Nine, below. It is sufficient to note at this point that Dr. Shorter had emerged from a graduate school which was the base of so much that was devious, insidious, evil and treasonous. It is entirely possible that Dr. Shorter was totally oblivious to what was swirling around him and that he was completely free on any taint from the Kissinger-Bundy influence. However, Dr. Shorter had been there and we would have to ask him about his experiences.[28]

Finally we were to note that it was in this general time frame that Dr. Kissinger produced his National Security Study Memorandum 200, as a guide for the in-coming President, Richard Nixon. NSSM 200 dealt with the great dangers posed to American National Security from the unfettered population growth in certain Third World countries, and how the United States would have to find ways to either decrease the birth rates or increase the death rates in the subject countries. And it was to be just one year later that, as we have seen, Dr. Donald M. MacArthur was to propose a new strategic weapons approach to the problem...develop two new pathogens, one which would disable and one which would kill, based upon the destruction of the human immune system! It was also the time when U.S. budget allotments to biological warfare research soared to over $125 million per year.

We turned up ten minutes early for our one hour interview with Dr. Shorter, in the church converted to University offices on College St., Toronto. Dr. Shorter arrived five minutes late, but was very courteous when he called us into his office.

Our first question caused him to furrow his brow, as if he could see no link between it and his book on CFIDS: "During your studies at Harvard did you meet, take any courses from ,attend any lectures by Dr. Kissinger or Dr. Bundy?..."No."

"As a professor of medical history have you read the London Times article of Monday, May 11, 1987, about the origin of AIDS?"..."I don't read the Times."

"Have you, perhaps, ever seen the CIA Document 1035-960 on how government can manipulate the media to discredit critics?" Dr. Shorter looked puzzled, so we added "Such as discrediting critics of the Warren Report?"..."I'm not into the JFK assassination. I know nothing about it."

"Do you believe that there are probably people who are engaged in efforts to lead public opinion about certain government positions? People one might call 'media assets'?..."Some colleagues...yes."

"In your studies of medical history have you looked at biological warfare?"..."I'm against biological warfare. I'm glad the U.S.A. never had to employ it in military action."

"Are you aware of any of the following U.S. Congressmen: George Mahon; Robert Sikes; Jamie Whitten; John Rhodes; Glenn R. Davis?" (All members of the House of Representatives who had met with Dr. MacArthur in the critical June 9, 1969 meeting)..."No. We only have a few minutes left- do you want to discuss CFIDS?"

Since only twelve minutes of our hour had passed we said "We thought we had an hour?"..."I'm sorry, but I have other business to attend to, so would you like to discuss CFIDS?"

"We prefer to try to relate our research to your position...Would you tell us what you, as a medical historian think about the evidence in Osler's Web that CFIDS is the 'mirror image' of AIDS? "That's nonsense."

"Are you familiar with the biological warfare tests over San Francisco in 1950?"..."No."

"Over Winnipeg in 1953?"..."No."

"Have you heard of the Skull Valley incident?"... "No."

"Are you aware of the June 9, 1969 meeting between certain congressmen of the U.S. and Dr. MacArthur of the Biological Warfare Branch of the U.S. Dept. of Defense?"..."I never heard of it."

"Would you like a copy of their conversation of that date?"..."No. It's not in the area of my study right now."

"In your book you emphasize 'middle-age women'..." Dr. Shorter nodded his assent.

"Is Onorio Antonucci a middle-aged woman?"... No reply

"How about the children in elementary school in Lyndonville, New York...they were aged from eight to fifteen?"...No reply, but Dr. Shorter looked meaningfully at his watch.

"We would like to read a few lines from your book (at this point we opened From Paralysis to Fatigue quoting lines with expressions such as 'trendy disease', 'disease-of-the-month', 'disease of fashion'. Dr. Shorter nodded each time, then we asked): "Do they not sound snide?"..."Yes, I meant that. I was aiming at the women with an imaginary disease."

On that note, we parted.

It was Dr. Shorter's chilling remark at the end of our 22 minute interview that told us all we needed to know about his book. He was, he said,"Aiming at the women…" History is supposed to be the record of what has happened over time. When one picks and chooses non-scientific anecdotes to make a case against the victims of a disease, one is not writing history, one is writing a polemic in support of a position one holds. What, really, is Dr. Shorter's position? Does it have anything to do with the need by certain people, such as Dr. Straus, to put a spin upon a disease which was designed to debilitate its victims? A disease such as Dr. MacArthur had described a way back in 1969 when Dr. Kissinger and Dr. Bundy and other right-wing fanatics were looking for a way to employ biological weapons against certain groups who posed a threat, real or imagined, against the strategic interests of America?

And, was one of those weapons the development of a genetically altered form of Brucella melitensis, a biological warfare agent which was sold to Saddam Hussein on May 2, 1985 by President Ronald Reagan? [29]

Here, Dr. Shorter may well have blundered into the truth, but of course, he would not recognize it. In his book he devotes two paragraphs to 'brucellosis',the chronic presentation of which has many features similar to chronic fatigue.[30] He may also have been unaware of the possibility that a particle of brucella nucleic acid known as a species of mycoplasma had been the subject of intensive U.S. Government biowar research. What Dr. Shorter also may not have known was that this pathogenic agent was being shipped to Iraq, and that scientific studies would suggest that the modified mycoplasma was, released as a biological weapon designed to incapacitate rather than kill its victims.

And, as we have noted, this is just what Dr. MacArthur had promised back in 1969!

Is Dr. Shorter a witting or unwitting media asset who is working with Stephen Straus and other U.S. government agencies to disguise the real nature of chronic fatigue syndrome? To answer this one must read his book, and then compare it with the reality that is becoming increasingly apparent: United States biological warfare researchers developed the CFIDS mycoplasma in a government or government controlled laboratory. They tested it on unsuspecting victims at Tahoe-Truckee High School and Lyndonville Elementary School, among other sites. The pathogen proved to be much more virulent than ever imagined and the disease is now loose in the world. Is this what happened? If it is, then we must embark upon a determined program to have the truth laid before the public so that we can use that base for further research to find the needed cure.

Whatever Dr. Shorter intended, besides his avowed intention to aim at 'the women with an imaginary illness', we must wait to learn. In the meantime we must seek to determine how effective his polemic was. Did it, indeed, hit the intended target? For that we must turn to a judicial decision reached by Madam Justice Rawlins in the Alberta Court of Queens Bench.(See Chapter Eight)

Science Magazine

Even in media which are supposedly objective reporters of established evidence, the effects of the official mythologies can be found. A case in point can be seen in the June 9, 2000 issue of Science magazine. Let us explain.

Every day over 6,000 people world-wide are dying of AIDS. And, as we have seen, the evidence that has been secured by courageous researchers such as the late Ted Strecker (he died mysteriously of gun shot wounds a few months after securing the document from the Pentagon) is beyond question: the AIDS pathogen was developed in laboratories across the United States by several of the world's top biological researchers and was deployed by the United States in several of the world's poorest countries under the direction of Henry Kissinger.

Despite the solid, unchallenged government-printed documentary evidence upon which we have based our major theses, as to the true source of AIDS, the establishment powers-that-be continue to promote a weird and fantastic tale of humans infected with a monkey virus. These powers, with their media assets such as the *New York Times, The Washington Post, Time,* etc. have kept up a steady stream of 'evidence' that they claim proves their story. Almost every six months there will be a new report from some obscure biological institution in Alabama or Mississippi or New Mexico about some research group which has found the AIDS virus in some monkey cadaver.

Well, on June 9, 2000,(a date exactly thirty-one years after Dr. MacArthur's Hearings before the Congressmen) a new piece of evidence was adduced by a group of mathematicians and microbiologists from New Mexico, England, Illinois and (you guessed it) Alabama, that 'proved' statistically that the 'Ancestor of the HIV-1 Pandemic Strains' had leaped from chimpanzees to humans in 1931! Nowhere in the story do they suggest the day, date and specific time…but if you asked for this information, they could probably come up with it. They had used 'parallel supercomputers'. If there is one thing that impresses the unwary (and uninformed) it is to be told that the computers say it is so.

The report of B. Korber, *et al.* was published in *Science*, V.288, #5472, on pages 1789-1802, and the media grabbed the story and ran with it. Papers across the nation, and probably much of the world, picked it up and trumpeted it to the masses. A member of our Common Cause Medical Research Foundation in Atlanta, GA., sent us a clipping from page A-16 of the *Atlanta Journal-Constitution* and another member from Ingersoll, Ontario, sent us a clipping from *The Toronto Star.* 'Study traces AIDS to 1930's' claimed the heading from Atlanta, while the Star informed its readers: 'HIV originated in Africa in 1931: Study.'

When our copy of *Science* arrived in the mail, we turned to page 1789 and read the evidence which so precisely established the year that some darn chimp had bitten some poor African. We first read the introductory abstract and were re-assured to read that the researchers had '…validated our approach by correctly estimating the timing of two historically documented points.' Great! We would be able, finally, to find a point that was documented, and we could then look up those documents and compare them with the government documents that indicated quite clearly that AIDS hadn't come from some monkey bite, but from some NIH laboratory. We were also somewhat concerned when we read that these scientists-mathematicians had employed "…a method that relaxed the assumption of a strict molecular clock…" Relaxing an assumption means that if something in your theory doesn't fit with some previously determined position, then ignore the latter!

As we struggled through the pages of mathematical jargon, we kept recalling the old computer GIGO dictum: 'Garbage in; garbage out'. At last, we reached the place in the text where the authors introduced their 'two historically documented points.' We carefully underlined the four sentences which we reproduce in full below:(the numbers in parentheses are endnotes from the original article)

"AIDS was first identified as a clinical syndrome in 1981 (47). Twelve AIDS cases were retrospec-

tively identified in 1978-79, and by the first quarter of 1983, there were already 1299 cases of clinical AIDS reported in the United States, spread over 35 states (48). In both Haiti and the United States, scattered cases of HIV-1 infection or AIDS were identified in the late 1970's with a handful of possible and probable cases noted in the United States and Haiti between 1972 and 1976 (48,49). Thus, our timing estimates for an ancestral sequence are plausible…"

We didn't feel challenged by the first claim, identified as endnote # 47…after all, our *Cambridge Factfinder* says right there on page 161 "1981 First reports of AIDS", so we could chalk that up for Korber, *et al.* We next turned to their next 'historically documented' point, and here we began to run into trouble.

First of all, we noted their dependence upon 'L.Gazzolo, *N. Eng. J. Med.* 311, 1252 (1984).' We were rendered a trifle uncomfortable by the fact that Gazzolo is listed in the "Special Virus Cancer Program", Progress Report #8, as one of the researchers working at Nixon's War on Cancer back in 1971. Given the strong evidence that the SVCP was a cover for the laboratory development of the AIDS pathogen that had been promised to the US Congress by the Pentagon in 1969, it struck us as a possibility that Gazzolo might well want to promote the idea that their handiwork had actually come into the world in 1931 when a green monkey or a chimpanzee or other simian species bit an African.{1}

However, we managed to suspend our disbelief in Gazzolo long enough to make our way to the Laurentian University Library where we dug out volume 311 of the *New England Journal of Medicine,* and read Gazzolo's 'historically documented' point. We received quite a shock when it turned out to be simply a letter to the editor! No peer review here. Then we received another surprise…one of Gazzolo's fellow signatories to the letter was none other than 'G. de-The'! Why, you may well ask, should we be bothered by this discovery? We were very bothered by the fact that G. de-The is also listed in the SVCP, Progress Report #8, and he has a total of 18 articles cited therein. He was, in other words, a major researcher in the program. Furthermore, on two of those articles, de-The collaborated with L. Gazzolo.

Our greatest shock came when we read this letter which the authors of the *Science* piece, so broadly reported by media assets throughout Canada and the U.S., had suggested was a historical document that validated their supercomputer-generated date when a chimpanzee bit a human being and gave the latter the world's first case of human AIDS. It is mind-boggling to report that the letter does not deal, as we are led to believe it does, with either Americans or Haitians. It deals, instead, with 211 residents of French Guiana who had immigrated to that country during the previous 10 years from Haiti. Furthermore, their blood had been drawn in 1983 by the Pasteur Institute, and had been tested, not for HIV, but for HTLV antibodies. This was very misleading!

Enter Jean W. Pape, et al.

Perhaps we'll do better when we refer to the next 'historically documented' evidence cited by Korber, et al, we mused, and we took down volume 309 of The *New England Journal of Medicine* and turned to page 945. Here, we had been led to believe, we would find solid evidence that as Korber and his colleagues had assured us, there was a 'handful of possible and probable cases [of HIV-AIDS] noted in the United States and Haiti between 1972 and 1976.'

Pape, *et al.* make no such a claim, despite their article being cited in *Science* magazine by Korber, *et al*. In fact, on page 949 of their article, Pape and his colleagues state quite unequivocally: "We do not believe that AIDS was present in Haiti before 1978."

Are the authors (skilled mathematicians and microbiologists) of this *Science* piece, who are so capable of relaxing scientific assumptions, and producing a date so specific as to when AIDS infected our human family, literacy-challenged? Or, are they, like Edward Shorter and Elaine Showalter, willing to misrepresent history to help cover the greatest crime ever committed against humanity?

You have to choose between the clearcut, specific US government document of June 9, 1969 and all of the media asset alternative evidence such as the piece under review.

Oh! Did we happen to mention that for the reported research, four of the authors had received funding from the NIH?

The authors wrote to the Editor of *Science* and pointed out the errors in their story, but, nearly two years later, we still have no reply.

The point again is clear. The mainstream media are willing to distort verifiable evidence in support of official mythology about the origin of AIDS and CFIDS.

Summary

Almost from the first outbreaks of chronic fatigue syndrome, the official agencies of the United States Government engaged in a campaign of misrepresentation, distortion, sabotage of research, and of put-down of the victims of CFIDS. There is also reason to believe that outright fraud was employed on occasion. In this endeavour, the CDC and the NIH were given strong support by certain professional journals such as *JAMA*, and by popular media such as CBS and Time magazine. The campaign to propagate an official line got a big boost in 1992 when Dr. Edward Shorter produced a polemic titled *From Paralysis to Fatigue*. The campaign of disinformation featured several persons, and resembled in several specific ways, the gross misrepresentation of the assassination of President John F. Kennedy. Names such as Rockefeller, Kissinger, Bundy, Jaworski and others recur throughout the history of the period when vast sums of money were spent by the United States Department of Defense to develop strategic biological weapons. Such weapons had to be tested upon someone, somewhere, and the Defense Department revealed that between 1947 and 1974, over 500,000 people were used as unwitting guinea pigs to test such pathogens. One pathogen promised by Dr. MacArthur to Congress (in secret, of course) was probably the modified brucella melitensis, which agent was later sold to Iraq by the Reagan Administration. This agent, according to the government's own documents, causes 'chronic fatigue, profuse sweating, loss of appetite, aching joints and muscles...' A clear description of chronic fatigue syndrome. If, indeed, this agent was tested and got out of control, there would be ample reason for people such as Stephen Straus to misrepresent, distort, put-down victims and even misuse research funds authorized by a part of Congress that was not privy to what certain congressmen were plotting.

Footnotes

{1} As we will develop in detail later in this work, the evidence is that in order to mask the research into the development of the AIDS/ CFIDS pathogens the US researchers conducted much of their research under the guise of looking for the cause and cure for cancer. They labelled the program "The Special Virus Cancer Program".

Endnotes

[1]. The authors quote this maxim from memory, and regret that its specific source has been forgotten.

[2]. Stephen E. Ambrose, *Eisenhower, Vol.2* (New York: Simon and Schuster, 1984) p.571

[3]. John M. Newman, *JFK and Vietnam* (New York: Warner Books, 1992) P.447. See also "The Twin Towers; Son of Tonkin, Great Grandson of the 'Maine'" able , V.1, #1 Nov.22, 2001. Executive Services, Box 37021, Ottawa, Canada. K1V 0W0. p.36

[4]. Seymour M. Hersh, *The Price of Power* (New York: Summit Books, 1983) p.303

[5]. Theodore Draper, *A Very Thin Line* (New York: Hill and Wang, 1991) p.353

[6]. Christopher Simpson, *Blowback* (New York, Weidenfeld & Nicolson, 1988) p.127

[7]. Robert J. Groden, *The Killing of a President* (New York: Viking Studio Books, 1993) p.32

[8]. Dan Rather, *The Camera Never Blinks,* (New York: William Morrow and Company, Inc. 1977)

[9]. We have used the careful, frame-by-frame analysis of the Zapruder film prepared by researcher, Martin Shackelford. This analysis is in the files of the authors.

[10]. Charles A. Crenshaw, M.D., *JFK: Conspiracy of Silence,* (New York: A Signet Book, 1992) p.79

[11]. Paul Mandel, "End to Nagging Rumours :The Six Critical Seconds" *Life,* December 6, (1963). P.52F.

[12]. Henry Hurt, *Reasonable Doubt* (New York: Holt, Rinehart and Winston, 1985) pp.407-410

[13]. *The Report of the Warren Commission,* New York Times Edition. Bantam Books, 1963) p.75

[14]. Harold Weisberg, *Selections From Whitewash* (New York: Carroll & Graf Publishers/ Richard Gallen, 1994)

[15]. David S. Lifton, *Best Evidence* (New York: Macmillan Publishing Co.,Inc., 1980)

[16]. John K. Lattimer, *JAMA* March 24/31, 1993- Vol.269, no. 12

[17]. Dick Russell, *The Man Who Knew Too Much* (New York: Carroll and Graf Publishers/ Richard Gallen, 1992) p.680

[18]. *Ibid,* p.680

[19]. "Lattimer Study Guide" from the *Second Annual Midwest Symposium of Assassination Politics,* State of Illinois Center, Chicago, April 1-4, 1993

[20]. Dr. Lattimer's statement appears in the work cited above, page 44. The 'Comments' are those of the authors.

[21]. Leon Jaworski, *Confession and Avoidance* (New York: Anchor Press/Doubleday, 1979)

[22]. Jaworski, *Ibid,* p.196

[23]. Leon Jaworski, *The Right and the Power* (New York: Reader's Digest Press, 1976) Ch.15

[24]. *Hearings before the Subcommittee on Health and Scientific Research of the Committee on Human Resources,* United States Senate. March 8 and May 23, 1977. Page 84

[25]. Edward Shorter, *From Paralysis to Fatigue* (New York and Toronto: The Free Press, 1992) p.323

[26]. Edward Shorter, *From Paralysis to Fatigue* (New York and Toronto: The Free Press 1992) pp.304-5

[27]. Johnson, *Ibid,* p.566

[28]. Walter Isaacson, *Kissinger* (New York: Simon and Schuster, 1992)

[29]. Congressional documents in the authors' files listing biological agents sold to Iraq before the Gulf War for use against Iran.

[30]. Shorter, *Ibid,* p.305

CHAPTER EIGHT

"WHEN I'M SICK, CALL A HISTORIAN"

If a medical historian actually studied the history of medicine and recorded that history, he could be regarded, like Dr. Johnson's lexicographer 'as a harmless drudge' who does no particular harm to anyone. However, when such a medical historian, writing from the sanctuary of a prestigious university, 'aims' his work at 'middle-age women with imaginary diseases', he must be called to account for his arguments. He must first be asked, what makes you so sure that the disease is imaginary? Dr. Shorter had attempted to demonstrate that such a claim was correct by first citing several anecdotal cases from history where patients, mostly women, were determined to have displayed symptoms of 'hysteria'.

He recounts how Mrs. King in 1705 and Mrs. Cornforth in 1713 and Jeanne-Marie de Viry in 1639 had manifested hysteric symptoms. Only now and then does he acknowledge in passing that factors other than psychogenic might have been at work in these patients. At one point he alludes to the tight corsets worn by many of the victims, and he notes that some persons believe that that particular article of apparel, working to limit breathing, bloodflow, digestion etc. may have been a causative factor. However, he doesn't have much regard for such suggestions. He moves relentlessly towards his thesis, that people, mostly women, are prone to psychosomatic illnesses which have some vague relationship to their lack of personal strength...or something. After several such anecdotes he then pronounces the truth about the condition of these sick women...they are play-acting. Mind you, some of their play-acting may be sub-conscious but, he declares from time-to-time, there is no physical basis for their symptoms. A typical such pronouncement is the following:

"These fits corresponded to some kind of model in the patient's unconscious mind of 'genuine' physical symptoms caused by demonic possession or by ungovernable reflexes." [1]

The suffering women are, according to Shorter, under some sort of stress but they have an out...in their minds, consciously or sub-consciously... they have a 'model' which they imitate. And, when they imitate this model they are pronounced as possessed...or whatever.

After several anecdotes from the eighteenth and nineteenth centuries, Dr. Shorter vaults his readers into the end of the twentieth century. In Chapter Eleven he blends his apparently self-taught skills in psychoanalysis into his mix of historic anecdotes and ersatz medicine and he states right off that the people sick with pain and chronic fatigue in the 1990's "have acquired the unshakable belief that their symptoms represent a particular disease, a belief that remains unjarred by further medical consultation." [2] It never occurs to the good doctor that the victims of this disease are suffering from something new in the world of medicine...a disease which, as Dr. Nicolson has pointed out,[3] is not to be discovered by the usual blood and tissue tests, but which requires very sophisticated testing not readily available to the general practitioner.

Dr. Shorter cannot be faulted for not being aware of the strides made in diagnosing CFIDS between the year his book appeared (1992) and the present. However, the fact that his mind was not open to the possibility that the victims of CFIDS were genuinely ill and that their disease was something new and extremely hard to pin down, is where he can be faulted as a scholar and as a human being. He wasn't able to listen, even second hand, to the words of the patients. A trait that he had learned from his role-model, Stephen Straus, and the 'disease detectives' of the CDC who went to Incline Village, Nevada, and read patient records, but didn't have an interest in meeting the patients. Dr. Shorter was a long way from Dr. Osler who had graced the University of Toronto by his presence a century before. But then, Dr. Osler was a doctor of medicine who wanted to help his patients, and Dr. Shorter is a doctor of philosophy in medical history who wants to get those "middle-aged women with imaginary diseases."

Dr. Shorter certainly does not make a very convincing case for his claim that chronic fatigue syndrome is 'imaginary'. As one reviewer put it:

"(Shorter) abandons the dispassionate tone of historical inquiry that gave the earlier chapters of his book such an authoritative air. Instead of judiciously presenting both sides of the issue, he becomes increasingly dogmatic, eager to persuade the read-

er of the correctness of his own position. (emphasis added…ed.) As a result, From Paralysis to Fatigue feels like an odd hodgepodge of a book; part medical history, part hypothesis, part diatribe." [4]

The next question that such a historian must be asked is: why 'aim' at anyone? A politician is free to select facts from the historic record to discredit the political philosophy of an opponent. A scientist is free to adduce certain facts about the actions of molecules in a vacuum and so challenge a theory advanced by another scientist. But does the person studying the history of a disease have the right to select anecdotes with a view, not to pointing out the truth about that disease, but to discredit its victims?

Wittingly or unwittingly, Dr. Shorter has taken up the anti-woman theme of Dr. Straus, and in the guise of writing medical history, has "aimed" a polemic at the victims of a disease which it seems clear is a disease that, for whatever their reason, the official 'health' agencies of the United States Government want to deny, discredit, and misrepresent.

We suggested above that such a polemic, if treated as just a theory by a historian who also pretends to be a psychoanalyst, would do no one much harm. However, when such a treatise is taken up by various persons, agencies and institutions in society and is used, as Dr. Shorter intended it to be, to discredit "middle-aged women with an imaginary disease" then his thesis and purpose must be challenged and repudiated. He is, after all, and this must be stressed, not a doctor of medicine. He is a student of the history of medicine. Jay A. Goldstein, MD, has bracketed Shorter with two earlier theoreticians who had found it difficult in their time to accept a new idea:

"Louis Pasteur's theory of germs is a ridiculous fiction. How do you think that these germs in the air can be numerous enough to develop into all these organic infusions? If that were true, they would be numerous enough to form a thick fog, as dense as iron."

—Pierre Pochet

"X-rays are a hoax."

—Lord Kelvin [5]

"In every large community there will be found at least one physician willing to play up to his patients' psychological need for organicity. Thus do the caregivers themselves contribute to their patients' somatic fixations, plunging youthful and productive individuals into careers of disability."

—E. Shorter

In Chapter One the story of one middle-age woman was presented. It was shown how Diane Martel had been bullied by her employer, superficially responded to by the Ontario Human Rights Commission, half-heartedly represented by her union and given the run around by the insurance carrier when she applied for disability benefits. The mind set of these people who had used her so badly had to have come from somewhere. In Chapter Three we traced the efforts of the CDC and the NIH to deny the existence of a disease and to foster the view that the victims of CFIDS were people with some sort of personal deficiency. Chapter Seven demonstrated how the media of America are used to translate official myths into popularly held views, and it appeared that, wittingly or unwittingly, Dr. Shorter had served as a 'media asset' in the advancement of the official mythology of chronic fatigue syndrome.

The tragedy doesn't stop there, for in a mind-boggling court ruling (alluded to in Chapter Two) the presiding Judge, The Honourable Madam Justice B. L. Rawlins drew heavily upon historian Shorter's thesis when she made her judgment in the case of Mackie versus Wolfe.[6]

Thus the path from government myth makers, through professional journals, through the mass media, through the scholarly tomes of the universities, to the incorporation of the official mythology into the law precedents of the land has been accomplished. The gross injustice of declaring suffering victims of an insidious disease to be something other than sick people is now in the law books of the nation. Thus, the system's capacity to create a myth that takes the place of a personal, thoughtful assessment of the reality of each individual's health, works. Score one for Stephen Straus and the myth makers.

To understand how a justice in the Court of Queen's Bench was able to arrive at the position she did, we must review her Reasons For Judgment and as we do so, we must test that reasoning against the facts of chronic fatigue syndrome as set out in the available literature.

Yvonne Mackie And Ronald Mackie,
Plaintiffs
And
Patrick Wolfe,
Defendant

"The injuries causally related to the accident were minor and the damages reflect that she (Mrs. Yvonne Mackie) would have lingering affects for

Justice Rawlins '6-8 months' appears arbitrary and wrong. Mark J. Pellegrino writes that "Fibromyalgia is a chronic and permanent condition for which there is no cure." [7] Dr. Goldstein cites several 'case studies' which demonstrate that the '6-8 months' affects do not apply to patients with fibromyalgia. It seems evident that up to this point in time, there is no cure for the disease, but, as Ismael Mena, MD, writes "...pharmacological interventions...are justified in their rationale, thus leading to treatment or amelioration of the crippling symptoms..." but such do not cure the patient.[8] Finally, the reader is referred to the results of a limited survey conducted by the authors in preparation for this work. It is significant that no respondent has ever experienced a 'cure'. Some have learned to live with their disability, some experience periods of reduced pain, some are on certain medications that ameliorate their symptoms...but none can be said to be 'cured'. It is the authors' opinion that Justice Rawlins is wrong in her claim that Mrs. Mackie would have lingering affects for approximately 6-8 months.

> *"With the exception of 5 months relating to chest pains and gall-bladder surgery, all the remaining time off work the Plaintiff attributes to the pain and discomfort she experienced from the motor vehicle accident which she says is fibromyalgia..."*
> (Rawlins, p.26)

The suggestion by Justice Rawlins that Mrs. Mackie has diagnosed herself..."which she says is fibromyalgia"... fits into the Shorter theme which recurs throughout Chapter Eleven of his book. He states at one point : "Many patients today have acquired the unshakable belief that their symptoms represent a particular disease, a belief that remains unjarred by further medical consultation." [9] Justice Rawlins was well aware of the fact that the diagnosis of fibromyalgia had been made by several qualified physicians, including Dr. McCain (page 31) ; Dr. Fink (page 43); and Dr. Verdejo (page 37)...although the latter used the term 'fibrositis syndrome'...an antecedent diagnosis of the same symptom ology. This hint of 'self-diagnosis' on the part of Mrs. Mackie suggests the view that the patient is a hypochondriac. Just what the Straus-JAMA-Shorter line has been urging.

Justice Rawlins severs the time that Mrs. Mackie was off work for what was diagnosed as a heart problem and for time lost due to a gall-bladder operation, from the illness diagnosed as 'fibromyalgia'. It is interesting to note that Diane Martel was initially believed to have a heart problem and was given an angiogram, as were several others who responded to our Survey. As we will later note, one characteristic of Brucella melitensis, used in the manufacture of biological weapons, is that it produces "...chronic fatigue, loss of appetite, profuse sweating when at rest, pain in joints and muscles, insomnia, nausea, and *damage to major organs.*" [10] Madam Justice Rawlins had no way to ascertain whether there was a relationship between CFIDS/ Fibromyalgia and both the heart and gall bladder problems at the time of her judgment. However, in hindsight and in view of what is now known, Mrs. Mackie's problems with her heart and gall-bladder were in all likelihood caused by her fibromyalgia.

"...the Difficulty He Had In Accepting Fibromyalgia"

When the chronic fatigue/ fibromyalgia syndrome burst upon the scene in 1984, and the victims went to their family physicians and explained their symptoms, their doctors were puzzled. The symptoms presented were numerous and varied greatly from one patient to another. Blood tests reflected few abnormalities. One of the most common variations from the norm was 'high Epstein-Barr virus antibodies'.[11] However, consensus was soon achieved among those doctors who were responding to their patients' distress that Epstein-Barr was not the ailment's cause, but simply a 'marker' that somehow or other was generated by the actual cause.[12]

Some doctors suspected that the genesis of the problem lay in the brain of their patients, and they had first ordered x-rays which revealed no apparent physical abnormality, and later they began ordering magnetic resonance imaging (MRI) which frequently revealed multiple punctate lesions in various parts of the brain. Later still, brain electrical activity mapping (BEAM) and positron emission tomography (PET) was turned to by doctors Jay Goldstein, Ismael Mena and Steven Lottenberg. BEAM and PET testing demonstrated a variety of physical abnormalities which tended to support the MRI results : something was not working right in the brains of chronic fatigue syndrome/fibromyalgia patients.

Other doctors who had a sufficient level of concern for their patients' well-being and a sufficient level of trust in the fact that by and large, their patients were genuinely ill, even if the diagnosis was difficult, were looking in other directions. For example, Susan Wormsley, a biochemist and flow cytometry expert at Cytometrics Laboratory in San Diego focussed her research on the immune system of the victims. And she discovered that the CFIDS patients had a significantly low ratio of suppressor cells, while AIDS patients had a significantly high ratio of suppressor cells. CFIDS was, Wormsley was to conclude, a "mirror image of Aids"!

However, while there was this relatively small number of doctors who, when told that there were no physical bases for CFIDS/Fibromyalgia, had responded by looking further, there was, tragically, a larger number of doctors, who, when their initial tests seemed to indicate that all was normal, responded by telling their patients:"It's all in your head".

It was, of course, this latter group who subscribed to the Stephen Straus line which, as we have seen, emanated from the CDC/ NIH through JAMA to the popular literature and to Dr. Edward Shorter in his *From Paralysis to Fatigue*. And in Madam Justice Rawlins' Court there appeared representatives of the two sides.

Madam Justice Rawlins certainly seems to have favoured the 'official mythology'. For example, when Dr. Glenn McCain was called to provide expert testimony, Madam Justice Rawlins writes: "I discounted the evidence of Dr. McCain because I find that he may have a personal and perhaps financial interest in *perpetuating* the existence of this condition (fibromyalgia)" (Rawlins, page 35.)

In other words, there is no such thing as fibromyalgia, but certain doctors who make money treating patients who think they have such a disease, will perjure themselves to keep their good thing going! Thus, a doctor who has specialized in the study and treatment of CFIDS/ Fibromyalgia, and who was one of the specialists who had developed the diagnostic criteria of fibromyalgia for the American College of Rheumatology, was not to be trusted as a witness for Mrs. Mackie. As Madam Justice Rawlins writes: "I have evidence to the contrary (of Dr. McCain's) which evidence I prefer." (Rawlins, Page 36.)

That preferred evidence was provided by Dr. Keith Pearce, a psychiatrist who testified on behalf of the Defendant. Dr. Pearce's testimony was to the effect that Mrs. Mackie was a 'hysteric' who was able to convert her psycho-social stress into acceptable physical symptoms.(Rawlins, Page 89). Then Dr. Pearce produced his piece de resistance…none other than Dr. Shorter's *From Paralysis to Fatigue*. Dr. Pearce 'referred to and accepted' Edward Shorter's views on hysteria as 'being authoritative on the subject.'And, it is evident, he was able to carry Madam Justice Rawlins along with him in that acceptance. Rawlins quotes Shorter when the latter 'deals with the phenomenon of the epidemic of chronic fatigue which he says (in one of those sweeping, generalized, but poorly supported pronouncements of his) has "gripped the imagination of all western society.') The present writers have never felt their imaginations so gripped, and in a random and rather unscientific survey of several friends and relatives, have been unable to find anyone else whose imaginations have been gripped by chronic fatigue syndrome. However, Madam Justice Rawlins 'found this particular excerpt to be quite helpful in understanding the progression of these symptoms to the onset of fibromyalgia…"

Justice Rawlins follows this statement with a four page summary of history professor Shorter's insights into just what it is that makes a victim of chronic fatigue syndrome tick. In this synopsis, Justice Rawlins includes direct quotes from Shorter's book with a number of the self-admitted snide expressions which Shorter had intended in order to aim "at the women with an imaginary illness." These expressions include such smart alec phrases as 'self-labelled sufferers', 'EBV became a disease of fashion', 'the yuppie flu','the first of a series of tactical re-labellings occurred.'

And Justice Rawlins seems wonderfully pleased with Shorter's 'pronouncements' to which we have noted he has a marked affinity. For example, on page 91 the Justice quotes her historian guide who had written: "In the mid-1989's EBV was warmly embraced as the explanations of one's difficulties…"

How very superficial and snide.

The fact is that when many victims of chronic fatigue began to feel ill, they went to their doctors. Several of these doctors asked for blood tests to assist them in making a diagnosis. When the results of these tests came back, most victims of CFIDS were found as we noted earlier, to have elevated "levels of antibodies to the Epstein-Barr virus." If Dr. Shorter had not been trying so hard to make a case for something, he would have reported this fact. And, he would have reported that in all probability, the doctor making the diagnosis would see this result and would then tell his patient "You have higher levels of Epstein-Barr antibodies in your blood than does the average person. Now, ninety percent of the world's population has such antibodies, but in your case the level is beyond the norm. The Epstein-Barr virus is generally regarded as the cause of mononucleosis, and since your antibodies are high, it would appear that your body is attempting to cope with what might be termed 'chronic mononucleosis-like syndrome'" [13]

Shorter cannot state such a business-like presentation because it does not do what he wants to do. He wants to 'aim' at the 'middle-aged women with an imaginary disease.' However, such middle-age women, together with all the men and children who were showing the signs of chronic fatigue, could not pick an elevated level of Epstein-Barr antibodies in their blood as a symptom from "some kind of model in the patient's sub-conscious". Their blood was tested. The blood showed an abnormality. That abnormality was an elevated level of Epstein-Barr antibodies! To say that the patients "warmly embraced" this objective test-finding is smart-alecky.

Justice Rawlins continues along the path staked out for her by Dr. Shorter. She writes: "Unfortunately…EBV fell out of favour as an illness with sufferers after it was determined by the Center (sic) for Disease Control in 1988 that there was a poor correlation between patients with EBV and those with chronic fatigue."

She almost got it right.

In her quoting of Dr. Shorter , Justice Rawlins makes a couple of errors. Not that that really makes a difference when one is quoting the historian who is demonstrating his mastery of both medicine and psychoanalysis. However, just to set the record straight, this is what Shorter had written : "…the correlation was poor between those patients *who had hematological evidence of chronic EBV infection* and those who had symptoms of chronic fatigue." [14]

What is the importance of what Justice Rawlins left out or, perhaps, overlooked? Patients with infectious mononucleosis were shown to have elevated levels of the Epstein-Barr virus. When persons suffering from CFIDS were found to have elevated levels of the same virus, it was at first interpreted to mean that the latter were suffering some sort of mononucleosis. However, it was soon recognized that the two were distinct diseases, and hence there was naturally, a poor correlation between them.

Justice Rawlins continues: "EBV was therefore

re-named chronic fatigue syndrome" and she quotes her authority:

> *"This renaming did not sit well with patient groups who promptly renamed the condition , CFIDS, chronic fatigue immune dysfunction, to better insist on its organicity." (Rawlins, Page 92).*

Thank you, Dr. Shorter, for this pronouncement. Actually, the words 'immune dysfunction' were suggested for the name because it had been recognized by several doctors who took their patients' health seriously that there was something in the latters' immune system that was not working.[15] There was also a feeling among the victims of CFIDS that the name based upon the symptom of 'fatigue' created a poor impression on those who were unfamiliar with it. After all, one doesn't speak of measles as "splotchy red rash syndrome".

Dr. Shorter was not alone in his campaign aimed at women with imaginary diseases. Justice Rawlins is able to report that the good doctor had someone else who shared his views…a Professor Donna Greenburg was quoted by Shorter as follows: "…it is the nature of chronic fatigue that (the diagnosis) will inevitably recruit subjects with depressive disorders…" and Justice Rawlins includes this distorted view. Actually, the record is very clear as Dr. Shorter and Dr. Greenburg could have determined, that it was after becoming physically ill that the victims of CFIDS began to show symptoms of depression. And, as one doctor said…" If I had suffered the way my patients have suffered, I'd be depressed, too."

The snide remark that chronic fatigue will "recruit subjects' continues the 'self-diagnosed' line. Neither Shorter nor Greenburg make any allowance for the fact that if a patient is suffering from a 'bone-crushing' fatigue, together with a mix of other symptoms such as nausea, insomnia, dizziness, memory loss, and so on, and such a patient goes to a doctor and he reports that blood tests are normal (except for an elevation of Epstein-Barr Virus antibodies) and the x-ray shows no abnormality, and that he has no name for whatever it is that is causing these symptoms, there will be an anxiety generated in the average person by the fear of the unknown.

Fibromyalgia Does Not Exist As A Physical Condition

There is much more like the above in The Reasons For Judgment delivered in the case of Mackie vs.

Wolfe. But the above sampling is enough to make the point. Despite the fact that several medical doctors testified that Mrs. Mackie suffered from fibromyalgia and that fibromyalgia was often triggered by a trauma of some sort, the Honourable Justice Rawlins was more impressed by the testimony of a psychiatrist whose principal authority was an historian who had never studied medicine, yet presumed to pronounce upon all victims of the disease. They are all, says Dr. Edward Shorter, suffering from an imaginary disease. And he manages to convince a Justice in the Court of Queen's Bench that his view should be given pride of place when someone seeks compensation for their suffering. And the Honourable Justice agrees and pronounces that "fibromyalgia does not exist" and that it is a "court-driven" ailment that has mushroomed into big business for plaintiffs.

Score another for Stephen Straus who has misrepresented data, misspent research money, mocked suffering victims, ignored physical data such as the punctate lesions shown by the MRI and the physical fading of fingerprints in several patients, withheld government grants to researchers who demonstrated any hint of belief in the physical basis of the disease, subjected patients to traumatic test procedures, then refused to tell what he had been looking for or what he had found. Stephen Straus who would probably have been the subject of a suit for malpractice by Susan Simon had she not been killed instantly in New York City. (See Chapter Three, Endnote 28)

ENDNOTES

[1]. Shorter, *Ibid*, p.97
[2]. Shorter, *Ibid*, p.295
[3]. Garth L. Nicolson, Ph.D. and Nancy Nicolson, Ph.D. "Chronic Fatigue Illnesses Associated with Service in Operation Desert Storm." *Townsend Letter for Doctors and Patients* May, 1996. pp.42-48
[4]. Quoted in: Johnson, *Osler's Web*, p.566
[5]. All quotations from Jay A. Goldstein, MD. *Betrayal by the Brain* New York-London :The Haworth Medical Press (1996) p.19
[6]. Mackie vs. Wolfe. Court of Queen's Bench of Alberta, Judicial District of Calgary. *Reasons for Judgment* of The Honourable Madam Justice B.L. Rawlins.
[7]. Mark J. Pellegrino. *Understanding Post-Traumatic Fibromyalgia* Columbus, Ohio: Anadem Publishing. 4. Further references to Dr. Pellegrino will not be endnoted.
[8]. Cited from the 'Foreword' in: Jay A. Goldstein, *Ibid*, xiv.
[9]. Shorter, *Ibid*, p.295
[10]. On page 38 of a report by the Senate Committee on Banking, Housing, and Urban Affairs on biological weapons sold to Iraq in the period 1985 to 1989. In the authors' files.
[11]. Johnson, *Ibid*, p.21
[12]. *Ibid*, p.46
[13]. Johnson, *Ibid*, pp.174-5
[14]. Shorter, *Ibid*, p.310
[15]. Johnson, *Ibid*, pp.404,405,514,518,585

CHAPTER NINE

THE CHRONOLOGY OF A HIDDEN WAR

The average reader is going to find it very hard to accept this chapter, for here we develop the chronology of a war that has been waged since 1945, but unlike the usual war, the ones that get written about in the average history book, this war has been largely hidden from the public view. It is only every now and again that the public gets a hint of what is going on, and as we have traced the growing public awareness of what chronic fatigue syndrome/fibromyalgia is and where it came from, we have caught glimpses of who is waging that hidden war. There have been no flags waving and no drums beating and no bugles sounding. Yet the war has been and still is being fought and casualties are still being suffered, and there has been a great price paid in both money and human lives.

What we reveal in this chapter is also hard to accept because it deals with something most readers haven't heard of before. It hasn't been heard of because those who are waging the hidden war as we have seen also control the major media, and the 'friendly elite...editors' referred to by the CIA in their document number 1035-950[1] can be counted upon to keep such stories from their readers and viewers. Furthermore, even if the major media were really free from their corporate controllers, the hidden war would not be reported because it takes place in secret places and the weapons used are silent and insidious. Yet the people waging this hidden war are real people in real places doing real things that have real consequences.

Despite their best efforts to keep their war hidden, some of the participants have been revealed. Dr. Donald MacArthur (Chapter Four) did not intend that the world would ever know what his researchers were up to in Fort Detrick in 1969. However, under the Freedom of Information Act his chilling revelations have leaked out. Even when his revelations to the congressmen were released to the public, most major media never reported what he had discussed, because they and he were parts of the military/industrial complex that has been waging the hidden war, and the less said, the better.

In this chapter our sources are very few because of the secrecy with which the hidden war has been carried out. But just because those waging this war have left very few traces of their activities does not mean that they have not been active. If one returns home after an evening out, and the house looks just as it did when it was left, one assumes all is right and that no crime has been committed. However, it is soon discovered that the stereo is missing. Police are called, but there are no finger prints, no sign of forced entry. All that tells the owner that a crime has been committed is the missing stereo.

So it is with the great crime against humanity that has been committed by the Dr. MacArthurs of this world. He met in secret with the right-wing Congressmen and they discussed how to create new synthetic pathogens...one which would disable its victims and one which would kill its victims. They didn't issue a press release about their plans. They didn't tell their constituents at the next election what they were spending $10 million on. They did it all in silence. And, as we shall see below, when they came up with their secret weapons they had to test them, and between 1940 and 1974 they tested them on over 500,000 unsuspecting citizens in the United States, and hundreds of thousands of other human beings in other countries...such as in Winnipeg, Canada.

No headlines in the Winnipeg papers: "U.S. Department of Defense sprays mystery toxin over City." All that was known was that on that day several citizens going to work or school or out shopping developed a cough or a sore throat or runny eyes. Those with asthma might have gasped for breath or those with a heart condition might have felt a tighter band around their chest. And as some of them visited a clinic or a hospital emergency room, there was someone silently and unobtrusively checking off numbers to 'quantitate' the results. And some politicians, elected to represent their constituents' best interests would be looking on silently. What the voters didn't know would hurt them...but they wouldn't know who it was that was doing the hurting. So, in this chapter we will point out the little hints that have crept out and we will note how all of these add up to an explanation for thousands of people suddenly finding their energy fading, their sleep non-restorative, their joints and muscles aching. They will know that something has happened to them to destroy their health, ruin their careers, often to cost them their families and their recreational activities. And they will go to doctors who cannot discover any physical clues about this mysterious illness and who will then tell their patients: *"It's all in your head."*

The victims will know that they are tragically disabled, just as Dr. MacArthur had promised, but it won't show on the surface, and only the most sophisticated tests will provide the objective physical evidence of the invading pathogen. In this chapter we will trace this hidden war, whose presence is revealed primarily in its casualties and in the way that the U.S. health agencies...the CDC and the NIH...have responded to their wounds. We will not attempt to indict war criminals upon the basis of these actions and our limited sources. Instead we will place the facts that our research has uncovered before you, and through you to the public, and ask all decent-minded, democratically oriented citizens to demand of their elected representatives that the full truth be revealed by way of a public enquiry where witnesses are called under oath and records produced and placed on the pages of history.

For example, we have already alluded to the fact that in February, 1953, someone in a position of power in the government of Canada gave the United States Department of Defense permission to fly a plane into Canada, and to spray a toxin over the City of Winnipeg. Then, persons assigned to the task monitored hospitals and clinics to determine how many citizens of that city reported symptoms which showed that they had been affected by the toxin. The U.S. Department of Defense could not test the toxin over an American city because, after a previous test over San Francisco in 1950, when at least one person was killed and several made ill, such tests were forbidden.

Who in Canada gave the Americans permission to spray the City of Winnipeg? What was the toxin that was being tested? Had there ever been a vote held where the citizens of Winnipeg had agreed to be guinea pigs for American biological warfare testing? And also of great importance is the question : How many in Canada, or even in Winnipeg ever heard of this atrocious invasion of the personal security of those affected?

As stated above, there have been great casualties in this hidden war. Among the casualties are many readers of this work...for the evidence is now clear:

the pathogens developed as biological weapons at Fort Detrick or by other research agencies under the direction of the Fort Detrick researchers include the pathogens which cause chronic fatigue syndrome and acquired immunodeficiency syndrome. If you suffer from CFIDS or AIDS you are just as much a casualty of war as a soldier who lost a leg landing on the beaches of Normandy on D-Day. And, the servicemen and women who became victims of the Gulf War Illnesses, are victims of the same biological pathogens that have destroyed the health of those who were afflicted with chronic fatigue syndrome/ fibromyalgia.

As the linkage between CFIDS and GWI/S has become clear, it also becomes clear why the health agencies in the United States, the Centers for Disease Control and the National Institutes of Health (who had according to Dr. MacArthur monitored the testing of new biological weapons) needed to co-operate in the cover-up of what had happened when certain pathogens being tested in Incline Village, Nevada, and Lyndonville, New York, proved to be much more infectious than had been anticipated and chronic fatigue syndrome had been let loose in the world.

How could an agency of the United States Government possibly admit that they had been a party to such a great crime against humanity? The fact of the matter is that they could not admit to their part nor reveal the activities of the Department of Defense which they had been monitoring. That is why they had to lie, misrepresent, commit fraud with research money, sabotage the research of independent researchers who might happen upon the truth, and recruit media assets to report through JAMA and the popular press an official mythology about chronic fatigue syndrome ("fibromyalgia does not exist") and about the spread of AIDS.(See Chapter Six). They had to keep their part in this evil enterprise from the public who, after all, they were supposed to be working to protect from disease, not to infect with disease.

This pattern of government health agencies participating with Department of Defense personnel in developing biological and chemical weapons and then helping with the cover-up is seen in the MK-ULTRA operation where:

"One of the largest supporters of 'behaviour research' was the Department of Health, Education and Welfare, and its subagency the National Institute of Mental Health. The subcommittee said

that HEW had participated in a 'very large number of projects dealing with the control and alteration of human behaviour.'" [2]

The NIMH was doing exactly what the CDC and other NIH agencies were to do when experiments were conducted in the development of the new synthetic pathogen which would 'disable' its victims...as Dr. MacArthur had promised the congressmen on June 9, 1969.

And, right from the beginning of their efforts to develop biological weapons all concerned strove to hide their role. As Peter Grose has written:

"From the start, therefore, CIA officers made no pretense that this project would be an innocuous matter of pure science. The research would have to proceed 'without the establishment of formal contractual relations,' Helms advised Allen (Dulles); the existence of signed contracts would reveal the government's sponsorship. Moreover, the scientists qualified to do research in this field 'are most reluctant to enter into signed agreements of any sort which connect with this activity, since such a connection would jeopardize their professional reputations.'" [3]

It was all part of the hidden war, and to set the stage for this chronology, we reproduce below a story from the *Delaware State News* which appeared on September 29, 1994. It is important to note that the horrifying facts revealed in this story came right from a congressional agency: The General Accounting Office. It is not a theory or a crack-pot day-dream. It is from the records of the agency which had to keep track of who was being paid public money to do what in the hidden war.

It is also important to note that as startling as the figure of 500,000 people being used as guinea pigs in the testing of biological, chemical and radiation weapons may be, the figures do not include those tests carried on in secret by the CIA and by the Pentagon under what the latter referred to as their "black budget".[4] Finally you should note that the figure of 500,000 covers just the time period between 1940 and 1974! How many people were victimized by those persons in secret places who were testing synthetic viruses and other pathogens after 1974? And the figure of 500,000 does not include human guinea pigs outside of the United States, such as the 400,000 in Winnipeg in 1953.

GAO LISTS GOVERNMENT EXPERIMENTS ON 500,000, 1940-1974
By Karen MacPherson. Scripps Howard News Service. Sept. 29, 1994

WASHINGTON – At least 500,000 people were used as subjects in Cold War era radiation, biological and chemical experiments sponsored by the federal government a congressional agency said Wednesday.

The General Accounting Office, in its first major overview of all defense-related human experiments, told a House subcommittee that the tests, conducted from 1940 through 1974, ranged from radiation to biological and chemical agents like mustard gas and LSD.

"This hearing reads like a chapter from a science-fiction novel," said Democratic Rep. John Conyers of Michigan, chairman of the House Government Operations Committee's legislation and national security subcommittee.

"There's something eerie about this. It is beyond most people's rational anticipation that their government could have been doing this," he said.

While many of the government's human radiation experiments have come to light over the past year, this is the first time Congress has been presented with an overview of all Cold War-era experiments.

GAO officials stressed that their work is preliminary, and that the numbers of experiments and people involved may rise as more information is made public by the Pentagon, the Energy Department, the CIA, NASA and other agencies.

Many of the Cold War tests were conducted in secret, while others involved the use of people without their consent or their full knowledge of the risks involved, the GAO said.

Some involved "vulnerable" populations, such as prison inmates and hospital patients.

Some of the tests were on individuals, such as Army and Navy skin tests during the 1940's with blistering agents and ointments on 60,000 people.

Other human experiments were done on a larger scale. From 1949 to 1969, for example, the U.S. Army conducted biological warfare tests that released radioactive compounds in 239 cities.

"The effects of government tests on participants' health have been difficult to determine," said GAO Assistant Comptroller General Frank Conahan.

"At the time of the tests, some people were clearly harmed," Mr. Conahan added, noting that available records show that people suffered immediate acute injuries in some tests, and that victims died in at least two tests.

"However, in other cases, possible adverse health effects related to the substances used were unknown or did not become apparent until years later."

Rep. Conyers said the hearing was designed to fill an important gap. A White House advisory committee created by President Clinton has been directed to focus only on human radiation experiments, leaving out hundreds of tests involving biological and chemical warfare agents.

"Radiation experiments are only part of the story," Rep. Conyers said. *"The only way to make sure that this doesn't go on anymore is to expose every part of it."*

GAO officials noted that federal agencies have devoted much attention, money and personnel to digging out information on human radiation experiments.

But far fewer resources have been focussed on gathering information about chemical and biological tests.

Defense Department officials agreed at the hearing that they hadn't spent as much time on the *biological* and chemical tests, but promised to step up their efforts.

Asked about the effectiveness of current federal protections for people involved in government-sponsored tests, Mr. Conahan pointed out that the federal government crafted such regulations in 1974.

But some federal health officials note that there is no mechanism to ensure that scientists are complying with the regulations, Mr. Conahan said, adding that GAO currently is studying the issue.(Emphasis added...Ed)

The American Establishment And The Hidden War

Well before the Second World War came to an end, there were a number of members of the 'American Establishment' who were getting ready to wage their next great battle...that was their anticipated battle against Communism. This Establishment had at its heart 'the New York financial and legal community' whose 'household deities were Henry L. Stimson and Elihu Root; its present leaders , Robert A. Lovett and John J. McCloy; its front organizations, the Rockefeller, Ford and Carnegie foundations and the Council on Foreign Relations; its organs, the *New York Times* and *Foreign Affairs.*" [5]

It was this group which President Dwight D. Eisenhower apparently had in mind when, in his final speech as President to the American people he had warned:

*"In the councils of government, we must guard against the acquisition of unwarranted influence, whether sought or unsought, by the **military-industrial** complex. The potential **for the disastrous rise of misplaced power exists and will persist.**"[6]*

It had been largely from this elite New York based group of the banking, legal, oil and industrial community together with a number of conservative academics that the American war time intelligence system, the Office of Strategic Services, had drawn its personnel.[7] Among their numbers were Allen Dulles, Richard Bissell, McGeorge Bundy, Arthur M. Schlesinger and others whose names were destined to crop up again when John F. Kennedy won the presidency and found himself in a life and death struggle against the forces of "darkness" which, he feared might "overtake the world." [8] And among those forces of darkness against which Mr. Kennedy had struggled silently and beyond the ken of the public were those people from the wartime intelligence service who had determined to recruit war criminals from Germany and Japan to help them develop chemical and biological weapons.

These war criminals who were recruited into the American defense system should properly speaking, have been placed on trial for their evil deeds. Consider, for example, the case of Otto von Bolschwing.

von Bolschwing had been appointed by the Germans as the SS and SD clandestine operations chief in Bucharest, Romania in 1941. In that post he organized an Iron Guardists attack upon the Jewish sector of Bucharest on January 20,1941.

"Hundreds of innocent people were rounded up for execution. Some victims were actually butchered in a municipal meat-packing plant, hung on meathooks, and branded as 'kosher meat' with red-hot irons. Their throats were cut in an intentional desecration of kosher laws. Some were beheaded. 'Sixty Jewish corpses (were discovered) on the hooks used for carcasses,' U.S. Ambassador to Romania Franklin Mott Gunther wired back to Washington after the pogrom. 'They were all skinned...(and) the quantity of blood about (was evidence) that they had been skinned alive.' Among the victims, according to eyewitnesses, was a girl no more than five years old who was left hanging by her feet like a slaughtered calf, her body bathed in blood." [9]

One would expect that such a murderer as von Bolschwing would be treated as the war criminal that he was; however, instead of being put on trial, he was hired by the American intelligence service from the end of the war until January, 1954 at which time "for reasons that are as yet unclear, the CIA decided to bring Otto von Bolschwing to the United States." [10]

Just what this war criminal did for democracy in the United States on the payroll of the taxpayers of that country, no one can learn. It is all top secret. However, telling von Bolschwing's story here is not meant to suggest that he was involved in the secret biological warfare work that was going on at the time. The purpose of presenting the facts about him is to make the point that the secret work of the intelligence services of the United States had absolutely no basis in common, decent morality. Otto von Bolschwing (nick-named the 'Butcher of Bucharest') is just one example of the many sick-minded people who found a lifetime of work in the hidden war being conducted by the U.S. military/industrial complex. If such a criminal could find work with those persons hidden from public view, it is very clear that others could be developing strategic war plans which would include the new weapons that Dr. MacArthur and his researchers were secretly working on.

Strategic Rather Than Tactical Weapons

On page 121 of Dr. MacArthur's June 9, 1969 testimony to the Congressmen, he makes the point that "The biological agents are considered strategic rather than tactical weapons..." [11] That is to say, the synthetic pathogens he envisions are designed for use in long term National Security goal achievement. And just what did those long-term goals include? Again, we have to fit together only the most elusive hints, for as with the case of Otto von Bolschwing, the details are carefully hidden from the public.

One clear strategic goal is to maintain the hold upon wealth and power by the Establishment we noted above, and by the military/industrial complex that Eisenhower had warned against. One important part of retaining such a strategic hold was the control of raw materials being drawn into the U.S. from Third World countries. This hold upon resources was being threatened by the fact that the population in the Third World supplier countries was growing and, as Henry Kissinger was to warn his patron, Nel-

son Rockefeller, when such happened, the supplier countries would want to retain more of their resources for their own use. Kissinger not only found a sympathetic ear among the Establishment who were nominally Republicans, but he also gained the active support of people in the Kennedy Administration such as Secretary of Defense, Robert McNamara. It was McNamara who once told a group of New York bankers that some way would have to be found to either lower the birth rate in these Third World countries, or "raise the death rate".

Although this strategic goal was strongly held among the Establishment, very little was said about it publicly. After all, how does anyone say openly that several million people in the Third World have to be killed off to protect the supply of raw materials to the United States? It is very challenging. Yet members of the Establishment have to be gently alerted to the problem so that the hidden war against the enemy...the citizens of Uganda, and Mali, and Thailand and the other countries identified by Kissinger in his NSSM 200 can be carried on without someone unwittingly alluding to a sensitive area.

One of the few such 'public' statements appeared in *Foreign Affairs* in an article by Jack Zlotnick [12] in July of 1961. We qualify the reference as 'public', because the views in this august journal are really not aimed at the readers of *Time* and *The New York Times*.

In his piece, Professor Zlotnick tries to put as positive a face upon his thesis as possible. He does not say that it is the increasing life span of Third World citizens that is the problem, but rather "The drop in the death rate is the core of the problem." Furthermore, he doesn't emphasize the reduced flow of goods to the U.S. as a major concern. He would have us believe that the Establishment figures in their clubs and on their golf courses, are concerned about the fact that these Third World citizens will not enjoy a higher standard of living:

"The Somalis might make automobiles if they adopt Detroit's technology, and might in time adopt Detroit's technology if they could accumulate the capital and skills. They can probably accumulate neither if they keep doubling in number every 20 or 25 years..."(p. 684)

It is not until page 685 that Zlotnick spells out the real point that he is trying to make:

"The problem (of population growth in Third World countries) perturbs some officials in Washington, where there is growing uneasiness about its

bearing on American security interests. There are also reservations about the expediency of taking the issue into consideration in reaching policy decisions."

Just who were those 'officials in Washington' who were uneasy? The author does not tell us, and we can only surmise who he might have had in mind. The most likely official would be Secretary of Defense, Robert McNamara. As we have remarked before, McNamara was a person who could in the view of John Kenneth Galbraith, (quoting George Ball) be 'on both sides' of a question at the same time.[13] Although McNamara was serving President John F. Kennedy, who had declared his opposition to any program of population control [14] and so one would assume be a supporter of the President's point of view, there is other evidence that in his typically insidious way, McNamara was working with those holding the opposing view. Such evidence is found in the record of the "Hearings before the Subcommittee on Health and Scientific Research of the Committee on Human Resources, United States Senate" dated March 8 and May 23, 1977. In this record we are told that:

"In May 1961 (note the year), the Secretary of Defense (McNamara) asked that the JCS: evaluate the potentialities of BW/CW, considering all possible applications. (emphasis added)…The JCS estimated that the cost for obtaining Secretary of Defense McNamara's complete spectrum BW/CW capability was about 4 billion dollars."

Thus, we have on another official record the fact that the Department of Defense was in 1961 considering programs of biological and chemical warfare that would cost the equivalent of the total federal income tax paid by 2,000,000 average American wage earners. Just what would that 4 billion dollars buy in the realm of biological and chemical weapons? From the same source we learn that "The development of vaccines for Q fever and Tularemia enabled work on Q fever and tularemia to proceed to standardisation as BW agents."

From this latter statement we learn something of great significance: it appears that only when the researchers have a defensive capability to a pathogen, that they will proceed to the production level of a biological weapon. This could suggest that before the mycoplasma that causes CFIDS was tested, there was already a known antidote for it! It is quite possible that hidden in the Department of Defense there already exists the information needed about how to

limit the ravages of the diseases known as CFIDS and AIDS.

We also learn that the development of the two vaccines cost $2.3 million. That leaves $3,997,700,000 still to be spent in McNamara's proposed budget! This fact has to be emphasized… someone, somewhere was doing something for that money! One of the questions which must be addressed is obvious: Upon what was the huge biological warfare budget being spent?

Part of the answer to that question might be found further on in Jack Zlotnick's *Foreign Affairs* article. On page 685 he informs us that: "In October 1959, the Senate Foreign Relations Committee published a report prepared by the Stanford Research Institute on 'Possible Nonmilitary Scientific Developments and Their Potential Impact on Foreign Policy Problems of the United States.' The report considered the two lines of attack on the *population problem*—increasing production and limiting births. The conclusion was that population pressures could become significant causes of social unrest and war, that 'some means of controlling population growth are inescapable' and that for this purpose the United States should provide funds to foreign agencies and *laboratories.*"

When one combines the essential thesis that limiting population growth in Third World countries was a problem for the United States, and the earlier recommendation by the "Draper Committee" to President Eisenhower that such population growth be treated as a *national security* matter with the huge biological warfare budget of Robert McNamaratwo further questions arise: how much money should be spent to limit population growth and what kind of program could accomplish that end?

At this point we must introduce another aspect of the McNamara factor…the kind of company he keeps.

On the surface McNamara is presented as a 'friend' of the Kennedy's. He may well have been such a friend. After all, Brutus was a friend of Caesar. But it is not McNamara's public friendships that we must look to; it is the friendships which he seems to have made less than public, and which are only discovered by careful research. In this latter class of friends we must place Alexander Haig who was appointed in February, 1962 'to a staff job in the murky reaches of the Pentagon'.[15] At one point he served in the top secret job of liaison between the Joint Chiefs of Staff and McNamara and he was in this critical job when the President was assassinated and some military officer in the Dallas-Sheraton Hotel reported to the Pentagon "That Secretary of Defense Robert McNamara and the Joint Chiefs of Staff are now the President"![16] Almost as if he thought that there had been a military *coup d'état*.

Haig also had more than a passing knowledge of the 'Miami Cubans' who have been suspected by many of having had a hand in the murder of Mr. Kennedy,[17] because after the Bay of Pigs fiasco, it had been Haig's job to integrate certain Cuban veterans into the regular U.S. Army. [18] Haig also had another unusual link...this one was with Eugenio Martinez who had served as a 'hit and run' saboteur against Cuba in 1963. Haig was one of the planners of these activities, many of which it appears, had been kept secret from Mr. Kennedy. Eugenio Martinez was later to turn up among the burglars who were caught breaking into the Democratic Party National Offices in the Watergate. However, besides his links with McNamara, the most critical links of Alexander Haig are those with Henry Kissinger when the former joined the Nixon Administration as Kissinger's deputy at the National Security Council. With this link in place, the circle is complete with population theorist and Rockefeller protege Kissinger tied to Robert McNamara who demonstrated a great concern for the need to 'increase the death rate' in Third World countries and Alexander Haig, the quintessential 'go-for' when unsavoury tasks had to be put into action.

It is important to note that it was very soon after Kissinger and Haig had joined President Nixon in their National Security Council roles that the budget for population control efforts increased dramatically.

It was also just six months later that Dr. MacArthur made his suggestions to the Congressmen. Again the question must be asked: what were the activities that were being bought with this money? And this, of course , brings us back to Dr. MacArthur's 'strategic' biological weapons program and the development of new pathogens for such strategic efforts. A new synthetic agent for which 'no natural immunity could have been acquired' [19] would provide the answer for the 'population problem' that had troubled the Eastern elite and the Foreign Affairs readership for several years. It would meet the so-called 'national security' concerns proposed by General Draper to Eisenhower, and expressed on several occasions by Robert McNamara. And, with Henry Kissinger, author of the NSSM 200 and the fears expressed therein about Third World countries whose populations were growing too fast, in a position to do something about it. The stage was set to commence the final solution to that problem. All they had to do was to get those two new pathogens into production and after a series of tests in isolated places, put them to work in the country's national security interests. Dr. MacArthur had proposed two pathogens with one to disable its victims and so cripple the economy of an 'enemy' and one to kill and so reduce the population in the fourteen countries Henry Kissinger thought needed some controlling.

Tests would, of course, have to be conducted and this meant that certain key people in the nations' health agencies, the CDC and the NIH, would have to be on side.

Summary

In the early part of the 1900's the so-called Eastern Elite demonstrated a growing concern about the dangers posed by unfettered population growth. The Rockefeller, Morgan, Dodge, Harriman and other wealthy families spent large sums of money on the study of the problem. Following the Second World War the military/industrial complex which to a considerable extent represented many of the same families, undertook to translate the concerns about population growth into action by linking the 'problem' to national security. The Report by General Draper to Eisenhower was the first step in this process. When President Kennedy succeeded Eisenhower, he played down the threat of population growth by emphasizing world economic development. This emphasis earned him further animosity from the Establishment and gave them one more reason for setting assassination plans in motion. In the meantime, Defense Secretary McNamara was urging the JCS to develop up to $4 billion worth of biological and chemical weapons.

When Nixon succeeded Johnson as President, the budget for population control was extended even further, and by June 9, 1969, the Director of Research for biological warfare was able to promise certain right-wing congressmen that within five to ten years he would be able to produce two new pathogens...one to kill for strategic purposes and one to disable. Both would be based upon pathogens which would be 'refractory to the immunological processes of the human body'. The hidden war was about to pass from theory and research into action, and in ten years time the casualties would begin to appear under the name of AIDS and CFIDS. And a new biological weapon would be added to the American arsenal.

ENDNOTES

[1].Robert J. Groden, *The Killing of a President* (New York: Viking Studio Books, 1993) p.144

[2]. W.H. Bowart, *Operation Mind Control* (New York: Dell Books, 1978) p.108

[3].Peter Grose, *Gentleman Spy–The Life of Allen Dulles* (Boston New York: Houghton Mifflin Company, 1994) pp.392-3

[4].Tim Weiner, *Blank Check: The Pentagon's Black Budget* (New York: Warner Books, 1990)

[5].Arthur M. Schlesinger, Jr. *A Thousand Days* (Boston: Houghton Mifflin Company, 1965) p.128

[6].Stephen E. Ambrose, *Eisenhower Vol. Two: The President* (New York: Simon and Schuster, 1984) p.612

[7].Anthony Cave Brown, *The Last Hero* (New York: Viking Books, 1984) P.173

[8].Schlesinger, *Ibid*, p.76

[9].Christopher Simpson, *Blowback* (New York: Weidenfeld & Nicolson, 1988)pp.254-5

[10].Simpson, *Ibid*, p.257

[11].Hearings, p.121

[12].Jack Zlotnick, *Foreign Affairs* Vol.39, July , 1961: "Population Pressure and Political Indecision". pp.683-694

[13].John Kenneth Galbraith, *A Life in Our Times* (Boston: Houghton Mifflin Company, 1981) p.471 (footnote)

[14].Zlotnick, *Ibid*, p.686. Zlotnick quotes Mr. Kennedy to the effect that: 'available resources of the world are increasing as fast as the population'. Hence, there was no national security threat as far as the President was concerned, in the population growth of Third World countries.

[15].Roger Morris, *Haig: The General's Progress* (Playboy Press, 1982) P.58

[16].Jim Bishop, *The Day Kennedy Was Shot* (New York: Greenwich House, 1983 edition) p.183

[17].Mark Lane, *Plausible Denial* (New York: Thunder's Mouth Press, 1991) pp.330-331. Lane does not mention that the message had dealt with the 'Miami Cubans' and their response to the assassination.

[18].Morris, *Ibid*, p.61

[19].Hearings, p.129

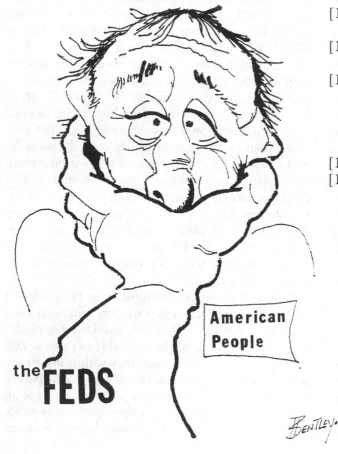

WAKE UP AMERICA!

American People

the FEDS

GULF WAR ILLNESS

WHAT GOES AROUND COMES AROUND

On the 6:30 pm edition of *ABC NEWS* of October 22, 1996, Peter Jennings reported that the Pentagon had made a 'damning admission'. According to Jennings, a Pentagon spokesperson had admitted that during the Gulf War of 1991, at least 20,000 and possibly more, Allied servicepeople had been exposed to nerve gas in March of that year.

Although this announcement probably came as a surprise to the average listener, it was no surprise to many others who for over five years have known that in the Gulf War some very evil acts had been committed by Iraq against the Allied Forces. Furthermore, as startling as the *ABC NEWS* story was, it didn't tell the true story nor the whole story. However, it was enough to let some people think that the growing phenomenon of the mystery illness called Gulf War Illnesses or Syndrome, was now accounted for. Jennings went on to present the Pentagon explanation…post-war demolition of Iraqi ammunition dumps containing 'chemical' weapons had polluted the air with nerve gas which had been spread by the desert winds to infect thousands of Allied servicepeople. The evidence, however, does not support this hypothesis. There is much greater evidence to suggest that certain military acts by the Iraqis were the source of the mystery illness. It was also probable that these acts accounted for the sudden stop of the Allied advance towards Baghdad and the rapid evacuation of the area by the Allies. These actions were kept hidden from the servicepeople affected and from the public at large. The reasons for such a deep conspiracy of denial and silence relate to the parallel conspiracy of denial and silence which followed the tragic spread of chronic fatigue syndrome and of acquired immunodeficiency syndrome.

The truth about what had happened in the Gulf War and in the epidemic of CFIDS/AIDS involved those people such as Dr. Donald MacArthur, who had been waging a hidden war on behalf of the military-industrial complex against any threat to its power and position of great privilege. And, when the consequences of their 'research' was evident in the destroyed health and lives of unwitting victims, the military had no choice but to attempt to cover-up their part in both disasters. And, for the cover-up to succeed the 'media assets' had to do their part by carrying the message to the public at large: these veterans of the Gulf War are not really sick; it's all in their heads. The message has a familiar ring to victims of chronic fatigue syndrome.

In the Gulf War, what had gone around came around in a mind-boggling series of events which threatened to expose the perpetrators of hidden evil to the world. And the perpetrators included more than Saddam Hussein who is a psychopath. They included the Pentagon (with its 'damning admission'), the American Establishment, the 'sympathetic media assets' (who during the War had been as controlled as any media ever were), and those researchers who over the years, had worked secretly to develop insidious new biological weapons. The truth about 'Gulf War Syndrome' had to be kept hidden and that truth was the fact that Saddam Hussein had used biological weapons the pathogenic components of which had been provided to him on May 2, 1986 by the United States, and which had been developed in Fort Detrick, Maryland by the Department of Defense biological warfare researchers. The growing number of veterans displaying all the symptoms of chronic fatigue syndrome were the unacknowledged casualties of the Gulf War and it was only to be after the numbers continued to grow that the Pentagon and its pliant 'media assets' had to start leaking out a graduated program of denial, distortion, misinformation and disinformation . The wheel was coming around.

But it wasn't just the wheel of biological weapons that had come around in Operation Desert Storm. The whole episode of the Gulf War was a coming around of a wheel initially pushed into motion by representatives of the American Establishment, as well as their British and French counterparts, some seventy years earlier when the collapse of the Ottoman Empire opened the way for the partition of the Middle East and the apportionment of pieces of it to various imperialist countries. It is a complex and convoluted story made all the more confusing by virtue of the fact that so much of what has happened transpired in secrecy. Because so much of what was done was unseen by the world, the consequences of these acts always came as a great surprise to the American and European public. And that which was done in secret by the likes of Allen Dulles, Frank Wisner, the 'Rockefeller interests', the 'Seven Sisters' oil companies, John J. McCloy, George Bush, Kermit Roosevelt and many others was violently anti-democratic and brutal.

Furthermore, the entire period from December 12, 1920 when Allen Dulles arrived in Constantinople [1] as a representative of the U.S. State Department to witness the dismemberment of the Ottoman Empire from that critical vantage point, and to protect the interests of American citizens, "largely missionaries and oil men[2] until 2:00 am on January 17, 1991, when the forces of Desert Storm launched their first air strikes against Iraq [3] is all of a piece. All the parts from the division of oil-rich Arab lands among foreign powers to the firing of Iraqi SCUD missiles armed with American biological weapons fit into a whole.

No part can be separated from another part without losing the logic of the tragic outcome. We say 'logic' because the apparently random acts of lunatic violence all grew out of what had been put in place over the years. One cannot comprehend nor condemn the brutality of the Iranian seizure of the American Embassy in Teheran on November 4, 1979 unless one first reflects upon the decision taken in the Eisenhower State Department 'to mount a coup' in Iran against Mohammed Mossadegh and return the discredited Shah to the Peacock Throne. A Shah whose principal credential for the job was his deep friendship with John J. McCloy, Nelson Rockefeller and Henry Kissinger. Neither can one understand how a lunatic such as Saddam Hussein could be allowed to purchase the components for biological weapons from the United States right up to the eve of the Gulf War unless it is taken together with the world view of Congressmen such as Robert Sikes of Florida, or Jamie Whitten of Mississippi, or George Mahon of Texas as revealed in their June 9, 1969 meeting with Dr. Donald MacArthur of the Biological Research Branch of the Department of Defense.

To take any one part of this wheel of many spokes and to try to understand it in isolation from the other parts of the wheel causes one to lose sight of the logic of history turning. To simply say that in 1945 the U.S. recruited into its defense establishment several Japanese war criminals, without fitting that act to the whole history of U.S. biological warfare research is to keep one from recognizing how that deed in 1945 can be related to the way Diane Martel was bullied by society because she was a victim of CFIDS. And to simply say on an ABC News broadcast that 20,000 veterans of the Gulf War have some mystery illness without fitting that illness to the May 2, 1986 sale of 'Brucella Melitensis' to Iraq is to keep oneself from recognizing the links between secret meetings in Washington and secret military deeds by Iraq in Desert Storm.

An Interlude About Negative Templates

We are dealing here, as at many other points in this study, with history that does not get into the standard history books. For some reason or other, many of the things that have happened and which we have discovered only by dint of long hours of research, are not recorded by the 'leading' historians of our time.

Professor Peter Dale Scott has advanced a wonderfully insightful hypothesis which he has called the 'negative template' to be employed for further investigation into any subject in history. Briefly, the point is this: find what is left out of an official account of some event and you will more than likely discover what is of profound significance.[4]

Just by way of one example: In his book about the Kennedy Presidency, which is widely regarded by most scholars as the touchstone of all histories of the one thousand days, Arthur M. Schlesinger, Jr., leaves several gaping holes about Mr. Kennedy's relationship with Israel.

When one turns to the index of A Thousand Days one looks in vain for 'Dimona' and when one turns to the index under 'Ben Gurion' one finds only a single reference to a one sentence, innocuous comment. Why, in view of the critical stress between Kennedy and Ben Gurion does Schlesinger choose to omit any hint as to the sources of that stress?

Kennedy had wanted the Israelis to stop work on the development of a nuclear capability and he had also wanted Israel to compensate the Palestinians who had been displaced from their homes, farms and businesses for their losses. And Ben Gurion was extremely angry at the President's pressure. Yet Schlesinger leaves out all references to the tension between the two. There is a very strong reason for Schlesinger's oversight which we will not develop at this point. It is cited only to illustrate the validity of Prof. Scott's 'negative template' hypothesis: what is left out is often far more important than what is put in. In the case of Mr. Kennedy's relationship with Israel, Prof. Schlesinger knew precisely what he had to leave out if he was to mask the reality of Ben Gurion's activities which followed.

End Of An Interlude

Allen Dulles –
An Overview Of An Underworld

There is a significant comment in one Dulles' biography: 'Allen discovered that only a thin line divided respectable high finance from a *shadowy underworld*'.[5](emphasis added) This thesis can be applied to every area of Allen Dulles' career, and is critical to this present study because we are trying to lead out into the light the whole background to the challenge faced today by people with chronic fatigue syndrome, acquired immunodeficiency syndrome and (now) Gulf War syndrome.

Decisions of great human consequence have been made in the shadows by people with no mandate from those whose lives have been affected in a very tragic way. In fact, those people who have been so affected have, generally speaking, no idea of just what decisions have been made by whom. Yet these decisions have destroyed their health, altered their life styles, affected them financially in a negative way, and in many cases have cost them friends and family. They have accepted their lot as something that has just happened in their lives and all that they can do is to bear their cross. And despite their very real suffering they can only look on with wonder and hurt when they are told by a Justice of a Canadian court "There is no such thing as fibromyalgia."

To give a more specific cast to the general thesis noted above, we can refer to the Gulf War. Why were there over 700,000 American, Turkish, British, French, Canadian and a variety of other national forces which attacked the Republic of Iraq in the months of January and February, 1991? [6]

On the surface the answer was simple: Iraq, under their apparently lunatic President, Saddam Hussein, had brutally attacked its neighbour, the Emirate of Kuwait. This was, as the media made clear, a repeat of what Adolph Hitler had done in Europe some fifty years before. It was only right and proper said the champions of democracy such as George Bush and John Major, that such naked aggression should be challenged by all freedom loving persons everywhere. The media in North America and in Britain and France, and to a lesser degree in other countries, took up the cry…for democracy, liberty, and justice the world should rally against the madman in Baghdad. That is what over 700,000 servicepeople from a significant group of nations were doing in January-February, 1991. And little did anyone suspect that in the coming conflict it would all come together: the secret machinations of a powerful elite centered upon the banking/oil/legal/military of the American Establishment and the biological warfare plotting of Dr. Donald MacArthur to develop two new synthetic pathogens for which no natural immunity could have been acquired. In the coming battle those who sponsored the evil, or at least their unsuspecting rank and file troops, would find themselves the target of their own mad schemes when a nucleic particle of 'brucella melintensis' (a mycoplasma species) would shower down upon Allied servicepeople. Servicepeople who were told by their politicians that they were in the Middle East for democracy, liberty and justice.

However, when one begins to peel that democratic onion one finds layer after layer of intrigue and sabotage to such an extent that when the peeling is finished there is no residue of democracy, liberty or justice. For example, on October 22, 1989 the Emir of Kuwait delegated his brother, Fahd Ahmed Al Fahd to meet with 'Judge William Webster, Director of the United States Central Intelligence Agency' on Tuesday, November 14, 1989.[7] Brigadier Fahd attended that meeting and later reported to the Emir that… "5. We agreed with the American side that it was important *to take advantage of the deteriorating economic situation in Iraq in order to put pressure on that country's government to delineate our common border…*" One may well ask which of the qualities of 'democracy, liberty, and justice' were apparent in this situation?

The Director of the CIA was an American who was not elected to his post. However, in a democracy such as the United States it was the reasonable right of the duly elected Government to appoint people to agencies of the government to carry out the will of the Administration. We must assume that Judge Webster was simply carrying out the general direction given to him by his boss, President George Bush. The question then arises, when did Mr. Bush tell the American people that, through the intermediary of the secret intelligence agency which he had once headed, he was going to connive with Kuwait in the latter's on-going border dispute with Iraq? The answer of course is clear: he never did tell his constituents what he was up to. Just as he had never told them about his drug-trading agreements while he was Vice-President.[8]

The pattern is very familiar, in fact it goes back at least as far as 1924 when Allen Dulles had tried to recruit people in the oil business as intelligence agents in various countries of the Middle East...including spies against Iraq. [9]

If one is prepared to overlook the secret intrusion of the US through its intelligence agency into the Iraq-Kuwait dispute over their common boundary, then one can go to the three basic principles of democracy, liberty and justice and argue that at least the people of Kuwait had the right to protest the violation of their natural borders.

But then another problem arises. Just where did Kuwait come from and by what traditional rights did they assert their claim to the oil-rich northern border area? The answer to that question continues the theme of power plays and border drawing that had absolutely nothing to do with the will of the Kuwaiti people. It goes back to 1913 when no one knew that there were any oil deposits anywhere near the Emirate. In that year Britain, who needed coal for its globe spanning fleet, coveted Kuwait because there were indications that the area had solid reserves of coal. Turkey, which felt itself exposed to danger in the anticipated struggles that some believed were bound to come as Germany dreamed of a Berlin to Baghdad railroad which would have to cross the path of Russia who in turn was looking for access to the Mediterranean, deemed it prudent to agree with Britain that Kuwait should be an autonomous district.

In 1916 Britain took the opportunity of the war to recognize the Emirate as totally independent of the Ottoman Empire...with Britain, of course, helping that tiny entity to survive and thus make its coal available to the Royal Navy. Iraq, which had been designated as a protectorate of Britain in 1916 under the British-French Sykes-Picot Agreement, had no say in the matter because there was no such nation until 1932, when it was granted independence as a monarchy. It was not until 1958 when a military revolt in Iraq created the present Republic, that any great interest was taken by anyone in just where the border between Iraq and the Emirate of Kuwait lay. And, by this time, the presence of vast oil deposits in the region made the question a critical one.

Britain helped keep the dispute in abeyance by declaring in 1961 that Kuwait was completely independent and that the northern boundary took in the disputed oil fields but was able to produce no real justification for such a claim. Despite being on very thin ice in their claim, Britain used its armed forces to ensure that Kuwait enjoyed its 'independence'. There was no hint of either democracy, liberty or justice in the whole affair, but that really didn't matter to Britain because with Kuwait independence came the latter's right to share its oil production with their patron- Britain.

If one were to examine the question of justice one would have to recognize that since the 19 million people of Iraq who enjoyed a Gross Domestic Product of only $1950 per capita while the 1.2 million people of Kuwait enjoyed a GDP of ten times that amount $19700 per capita. [10] Justice really didn't enter into the matter.

Since it is obvious to any objective student of history that the 700,000 servicepeople (who it would turn out were to be the victims of a biological attack and to be largely betrayed by their own governments) were gathered in Saudi Arabia in January, 1991, ready to risk their lives and their health to drive Iraq from Kuwait that democracy, liberty and justice had nothing to do with the struggle. One has to ask again, what were they doing there?

The answer is to be found in one word: oil. Iraq wanted a large share of Kuwaiti oil wealth, and if this were to be achieved, then Iraq would be able to even out the gross discrepancy between the GDP of Iraq and that of Kuwait. But that wasn't really their goal. The goal of Iraq was to make itself the undisputed leader of the oil rich Middle East. As the leader of that critical area Saddam Hussein would be able to exercise very significant strength in his dealings with the oil-hungry United States and Europe. And that is where George Bush and John Major and Francois Mitterand drew their line in the sand. The battle was joined at 2:00 am, January 17, 1991 (Baghdad Time) when the air attacks began.

HE MAY BE LUNATIC, BUT HE'S NOT NUTS

Many people puzzle over the question: Who gave Saddam Hussein the idea that the United States would stand by and allow Iraq to seize Kuwait with its huge oil reserves?

The answer is simple: The United States.

The slow but steady movement of United States support for Saddam Hussein may be said to have begun on September 22, 1980 when Iraq invaded Iran. The United States was in the midst of a struggle with the latter country holding American Embassy personnel as hostages, and President Carter felt that the Iraqi attack might persuade the Ayatollah Khomeini that "it would be in (Iran's) best interest to release the prisoners in order to restore some of their standing in the international community, bring an end to our economic boycott, and gain the use of their confiscated billions of dollars." [11] Although this hope was to be quickly dashed, the profound hostility towards Iran led to a softening American attitude towards Saddam Hussein and Iraq.

By 1982, when Iran had surprised most of the military pundits around the world by first holding the Iraqi incursion and then beginning to gear itself for a counter-attack which could well have over-run Iraq, the United States had to translate their vague pro-Iraqi feelings into something more tangible. By mid-June of that year a decision was made in the Reagan White House to communicate with Saddam Hussein and to tell him that the U.S. government "wanted to offer Iraq some assistance in the war with Iran." [12] The help would consist of sending an American intelligence officer to Baghdad with satellite photography and maps which would show Iraq where the Iranian attack was going to occur. The Iraqis quickly accepted the entire package, and the Iranian attack was defeated with heavy casualties... thanks to the United States who was still publicly condemning Saddam Hussein and his "murderous regime."

Despite the set-back to Iran, something further had to be done to bolster Saddam Hussein, and that help came on February 8, 1985 and on several dates thereafter up until November 28, 1989 when the United states shipped a startling array of biological pathogens which could be deployed against Iran. Pathogens which had been developed following the June 9,1969 Hearings between the Pentagon and the Congressional Representatives. Again, the transactions were completed under cover but "pursuant to application and licensing by the U.S. Department of Commerce." [13] We should note in passing that the shipments included 'Brucella melitensis Biotype 1 and 3'. This pathogen can cause "chronic fatigue,

loss of appetite, profuse sweating when at rest, pain in joints and muscles, insomnia, nausea, and *damage to major organs."* We will be returning to this shipment, whose effects are practically identical to the presenting symptoms of Gulf War Syndrome, at a later point.

By 1988 with over a million Iraqis and Iranians dead, the two nations reached a final stalemate and in July both declared victory and hostilities ceased. Saddam Hussein would not have survived had it not been for the help received from the Reagan and Bush administrations. But the consequences of the eight years of war had been catastrophic for Iraq; the country was on the brink of a total economic collapse, and ironically, it was the United States which again came to the rescue. Iraq became the "biggest user in the world of the American Community Credit Program" wherein surplus U.S. stocks of corn, rice, flour and so on which had been bought up with taxpayers' dollars as a part of farm price support programs were shipped to countries who could not afford their purchase.[14]

Two years later the Bush administration moved the support for Saddam Hussein up another notch. On February 12,1990, Bush sent John Kelly to Baghdad with this mind boggling message for Hussein: "You are a force for moderation in the region, and the United States wishes to broaden her relations with Iraq." [15] Unfortunately, Hussein's public utterances did not carry that tone of 'moderation' to the rest of the world.

On April 2, less than two months after receiving John Kelly, Saddam Hussein made a speech in which Israel was his major target of criticism and in that speech he made this remarkable statement: "Whoever threatens us with atomic bombs (ie Israel...Ed) will be exterminated with *chemical weapons."* [16] Then he made another point of critical significance: Iraq now possessed "the binary chemical weapon"? It is important to make the point that Dr. MacArthur in his June 9,1969 testimony to the congressmen had introduced this concept as a target for American research:

Dr.MacArthur: ...if we go to this binary concept...
Mr.Sikes: How do you spell the term 'binary'?
Dr.MacArthur: 'B-I-N-A-R-Y' (Hearings p.142)
However it was spelt, Iraq now possessed the device, and there are many guesses as to where they got it. But this question is not nearly as significant as the reply made by George Bush when he was advised what Hussein had said. Bush replied,"I suggest that such

statements about chemical or biological weapons be forgotten." [17]

Saddam Hussein had not mentioned 'biological' weapons! What was George Bush thinking about? Obviously he knew something about Iraq's biological capabilities that the public did not know. The latter had no idea that both Reagan and Bush had been supplying Iraq with biological weapons for several years.

Equally significant was the decision of George Bush not to call for any sanctions against Iraq in response to Hussein's tirade against Israel. In fact, possibly influenced by his strong Christian principles, Bush appears to have favoured the idea that a 'soft answer turneth away anger', for just ten days later he sent five Senators, led by Robert Dole, to see Hussein on April 12.

The Dole delegation began with a letter apparently prepared in their talks at the White House before they had left. It was read to Hussein by a translator and it continued that puzzling Bush reference to 'biological weapons' to which Hussein had never alluded: "…your desire to equip yourself with chemical and biological weapons, far from strengthening your country's security, exposes it to serious dangers." [18]

Saddam responded to the letter and Dole's conciliatory remarks by complaining that there was a media campaign being carried on in the U.S. against him.

"'Not from President Bush,' Senator Dole cut in. 'Yesterday he told us he does not support this.' The person responsible for the Voice of America editorial that had offended Saddam 'has been fired,' Dole declared." [19]

"On April 25, as an indication of this new-found peace of mind, George Bush sent a message of friendship to Saddam Hussein…" [20]

Saddam Hussein must have been greatly heartened by the Bush decision against sanctions; by the Dole delegation with their warm message; and, finally, with the April 25 letter from the President. There seemed to be no indication that the U.S. was worried about his sabre rattling. By July 24 Hussein was so confident about the U.S. position that he moved two Iraqi army divisions up to the Kuwaiti border. Then he waited for a response from the world… especially the United States. That response came the next day when he received the American Ambassador to Iraq, April Glaspie.

Poor Ms. Glaspie. She now claims that the gist of what she carried to Hussein was what she had received from the Bush administration. And what was it that she told Saddam Hussein just the day after he had moved his army to the border of Kuwait? First, she assured him that "I have a direct instruction from the President to seek better relations with Iraq." Later she literally gave Saddam the green light to continue in the direction he seemed to be heading:" …we have no opinion on Arab-Arab conflict, *like your border disagreement with Kuwait."* [21] In testimony before Congress in March, 1991, she claimed to have warned Hussein repeatedly not to use force against Kuwait. When the cables between the White House and the Ambassador were declassified in July, 1991 they told a different story. The cables suggested that Ms. Glaspie's did not contain any warning to Iraq, and led Senator Alan Cranston to declare that Glaspie had "deliberately misled Congress." [22]

It appears Saddam Hussein had indeed received what amounted to a green light and he followed this meeting with the movement of several more units to the Kuwaiti border. Then, while his army sat poised on that border, John Kelly of the U.S. State Department was asked by a reporter on July 31: "If…Iraq crossed the Kuwaiti border…is it correct to say that we have no treaty, no commitment, which would oblige us to use American forces?" Kelly replied: "That's right".

"John Kelly's statements were broadcast on the World Service of the BBC and were heard in Baghdad. At a crucial hour, when war and peace hung in the balance, Kelly had sent Saddam Hussein a signal that could be read as a pledge that the United States would not intervene."[23]

Who had given Saddam Hussein the idea that he could invade Kuwait with impunity? The United States.

Two days after Kelly's ambiguous reply to the reporter, Saddam Hussein invaded Kuwait and in forty-eight hours he had total control of the Emirate, and followed up his success there by moving several parts of his army up to the border of Saudi Arabia.

The wheel of intrigue, secret manoeuvring, secret deals, secret development testing and finally sales of biological weapons to lunatic dictators, was coming full circle with Desert Shield and Desert Storm and when SCUD missiles laden with 'Brucella melitensis' exploded over the heads of the Allied defenders of democracy, liberty and justice, Dr. Donald MacArthur's evil seeds came to fruition and the 'incapacitants' that he had promised Mr. Sikes of Florida, Mr. Whitten of Mississippi , Mr. Andrews of Alabama, Mr. Flood of Pennsylvania, Mr. Slack of West Virginia, Mr. Addabbo of New York, Mr. Evans of Colorado, Mr. Davis of Wisconsin, Mr. Rhodes of Arizona, Mr. Minshall of Ohio and Mr. Lipscomb of California all under the Chairmanship of George Mahon of Texas, did their promised evil and the sons and daughters of many of the constituents who had voted for these right-wing hawks breathed in the contaminated air.

But there were still a couple more spokes to go before news of Gulf War Illnesses began creeping into the media. The illnesses, like chronic fatigue syndrome before it, were strenuously denied by the Pentagon through people such as Deputy Director of Health Services, Stephen C. Joseph who had a murky background as a health control official in New York, and by various others in the NIH and CDC.

I Pledge To You; There Will Not Be Any Murky Ending [24]
President George Bush, November 1990

The ending of Desert Shield and Desert Storm is certainly not murky as far as who is in and who is out of power. Saddam Hussein is as of the time of writing, still running Iraq with an iron hand. His erstwhile foes, however, have not fared as well. George Bush Sr., Margaret Thatcher, Yildirim Akbulut, Francois Mitterand, Mikhail Gorbachev, and Brian Mulroney were all packed off to an early retirement by their party or their electorate. Which leader(s) survived the Gulf War is not murky, but why Saddam Hussein is the one who prevails is certainly murky. How can it possibly be that this psychopathic lunatic still sits at the head of his Cabinet table wearing his neatly tailored uniform with his armed bodyguard standing behind him, while George Bush Sr. has so much idle time that he can travel up to Canada to go fishing with Premiers Clyde Wells of Newfoundland and Mike Harris of Ontario?

To find the answer to that question we must examine the unusual Saddam Hussein-George Bush exchange over chemical cum 'chemical-biological' weapons of April 2, 1990, and the way that the Gulf War finally ended...not with a bang but a whimper.

Biological weapons are the poor nation's nuclear bomb. According to a chilling scenario by microbiologist Larry Wayne Harris whose twenty-seven

year career includes nine years with CIA- Biological Warfare units, eleven people starting with one vial of Plague could kill 400,000 New Yorkers in approximately three weeks.[25]

On November 2, 1974, Iraq established its first bacteriological laboratory when it signed a contract with the Paris-based Institut Merieux.[26] Over the following five years their program in biological weapon development was complemented by a chemical weapon component. Under the latter the Iraqis were able by 1980 to produce 1,000 tons a year of organic phosphorus compounds which form the basis of nerve gases such as Sarin and Tabun. [27]

In their biological weapons development quest Iraq got a big boost in 1985 when the United States began exporting biological materials 'which were not attenuated or weakened and *were capable of reproduction'!* Among these biological components were those capable of either killing a victim or of disabling him. The details of this absolutely stupid transfer of agents capable of causing death from anthrax or clostridium perfrigens (the 'flesh eating disease' that almost killed Lucien Bouchard) or of causing disablement from Brucella melitensis. Which as we noted earlier causes an array of symptoms which are identical to those of chronic fatigue syndrome and of Gulf War Illnesses.

To summarize the U.S. support of Iraqi biological warfare capabilities we must note the following:

1. Shipments started in 1985 (under the Reagan administration) and continued until November 28, 1989 (under the Bush, Sr. administration) thus, for most of the years when George Bush was publicly condemning Saddam Hussein, his administration was secretly approving the shipments of deadly biological agents to Iraq.

2. On page 49 of the Reigle Report, the following statement occurs: "Biological agents cannot be detected by the human senses. A person could become a casualty before he is aware he has been exposed to a biological agent."

3. On page 38 of the same Report there occurs this description of the symptoms caused by 'Brucella melitensis': "...a bacteria which can cause *chronic fatigue,* loss of appetite, profuse sweating when at rest, pain in joints and muscles, insomnia, nausea, and *damage to major organs,* Compare these symptoms with those of the veterans suffering from Gulf War Illnesses. In the latter list you will note chronic fatigue, pain in joints and muscle spasms, insomnia(ie 'sleep difficulties'), and nau-

sea. Finally, compare both of these partial lists with the symptoms of chronic fatigue syndrome as listed (partially) in the Index of *Osler's Web*: aching joints, chronic fatigue, non-restorative sleep (ie insomnia) and apparent damage to various major organs.

4. On page 45 of the Reigle Report, it is to be noted that the Centers for Disease Control began keeping records of the export of certain pathogens on October 1, 1984. Thus they would be in a critical position to identify the fact that Gulf War Illnesses were actually manifestations of agents which they knew had been exported to Iraq. When they failed to come right out in 1991 and point out that the Gulf War Illnesses was essentially CFIDS and that both were caused by Brucella melitensis, they were continuing the cover-up that they had instituted in 1984 when they began their myth creation that CFIDS does not exist. That it was 'all in the head' of the victims.

When, on April 2, 1990, Saddam Hussein declared that he would use *chemical* weapons and George Bush urged him not to talk about *'chemical-biological'* weapons each knew what the other was talking about because the U.S. had provided the biological capability and had also probably provided the binary delivery system for chemical attack weapons to Iraq.

One more spoke and the wheel will be full circle.

Most Of The Scuds Are Exploding Harmlessly In The Air

Much was made of the apparent fact that the modified Iraqi SCUD missiles could seldom make it to their targets in one piece. One account puts it this way:

"The Iraqi-modified SCUDS were poorly constructed. Moreover, in doubling the range of the original SCUD (in the 'Al Hussein' version), the Iraqis made the speed of the SCUD as it plunged to earth twice what the missile was originally designed for. The additional stresses generated by this greater speed caused most SCUDS to break up at about the same time the Patriot radar picked them up." [28]

Several eye-witnesses reported such relatively harmless SCUD incursions into their areas, and many commentators found the failure of the SCUD surprising and to a degree humourous. However, one must not forget what both Saddam Hussein and George Bush knew. Both were well aware of the fact that an apparently harmless explosion of a

SCUD could shower down a invisible mist of Brucella melitensis which, while not fatal, would disable thousands of servicepeople exposed to it over an area of up to 3,600 square kilometres.

There were many other accounts about 'chemical-biological' weapon attacks which were later decreed to have been false alarms.

In all probability many of such alarms were not false. The 'harmlessly' exploding SCUD was showering its cargo of made in America Brucella melitensis, shipped to Iraq on May 2,1986, down upon the service men and women who believed that they were in the Gulf War in the defense of democracy, liberty and justice. George Bush,Sr. and Saddam Hussein knew better. Both knew that there was a great power struggle going on and in that power struggle both knew that Saddam Hussein had biological weapons and that one of those was brucella melitensis. The biological agent that had been developed in Fort Detrick, Maryland after Dr. Donald MacArthur committed his Research Branch to that task on June 9, 1969. On page 144 of The Hearings, the good doctor promises to be working upon: "viruses and bacteria...mutated to new forms resistant to vaccines," (Para.6) and "Large area incapacitating weapons systems."

But the worst was still to come.

Both Saddam Hussein and George Bush,Sr. also knew that not only had there been several shipments of CFIDS-inducing brucella melitensis shipped to Iraq, but there had been many more shipments of the deadly anthrax. Seven known shipments have been recorded.

The SCUD missiles apparently breaking up harmlessly over the Desert Storm forces could just as easily carry 'bacillus anthracis' as 'brucella melitensis'. The big difference was, when the latter showered down upon the Allied forces they wouldn't be aware of what had happened to them for several weeks. Indeed, some could carry the pathogen in a latent form for up to five or more years. Then following a trauma (physical or psychological) they could manifest the symptoms of chronic fatigue syndrome. And the CDC could continue to deny that they were sick, using the myth they had created when several human guinea pigs upon whom the initial tests had been made demonstrated that the modified pathogen was far more infectious than had been imagined. In the meantime, the Health Services Deputy Director, Stephen C. Joseph would be already to deny that returning servicepeople who complained of chronic fatigue, aching joints and muscles, nausea etc. were really sick.

However, if the next few SCUDS came over laden with 'bacillus anthracis' the results would be dramatically different. The disease "begins abruptly with high fever, difficulty in breathing, and chest pain. The disease eventually results in septicaemia (blood poisoning), and the mortality is high." If this began to happen to a significant portion of the seven hundred thousand Desert Storm forces, what would George Bush do then…and what would he say to the American people who had just witnessed such a triumphant victory over the forces of Saddam Hussein?

There was no alternative. Desert Storm had to stop dead in its tracks and, as rapidly as possible, they had to head for home. Joel Bainerman sums up the questions the world was asking:

> *"The mystery of the Gulf War lies in the President's actions: Why did he order General Schwarzkopf to cease the ground attack after only 100 hours and not destroy Saddam Hussein when he had the chance? How could that man the American people were told was as evil as Hitler was allowed to remain in power? Why instead of being dead or deposed, does he still pose a threat to his neighbours?"[29]*

When the SCUD missiles began exploding 'harmlessly' over the forces of Desert Storm, the wheel had come full circle.

Now it is beginning another circle. What goes around, comes around.

There were 390 Americans who had been killed and 458 wounded in action. There were 510 allied casualties. Lt. Richard was not given the benefit of the doubt and like so many of her comrades in arms she too was denied fair and just treatment. That was by official count. But what about the mystery illness now being called Gulf War Illnesses? "Well," said Deputy Director of Pentagon Health Services, Dr. Stephen C. Joseph,"It's all in their head."

Like chronic fatigue syndrome and fibromyalgia before it, and just as Justice Rawlins had ruled in her courtroom: "Fibromyalgia does not exist" and neither does Gulf War Syndrome.

But George Bush, Colin Powell, Saddam Hussein, Stephen Joseph and the CDC all know better.

SUMMARY

Following the collapse of the Ottoman Empire in World War One, the victorious nations of Europe and the United States began a great power game aimed at controlling the vast oil wealth of the Middle East. No thought was given to the welfare or rights of the people who had lived in the area for thousands of years. All that mattered was to engage in secret manoeuvres to possess the wealth extracted for the use of a relative handful of people in what are referred to as the 'developed nations.' To achieve control, plots and counterplots were hatched and various puppet governments set up by the real masters. Such puppet masters were armed to the teeth so that they could maintain their hold on power. When Mohammed Mossadegh of Iran staged the closest thing to a populist revolt by nationalizing the oil wells and deposing the Shah, the United States through the agency of Allen Dulles' CIA 'mounted a coup' in Iran and returned the Shah to his peacock throne. Without any semblance of democratic participation open to them, many in Iran turned to the Islamic Fundamentalist, The Ayatollah Khomeini, to rid them of foreign domination. When the Shah fled a second time, and the Iranians seized American Embassy personnel as hostages, the U.S. began to secretly assist Iraq as a bulwark against Iranian led Islamic fundamentalist expansion.

The U.S. aid included components for deadly biological weapons that had been secretly developed in the U.S. between 1945 when they recruited Japanese war criminal Gen. Ishii Shiro, to the present. Saddam Hussein was provided with brucella melitensis which essentially causes the incurable chronic fatigue syndrome and bacillus anthracis which could kill hundreds of thousands of victims. Hussein fired at least six SCUD missiles (and probably up to twenty-four) which showered the Desert Storm forces with brucella melitensis. He was poised to fire more armed with anthrax when after 100 hours of battle, George Bush stopped the war and began an immediate withdrawal.

Over the following weeks troops exposed to brucella melitensis began to manifest symptoms of chronic fatigue syndrome, labeled in their case, Gulf War Illnesses. The Pentagon, like the Centers for Disease Control and the National Institutes of Health before them, could only respond by declaring that the veterans were not ill. However, the disease is significantly contagious and family members, fellow employees, and other service personnel are going to be manifesting symptoms for several years.

EndNotes

[1].Peter Grose, *Gentleman Spy* (Boston, New York: Houghton Mifflin Company, 1994) p.76

[2].*Ibid*, p.76

[3].Pierre Salinger and Eric Laurent, *Secret Dossier* (New York: Penguin Books, 1991) p.211

[4].Peter Dale Scott, *Deep Politics and the Death of JFK* (Berkeley and Los Angeles: University of California Press, Ltd., 1993) p.60

[5].*Ibid*, p.101

[6].James F. Dunnigan and Austin Bay, *From Shield to Storm.* (New York: William Morrow and Company, Inc., 1992) p.401

[7].Salinger and Laurent, *Ibid*, pp.239-241

[8].Joel Bainerman, *The Crimes of a President* (New York: Shapolsky Publishers, Inc., 1992) p.21

[9].Grose, Ibid, p.87

[10].Davis Crystal, *The Cambridge Factfinder*, pp.259, 269 respectively

[11]Jimmy Carter, *Keeping the Faith* (London: Collins, 1982) p.559

[12].Howard Teicher and Gayle Radley Teicher, *Twin Pillars to Desert Storm* (New York: William Morrow and Company Inc., 1993) p.207

[13].*Senate Committee on Banking, Housing, and Urban Affairs. Report on U.S. Exports of Biological Materials to Iraq.* pp.36-50

[14].Salinger and Laurent, Ibid, p.9

[15].*Ibid*, p.4

[16].*Ibid*, p.20

[17].*Ibid*, p.21

[18].*Ibid*, p.23

[19].Timmerman, *Ibid*, p.381

[20].Salinger and Laurent, *Ibid*, p.25

[21].*Ibid*, pp.57,58

[22].Joel Bainerman,*Ibid*

[23].*Ibid*, p.69

[24].Rick Atkinson, *Crusade* (Boston * New York: Houghton Mifflin Company, 1993) p.497

[25].Larry Wayne Harris, *Bacteriological Warfare: A Major Threat to North America*

[26].Timmerman, *Ibid*, p.20

[27].*Ibid*, p.35

[28].Dunnigan and Bay, *Ibid*, p.185

[29].Bainerman, *Ibid*, p.211

[30].Atkinson, Ibid, p.492

A CASE STUDY IN GULF WAR ILLNESSES

The following presentation is re-produced with the approval of Ms. Louise Richard.

Ms. Richard, a member of a long-time distinguished military family, had been a Lieutenant in the Royal Canadian Navy. She had served in the forward battle area during the Gulf War and had come under attack by SCUD missiles and a few days later she began to experience nausea, headaches, extreme fatigue and other symptoms which have now become associated with Gulf War Illnesses. Despite all of the above, the Canadian Military treated Lt. Richard as if she were a malingerer and claimed that she was not really ill. A response typical of that meted out to Gulf War veterans in both Canada and the United States and reminiscent of the psychobabble used to describe ME/FM/CFIDS victims!

The authors have been honoured during the process of researching this book to come to know Ms. Richard and to work with her in her on-going struggle with the bureaucrats in the Canadian Military and the Veterans Administration. It was during this period that the following "Intervention" was prepared and submitted to the Veterans' Review and Appeal Board by the authors.

REFERENCE

LOUISE M. RICHARD
OTTAWA, ONTARIO
FILE:
SERVICE: Fxxxxxxxxx
DECISION: 6239575

TO:
VETERANS REVIEW AND APPEAL BOARD

Submitted by:
Donald W. Scott, MA., MSc.
President,
Common Cause (Medical Research) Foundation

THE MYCOPLASMAS

Writing specifically about *Mycoplasma pneumoniae*, Stephen G. Baum, M.D. suggests that "This disease is under diagnosed because the organism is difficult to grow,[and] there is general unfamiliarity with the syndrome..."[30] This view can reasonably be extended to all the mycoplasmas isolated from human beings including *M. orale; M. salivarium; M. hominis; M. arthritidis;* and *M.fermentans*.[31] These two handicaps to the diagnosis of diseases whose etiological basis lies in the class Mollicutes has led many researchers to suggest that many human victims have been poorly served by the medical profession,[32] since a significant number of doctors often lack even a rudimentary knowledge of the organisms,[33] as was demonstrated recently by a doctor in the Canadian Armed Forces.

Thus, those who have the tragic experience of contracting any of the diseases now known to derive from the mycoplasmas, are victims two times over: first, they are victims of the disease and second, they are often victims of misdiagnosis.

MYCOPLASMA FERMENTANS (INCOGNITUS STRAIN)

However, not every medical professional is unaware of the nature, scope, and seriousness of the mycoplasmas as disease agents. I attach herewith (as Appendix One) four pages from the Course Calendar of the United States Military Institution known as the *'Uniformed Services University of the Health Services'* for the academic year 1993-1994. These pages deal with the study unit of the Department of Microbiology, 'Sect lll. Bacterial'.

Some of the salient features of this course unit need to be noted in this submission.

Under "Clinical and Pathologic Changes" (page one) the following statement is made:

"The most serious presentation of M.fermentans infection is that of a fulminant systemic disease that begins as a flu-like illness. Patients rapidly deteriorate developing severe complications including

*adult respiratory distress syndrome, disseminated
intravascular coagulation, and/or multiple organ
failure.*

*"The organs of patients with fulminant
M.fermentans infection exhibit extensive necroses.
Necrosis is most pronounced in lung, liver, spleen,
lymph nodes, adrenal glands, heart, and brain."*

Such statements in a course unit of the Uniformed
Services University of the Health Sciences must be
given substantial weight in evaluating the extent of
disability in any patient who tests positive for *M.
fermentans.*

Mycoplasma Fermentans Morbidity And Mortality

Major T. Cook, in his aforementioned Memo to General Baril, makes the following startling statement:

*"M. fermentans...causes, at most, a chronic illness
arising late after exposure rather than an acute,
disabling or fatal one..."[34]*

I suggest that such a statement is startling since it
is contradicted by Dr. Shyh-Ching Lo who is quite
possibly the world's leading authority on mycoplasmas,[35] and by other well-qualified researchers
such as those cited below.

In 1993 Dr. Lo placed the following statement
on file with the United States Patent Office:

*"Six patients from six different geographic areas
who presented with acute flu-like illnesses were
studied. The patients developed persistent fevers,
lymphadenopathy or diarrhea, pneumonia, and/or
heart, liver, or adrenal failure. They all died in
1-7 weeks.*

*"...The clinical signs as well as laboratory and
pathological studies of these patients suggested an
active infectious process, although no etiological
agent was found despite extensive infectious disease
work-ups during their hospitalization.*

*"Post-mortem examinations showed histopatho-
logical lesions of fulminant necrosis involving the
lymph nodes, spleen, lungs, liver, adrenal glands,
heart and/or brain. No viral inclusion cells, bacteria, fungi, or parasites could be identified in these
tissues using special tissue stains. However, the use
of rabbit antiserum and the monoclonal antibodies raised against M. fermentans incognitus, the
pathogen shown to cause fatal systemic infection in
primates, revealed M. fermentans incognitus antigens in these necrotizing lesions."[36]*

To learn that six patients died of an infection caused
by *M. fermentans* raises the question : how is it that
a potentially fatal disease can go undiagnosed? The
answer lies in the facts adduced earlier in this submission: since the organism is difficult to grow and since
there is a general unfamiliarity with the syndrome,
the attending physicians are often inclined to record
the cause of death as 'congestive heart failure' or
some other more frequently seen illness.

However that may be, the research reported by Dr.
Lo should lay to rest the erroneous viewpoint that *M.
fermentans* "...causes at most, a chronic illness." And
it should also be enough to make it unnecessary for a
potential victim to die before an autopsy will reveal
the full extent of the damage sustained.

Since mycoplasmas are organisms with no cell
wall, but consist of bacterial molecules linked by a
membrane filament, they do not have the capability
to ingest nutrient and oxygen and hence manufacture their own growth requirements. Instead, they
"...incorporate *preformed* sterols from the growth
medium [the cell which they have invaded- Ed] into
their cytoplasmic membranes."[37] In the process of
building themselves up with the preformed sterols of
their host, they diminish and ultimately destroy the
latter.

When the host cell is killed by its parasitic invader,
it ruptures and hence releases its remaining nucleic
acids into the blood.

It might be helpful at this point to quote Dr. Lo's
full definition:

*"Mycoplasma is a genus of cell wall-less sterol-re-
quiring, catalase-negative pathogens commonly
found in the respiratory and urogenital tracts of
man and other animals. The cells of Mycoplasma
are typically non-motile and pleomorphic, ranging
from spherical, ovoid or pear-shaped to branched
filamentous forms."[38]*

Polymerase Chain Reaction

Besides reporting upon his experience with the six
fatal cases of *M. fermentans* -infected patients, Dr.
Lo reported that:

*"A polymerase chain reaction (PCR) assay to
detect M.fermentans was designed on the basis
of specific nucleotide (nt) sequences found at one
terminus of the cloned incognitus strain of M. fermentans DNA psb-2.2.. The PCR assay detected
very specifically the mycoplasmas of M. fermentans
species but not other human or non-human myco-*

plasmas, bacteria or eucaryotic cell DNA that we tested."[39]

The PCR tests are clearly the most reliable way to diagnose the presence of a mycoplasma infection:

"PCR provides the potential for early and reliable diagnosis of this infection. Garret and Bonnet developed an assay that amplified a 144-bp segment of the M.pneumoniae genome. Others have used primers that amplify unique sequences from 16S rRNA and P1 adhesion protein..." [40]

It must be stated with emphasis that using this PCR diagnostic technique, it has been determined that Lt. Louise Richard tests positive for the *M. fermentans-incognitus* strain. One must ask why it is that Lt. Richard had to seek out and utilize this cutting-edge technology on her own?

The Misdiagnosis Of *M. fermentans*

"Some of these patients who are infected with M.fermentans incognitus will be patients who have been diagnosed as having AIDS or ARC, Chronic Fatigue Syndrome, Wegener's Disease, Sarcoidosis, respiratory distress syndrome, Kibuchi's disease, autoimmune diseases such as Collagen Vascular Disease and Lupus and chronic debilitating diseases such as Alzheimer's Disease." [41]

This very significant statement by Dr. Lo must be given careful consideration if we are to understand the etiology and disabling features of mycoplasma-instigated diseases. I will, therefore, comment briefly upon each of the 'mis'-diagnoses listed.

Aids Or Arc, Chronic Fatigue Syndrome

Many researchers have been aware for nearly fifteen years that there is some linkage between AIDS and CFS. This is well demonstrated in *Osler's Web* by Hillary Johnson:

"Wormsley's results showed that four of five Tahoe patients did have abnormal helper-suppressor ratios. But, unlike the ratios in AIDS sufferers, they were low in the number of suppressor cells. Instead of one-to-two or one-to-three, which are typical of healthy people, the Incline patients had helper-suppressor ratios of five-to-one, ten-to-one, and higher. It was the mirror image of AIDS."[42]
[emphasis added]

Dr. Lo, by pointing out that there is a common factor between AIDS and CFS in that both present with *M. fermentans* when tested by PCR, narrows

the linkage to some factor in the"... sera from suspected patients."

Wegener's Disease

Given the marked similarities between the symptoms of Wegener's Disease (Coughing, breathing difficulty, chest pain, and blood in the urine...loss of appetite, weight loss, weakness, fatigue, and joint pains)[43] it is understandable why patients with infections due to *M. fermentans* are sometimes diagnosed as victims of Wegener's Disease.

Organ involvement in WD also has close parallels to those involved in *M. fermentans* infections.[44] It should also be noted that Wegener's Disease is described as "...a distinct clinicopathologic entity of *unknown etiology*"

Sarcoidosis

"Sarcoidosis may be defined as a disease of unknown etiology, characterized histologically by non-caseating granulomas in multiple tissues..."[45] Although possessing certain distinctive features, sarcoidosis has more in common with Wegener's Disease and M.fermentans infections than it has differences. Among the more significant of the similarities is the broad range of body systems affected by the disease. [46]

Respiratory Distress Syndrome

Although Dr. Lo does not specify to this effect, he probably intended to limit his reference to RDS to the adult rather than the infant condition.

In adults the condition affects people whose lungs have been damaged by disease or injury. Since the etiology of the latter is self-evident, we need only consider those whose symptoms have no known etiology. In the latter "...the disorder is caused by a stiffening of lung tissue and an increase of fluid in the tissue between the alveoli..." [47]

It is the latter condition that bears the strongest similarity to the lung damage experienced by many patients infected with M.fermentans.

Collagen Vascular Disease

Collagen, which comprises about one-fourth of the body's total protein, [48] is essential in the building and the maintaining of the body's structure. All tissues and muscles, as well as the matrix of collagen forming the bones, provide the framework within which the heart pumps, the blood circulates, the brain receives and transmits energy...in other words the structure within which life is expressed.

The fact that Dr. Lo includes 'collagen vascular disease' in his list of M.fermentans diseases often diagnosed as one of the CVD variants warrants our careful consideration, for included in these diseases are *rheumatoid arthritis,* systemic *lupus erythematosus, polyarteritis nodosa, scleroderma,* and *dermatomyositis.*[49]

It must also be noted that like most of the other diseases specified, it is said of all of the CVD's that "...the etiology is unknown."

Alzheimer's Disease

Dr. Lo's classification of AD as a 'chronic debilitating disease' must be regarded as extreme understatement. Furthermore, what he intended to be included in his reference to 'diseases such as' must be a matter of individual conjecture. In this submission it is assumed that he would include multiple sclerosis, Huntington's, and Parkinson's.

Again it should be noted that all of these are said to be diseases whose etiology is unknown. However, the fact that Alzheimer's, multiple sclerosis, Huntington's and Parkinson's all present with necrotizing lesions, and that M.fermentans was revealed in these lesions would suggest that *M. fermentans* may well turn out to be a common initiating disease factor.

Appendix Two

In order to emphasize the significance of M.fermentans in all of these diseases which are characterized by cells in a range of organs which are dying from an unknown cause, I append six representative drawings from Dr. Lo's Patent Application.

Fig. 1 C shows the colony morphology of M.fermentans incognitus

Fig. 1 D shows the colony morphology of the prototype strain (PG18) of *M. fermentans.*

These two drawings reflect the growth characteristic of the mycoplasma referred to by Dr. Lo:

> "Using a S radiolabeled psb-2.2 M.fermentans incognitus DNA probe, strong labelling of clusters of cells **at the margins** of necrosis of the affected tissues was observed."[emphasis added] [50]

This observation may well be explained by the fact that "gradation in the histologic findings from the center to the lesion edge suggest that the lesions expand by concentric outward growth,[51] creating the 'fried egg' look frequently seen. The presence of the mycoplasma on the leading edge of the concentric circle is significant since it suggests that it is indeed the mycoplasma that is doing the damage and that it is not just an "accidental bystander"[52] as has been suggested by some who would discount the role of *M. fermentans.*

Fig. 21A shows the M.fermentans incognitus-induced histopathological changes of fulminant necrosis in the spleen of a patient without AIDS dying of an acute systemic disease.

Fig. 21B shows the advancing margin of Fig. 21A.

Fig. 21C shows M.fermentans incognitus-induced histopathological changes of fulminant necrosis in the *lymph-node* of a patient without AIDS dying of an acute systemic disease.

Fig. 21D shows M.fermentans incognitus-induced histopathological changes of fulminant necrosis in the *adrenal gland* of a patient without AIDS dying of an acute systemic disease.

These drawings are critical since they demonstrate in a very compelling way that the M.fermentans is emphatically not just the innocuous 'bystander' as suggested by some researchers referenced above. Also, since they reveal damage to the spleen, lymph-nodes, and adrenal glands , the pathogenic qualities of the mycoplasma are evident.

The Sickle Cell Model

Sickle cell anaemia provides a strong model for certain features of the diseases deriving from M.fermentans, and these features should be reviewed carefully. Before doing so, however, it is useful to note that links between sickle cell disease and mycoplasma diseases have been noted for some time in a variety of research. Two examples can be cited:

> "Patients with sickle cell disease are also prone to severe infection with M.pneumoniae".[53]
> "M.pneumoniae can be isolated from the pleural fluid in more severe cases. In children, especially those with sickle cell anaemia or other underlying diseases, effusions are often extensive." [54]

Sickle cells get their name from the fact that under certain circumstances which include genetic, hormonal, environmental, and other factors, red blood cells lose their normal 'donut' shape and convulse into a sickle shape. Although the term 'sickle cell' suggests a single disorder, it is actually more aptly described as a "catch-all for the clinical disorders produced by haemoglobin (Hb) S."[55] "Apparently diverse disorders are grouped together because they share two basic processes- vascular occlusion and haemolysis- which are produced by the sickling of red blood cells."

It is to be noted that these two processes (among others) are factors in the diseases instigated by the various mycoplasmas. It is, therefore, useful to review the mechanics of the sickle cell diseases in order to better understand the mechanics of the mycoplasma disorders.

"Sickle cell disease is a condition in which certain red blood cells become rigid, elongated, and sickle-shaped. As the stricken cells move through the body, they become lodged in tight spots, cutting off the flow of blood-and thus oxygen. The oxygen-starved area becomes swollen and tender, and causes a throbbing pain..."[56]

The principal factor in causing the normal red blood cell to convulse into its sickle shape is genetic. The beta chain of human haemoglobin consists of 146 amino acids. Normally, the sixth position is glutamic acid; however, in some individuals there is a valine substitute for the glutamic acid. This is the genetic pre-disposition to sickle cell disease. [57]

The improperly encoded red blood cells will continue in their functioning until they encounter an internal area of reduced blood pressure, with the area between the lungs and the left atrium being the most significant. When the pressure is lowered the valine in solution will precipitate and cause the cell to convulse. This primary disease factor will be succeeded by secondary factors when the distended cells block the vascular system and by tertiary factors when the organs are deprived of oxygen and nutrient.

This three stage presentation of damage is very significant to note.

The Sickle Cell Phenomenon And The Mycoplasma

Convulsing to a sickle shape is the distinctive feature of SC diseases. However, extensive research has demonstrated that there are other variants of the surface topography of erythrocytes that can occur

and have been observed in patients with mycoplasma infection.[58]

This same phenomenon was studied by other researchers with an emphasis upon the changes induced by amphipathic drugs acting upon the membrane of intact cells.[59]

Appendix Three is meant to summarize the effects upon the vascular system when the red blood cells are hardened, distended or misshapen due to internal and external factors. This primary factor creates the basis for the secondary factors of impeded blood flow and reduced nutrient/oxygen supply.

The first and second pages depict the shape changes in sickle cell disease and in mycoplasma diseases. The latter is based upon the sample and analysis of blood provided by Louise Richard to Dr. Les Simpson (cited above). As will be demonstrated this vascular damage accounts for several of Ms. Richards symptoms as shown on page five of Appendix Three.

The Mycoplasma And Blood Morphology

Based upon the characteristics of the Mycoplasma as summarized above, and upon the consequences for its host cells, the following hypothesis can be advanced.

Primary Damage

The mycoplasma, being non-motile and incapable of manufacturing its own cytoplasmic membranes, once introduced into a human or other animal, can penetrate the wall of a host cell. Here it takes up *preformed* sterols from its host for its on use. It will grow in any of its pleomorphic varieties until it kills its host. Because it grows by incorporating the preformed host sterols, it will be found on the periphery of the lesion and, there will be no bacteria or virus evident to explain the cell necrosis.

The host cell when killed, ruptures and dumps its remaining nucleic acids into the blood. Included in the dumped nucleic acids is its glutamine, and, "...glutamine, when not used for the fabrication of proteins, is used as the currency of ammonia."[60] The free glutamine tends to seize the ammonium ion from any molecule of urea that it encounters and so release the cyanate ion into the blood.[61]

Secondary Damage

The free trace cyanide is then liberated to do a variety of secondary damage to the body which is summarized on Appendix Four: Glutamate and Urea. However, there is another level of damage done in the Krebs's cycle at the electron transport chain when at complex IV, cytochrome c oxidase, the trace cyanide frequently inhibits the electron transport.[62] This interference with energy uptake by the cells presents as a condition of extreme fatigue, and may even be a factor in the growth of cancers as recently suggested by Charles Graham, et al.[63]

Furthermore, the red blood cells, subject as are all other cells of the body to invasion by the mycoplasma, has its membrane sterols taken up with a consequent severe impact upon its cytoplasma and hence its ability to transport oxygen.

Tertiary Damage

Over varying periods of time the various affected body organs deprived of oxygen and nutrient by the impeded blood flow will degenerate until they fail completely. This can be seen in the previously referred drawings: 21A, necrosis in the *spleen;* 21C, necrosis in the *lymph-node;* 21D, necrosis in the *adrenal gland*. Similar evidence can be adduced for necrosis of the beta cells in the pancreas; for necrosis of target cells in the left ventricle accompanied by myocardial fibre hypertrophy and myofiber disarray such as can be seen in Alzheimer's and multiple sclerosis.

Mycoplasma Summary

Mycoplasmas as cell wall-less organisms which incorporate preformed sterols from its host, destroys its host in a process of fulminate tissue necrosis. This process presents in the patient as the primary stage of illness as flu-like symptoms.

The killed host cell ruptures and dumps its nucleic acids into the blood. One of these acids, glutamine, seizes the ammonium ion from urea and liberates the cyanate ion. The cyanate then has the potential to do a protean range of damage to every body system and organ. The damage will vary depending upon factors such as genetic predisposition and the health of the patient's immune system.

In respect to the latter, Dr. Lo suggests that:
"It is believed that infection of M.fermentans incognitus either has concomitantly caused damage to key components of the hosts' immune system, or this pathogen has special biological properties which enable it to elude immunosurveillance of the infected hosts."[64]
Our research suggests there are some of both properties.

This process represents the secondary stage of damage, and presents as cognitive impairment, alopecia, respiratory distress, Raynaud's phenomenon, irritable bowel syndrome, various skin lesions etc.

Over time, the prolonged deprivation of adequate nutrient and oxygen to the major organs will present with brain lesions (usually in the pre-frontal lobe area and identifiable by magnetic resonance imaging as 'unidentified bright objects') kidney failure, liver failure, heart distress (usually detected by Holter 24 hour ECG revealing flattened or inverted T-waves), menstrual dysfunction and/or endometriosis, bone damage and consequent red blood cell depletion, etc. This is the tertiary stage of damage.

Ms. Louise Richard

Ms. Richard has tested positive by PCR for *Mycoplasma fermentans incognitus* strain. She has also been diagnosed with a very high percentage of hardened and flattened red blood cells.

In view of the capacity of the mycoplasma to invade cells and incorporate preformed sterols into itself from its host, and the fact that the hardened and flattened red blood cells impede the passage of blood and the supply of oxygen and nutrients to all major organs, it follows that the severe health problems that Ms. Richard has experienced since serving in the Gulf War are related to that service.

A review of her health status is appropriate, together with such comment as the foregoing submission reasonably suggests. I will first refer to actual diagnoses (together with any treatment which resulted), then relate these to the positive tests for mycoplasma and damaged red blood cells.

Asthma

It is acknowledged by E.D. Callaghan, Pension Services, in his letter of 05 October, 1998, that:
"During your Persian Gulf service, there is medical evidence that you had respiratory problems which were diagnosed as Asthma in 1995. You were granted pension entitlement for your Asthma in 1996"
It is important to recognize that "Clinicians and investigators have had difficulty over the years assigning a single, concise definition to the disorder known as asthma. The inability to define asthma largely reflects our insufficient knowledge of its fundamental pathogenic mechanisms as well as confusion about

whether asthma is really a single definable disease with a unique pathogenesis or multiple disorders with common manifestations."[65]

In view of the fact that *M.fermentans* is "...a well established pathogen of the respiratory tract"[66] and that the symptoms evident from mycoplasma infection include respiratory distress, difficulty in breathing, respiratory mucosa, etc. I suggest that Ms. Richard does not have asthma in the usual limited sense. Instead, her extreme difficulty at times in catching her breath and other indicators of respiratory distress represent one of the most ubiquitous signs of mycoplasma infection.

Alopecia

Very soon after her Persian Gulf experience began, Ms. Richard began to experience extreme hair loss. It was not a case of hair loss in the usual sense, but of the loss of hair by the handful. Today Ms. Richard is completely bald.

In his summary of diseases related to the M.fermentans, Dr. Lo had noted "Lupus".[67] One of the more common of the lupus symptoms is alopecia.[68] I suggest that the hitherto unexplained loss of hair by Ms. Richard is clearly attributable to the M.*fermentans incognitus* that Dr. Lo identified in the patient he referred to.

Uterine Bleeding And Total Abdominal Hysterectomy

For four years following her return from the Persian Gulf, Ms. Richard experienced prolonged and painful menstrual periods. It was not simply a matter of a heavy flow, but of a heavy flow punctuated by the passage of large clots which in retrospect were probably portions of the endometrium. This condition worsened to the point where it was deemed necessary by her physician to perform a total abdominal hysterectomy.

There are several well-researched, peer-reviewed articles in the literature that clearly establish mycoplasma infections as a cause of genitourinary problems.[69] Prior to her Persian Gulf experiences, Ms. Richard reports a normal and healthy menstrual cycle. It was only after her GW service that her menstrual periods became progressively worse, culminating in the tragic total hysterectomy of 1995.

Given the evidence in the literature and the appropriate time frame involved, I suggest that Ms.

Richard's genitourinary problems stem directly from her mycoplasma infection.

I further submit that the skin rashes she experiences in the genital area are totally compatible with the symptoms noted by Dr. Lo in respect to dermatological evidence of M.fermentans incognitus.

Raynaud's Syndrome And Carpal Tunnel Syndrome

Ms. Richard experiences tingling and numbness in her hands and feet. She has been diagnosed with both Raynaud's Syndrome and Carpal Tunnel Syndrome (Bilateral). Both these signs and diagnoses are compatible with the reduced blood flow caused by the flattened and distended red blood cells as diagnosed by Dr. Les Simpson. The Carpal Tunnel plaque build-up is typical of mycoplasma plaque accumulations in various focal points.

Gastrointestinal System

Dr. Lo has detailed the major symptoms of six patients who tested positive for *M.fermentans* incognitus. Most of these patients reported diarrhea, malaise, vomiting, nausea, and other symptoms reflecting damage to the gastrointestinal system.

Ms. Richard reports diarrhea, abdominal cramps, irritable bowel syndrome, nausea, heartburn, and reflux. The fit is most precise and suggests very strongly that the *M.fermentans* has invaded her gastrointestinal system and is progressively damaging infected cells.

Such a hypothesis is in keeping with the observation by Embree, *et al*[70] who cite the mycoplasma as a pathogenic agent in "...anorexia, nausea, vomiting, and diarrhea."

Cardiovascular

Two of the six patients referred to by Dr. Lo had cardiovascular problems clearly related to the degeneration of cells in the muscle of the left ventricle.

Ms. Richard experiences irregular heart beats, hypotension, dizziness, and frequent loss of balance. Again, all of these symptoms can be logically attributed to muscle damage in the heart...possibly in the left ventricle. Although she has not reported symptoms to this effect, I would surmise that she has a mitral valve prolapse.

SUMMARY

Ms. Richard left Canada as a healthy, well-adjusted medical professional to serve her country in the Persian Gulf War.

Within a very few months of her arrival in the war theatre she began to experience a protean range of symptoms including Alopecia, asthma, gastrointestinal problems, menstrual problems, Raynaud's Syndrome and Carpal Tunnel Syndrome, as well as cognitive impairment and cardiovascular symptoms.

This full range of disabling symptoms is completely compatible with the course of mycoplasma infections as presented by Dr. Shyh-Ching Lo and many other medical professionals who have taken the time and made the effort to inform themselves about these infections and their secondary and tertiary consequences.

Among the secondary effects are the hardening and flattening of the red blood cells. Ms. Richard made the effort to have the blood test by Dr. Les Simpson...a test that has been reported upon favourably in several peer-reviewed journals. This abnormal red blood morphology is obviously causing Ms. Richard a variety of painful conditions.

Additional evidence that Ms. Richard's blood morphology is abnormal and suggestive that some infectious agent is doing damage can be seen in the blood test she had at the Ottawa Civic Hospital on Feb. 20, 1998 as ordered by Dr. Mickelson Ross. The 'Cumulative Report' identifies FIVE categories of abnormality: i. low aspartate aminotransferase ii. high mean platelet volume iii. low mean corpuscular haemoglobin iv. & v. low HB and HCT count. In addition Ms. Richard's mean corpuscular volume is borderline low. All of these abnormalities should be evaluated in reference to her positive test for *M. fermentans*.

In the 05 October 1998 letter from Pension Services, it is stated that:

> "...a Departmental Medical Consultant confirmed that no disability from your Mycoplasma is recorded."

This is a most superficial comment. Nowhere in the letter to Ms. Richard is there any indication that all of the signs and symptoms which are reasonably attributable to her M.fermentans incognitus infection have been taken in to account.

Finally, I want to refer to a speech made in Halifax on August 17,1998 by the Honourable Fred Mifflin, Minister of Veterans Affairs. Mr. Mifflin states on page 3:

> "As far as Gulf War illnesses are concerned, I do want to re-assure you of one thing. As we wrestle with pinning down a precise diagnosis of the ailments suffered by many of the Allied forces, we want to make sure that Canadian Gulf War veterans continue to receive all benefits that are their due.

> "As for entitlement to Disability Pensions, these veterans, like all veterans, will get every consideration for entitlement. It is important to note that we continue with the policy that we ensure the benefit of the doubt, **is resolved in favour of the veteran, and give significant weight to supporting statements made by medical examiners and clients.**"

I suggest that any decision to the effect that "no disability from your Mycoplasma is recorded" is in total disagreement with the facts. Ms. Richard's well established medical records taken into consideration with the documentation I have referred to and append herewith demonstrate that the mycoplasma infection is in precise accord with the evidence.

In conclusion allow me to state that I am here at my own expense. I charge no fee, and am here as a veteran myself of over seven years in the Royal Canadian Navy because I want to see justice done for our veterans who have served when asked.

Actually, to a very great extent, Ms. Louise Richard has literally given her life for her country. She may be alive and able to appear at this hearing, but she has endured much with her hysterectomy and her neuro/systemic degenerative symptoms, and the protean range of mycoplasma infections; but her life has been robbed of many of the dreams and accomplishments that she will never achieve because of her war-inflicted disabilities.

Respectfully submitted, I am
Yours sincerely,

Donald W. Scott, M.A., M.Sc.
President:
The Common Cause (Medical Research) Foundation

Military Decorations:
1939-1945 Star; Atlantic Star; Burma Star with Clasp; Canadian Volunteer Service Medal; Victory Medal.

Endnotes

1. Stephen G. Baum, M.D., "Atypical Pneumonia" in: Rex B. Conn, M.D. Editor *Current Diagnosis 8* (Philadelphia; W.B. Saunders Company, 1966) p.373

2. Gail H. Cassell, M.S., PhD, and Barry C. Cole, PhD "Mycoplasmas as Agents of Human Disease". *The New England Journal of Medicine*, Vol. 304. (Jan. 8, 1981) pp.80-89

3. "Severe Mycoplasma Disease - Rare or Undiagnosed?" *West. J. Med.* Vol. 162(2), (Feb.1995) pp.172-5

4. An example of this can be seen in a Memorandum dated 'Aug 98' from Major T. Cook, M.D. FRCPC, Head Medical Services, Can. Armed Forces, to the Chief of the Defence Staff, General J.M.G. Baril. In this Memo, Maj. Cook stated "These organisms were first identified and classified in the 1960's" (page 1). Actually, the term 'mycoplasma' was first used by B. Frank in 1889, and there was a period of time when the organisms were "...referred to as *pleuropneumonia-like organisms* (PPLO)." In 1967 the reference to PPLO gave way to Mollicutes which were further categorized into three families (i. Mycoplasmataceae; ii. Acholeplasmataceae; and, Spiroplasmataceae)

5. August 1998 Memorandum of Major T. Cook to General J.M.G. Baril, p.2

6. In such a complex area as evaluating the degree of expertise one possesses in any particular field of science, there is always room for disagreement. However, since Dr. Shyh-Ching Lo was the applicant of record for United States Patent Number 5,242,820 on September 7, 1993, and since this was a patent for *"Pathogenic Mycoplasma"*, I think my categorization of Dr. Lo is reasonable.

7. Dr. Shyh-Ching Lo; "Pathogenic Mycoplasma". United States Patent Number 5,242,820. Sept. 7, 1993 p.43

8. Wesley A. Volk and Jay C. Brown: *Basic Microbiology* (Addison Wesley, Longman, Inc., 1997) p.17

9. Lo, *Ibid*, p.2

10. Lo, *Ibid*, p.18

11. Wm. B. Coleman & Gregory J. Tsongalis, Eds.,: *Molecular Diagnostics* (Totowa, New Jersey; Humana Press, 1997) p.347

12. Lo *Ibid*, p.20

13. Hillary Johnson: *Osler's Web* (New York: Crown Publishers, Inc., 1996) p.95

14. Peter Morgan, M.D.: *Home Medical Encyclopaedia* (Montreal; Reader's Digest, 1992) p.1075

15. Conn *Ibid*, p.1144

16. Conn *Ibid*, p.382

17. The broad range of body systems affected by the various mycoplasmas can be seen in the title of an article in the *Canadian Medical Association Journal* of October, 1968: "The Protean Manifestations of Mycoplasma Infections in Childhood" by Turner, et al. But an even more compelling case for the protean range of the disease can be seen in the article by Cassell and Cole, referenced in endnote #2 above.

18. Peter Morgan, M.D. *Ibid*, p.867

19. David S. Goodsell: *Our Molecular Nature* (New York; Copernicus, 1996) p.94

20. David S. Goodsell: *Our Molecular Nature* (New York; Copernicus, 1996) p.94

21. Lo *Ibid*, p.44

22. Joseph B. Martin, M.D., PhD: *Molecular Neurology* (New York: Scientific American, Inc. 1998) p. 206

23. Robert Gallo, *Virus Hunting* (A New Republic Book, 1991) p.45

24. Conn *Ibid*, p.373

25. Gail H. Cassell, M.S., PhD and Barry C. Cole, PhD *Ibid*, p.81

26. Conn *Ibid*, p. 542

27. Patricia Barnes-Svarney: *Science Desk Reference* (New York; Macmillan, USA, 1995) p.191

28. Adapted from Wayne M. Becker and David W. Deamer: *The World of the Cell* (The Benjamin/Cummings Publishing Company, Inc.1991) p. 459

29. Simpson, L.O., Shand, B.I., Olds, R.J.: "Blood rheology and myalgic encephalomyelitis: A pilot study" *Pathology* Vol. 18. (1986) pp.190-92

30. Fujii, T., Takashi, S., Tamura, A., Wakatsuki, M., Kanaho, Y: "Shape changes of human erythrocytes induced by various amphipathic drugs acting on the membrane of the intact cells." *Biochemical Pharmacology*, Vol. 28. (1979) pp.613-20

31. Goodsell, *Ibid* p.12

32. Becker and Deamer, *Ibid* p.10

33. *Ibid*, p.297

34. Charles H. Graham, Jennifer Forsdike, Carolyn Fitzgerald, and Shannyn MacDonald-Goodfellow: "Hypoxia-mediated stimulation of carcinoma cell invasiveness via upregulation of urokinase receptor expression". *International Journal of Cancer*, Vol.80. (1999) pp. 617-23

35. Lo, *Ibid*, p.14

36. David S. Prince, M.D. and James E. Fish, M.D.: "Asthma in Aduklts" Conn: *Ibid*, pp.353-359

37. Joanne E. Embree, M.Sc., Juan A. Embil, M.D., PhD, FRCP[C]: "Mycoplasmas in diseases of humans" *CMA Journal*, Vol.123. (July 1980) p.105

38. Lo, *Ibid*, p.20

39. Peter Morgan, M.D. *Ibid*, p.88

40. To note just two:

Gnarpe, H. and Friberg, J.: "Mycoplasma and human reproductive failure" *American Journal of Obstetrics and Gynaecology*, Vol.114, (1972) p.727

and

Schoub B.D., Jacobs, Y.R., Hylen, E., et al. "The role of mycoplasma in human infertility." *South African Medical Journal*, Vol. 50 (1976) p.445

41. Embree, et al, *Ibid*, p.107

COMMENTARY

Despite the fact that we had cited the most recent authorities on the mycoplasma and human diseases and had clearly linked these to Lt. Richard's medical situation, the Veterans and Pension Review Committee denied her application. This despite the further fact that according to veterans administration policy in any case where a doubt existed, the benefit of the doubt was to be given to the veteran.

Lt. Richard was not given the benefit of the doubt and like so many of her comrades in arms she too was denied fair and just treatment. That was by official count. But what about the mystery illness now being called Gulf War Illnesses? "Well," said Deputy Director of Pentagon Health Services, Dr. Stephen C. Joseph,"It's all in their head."

Like chronic fatigue syndrome and fibromyalgia before it, and just as Justice Rawlins had ruled in her courtroom: "Fibromyalgia does not exist" and neither does Gulf War Syndrome.

But George Bush, Colin Powell, Saddam Hussein, Stephen Joseph and the CDC all know better.

SUMMARY

Following the collapse of the Ottoman Empire in World War One, the victorious nations of Europe and the United States began a great power game aimed at controlling the vast oil wealth of the Middle East. No thought was given to the welfare or rights of the people who had lived in the area for thousands of years. All that mattered was to engage in secret manoeuvres to possess the wealth extracted for the use of a relative handful of people in what are referred to as the 'developed nations.' To achieve control, plots and counterplots were hatched and various puppet governments set up by the real masters. Such puppet masters were armed to the teeth so that they could maintain their hold on power. When Mohammed Mossadegh of Iran staged the closest thing to a populist revolt by nationalizing the oil wells and deposing the Shah, the United States through the agency of Allen Dulles' CIA 'mounted a coup' in Iran and returned the Shah to his peacock throne. Without any semblance of democratic participation open to them, many in Iran turned to the Islamic Fundamentalist, The Ayatollah Khomeini, to rid them of foreign domination. When the Shah fled a second time, and the Iranians seized American Embassy personnel as hostages, the U.S. began to secretly assist Iraq as a bulwark against Iranian led Islamic fundamentalist expansion.

The U.S. aid included components for deadly biological weapons that had been secretly developed in the U.S. between 1945 when they recruited Japanese war criminal Gen. Ishii Shiro, to the present. Saddam Hussein was provided with brucella melitensis which essentially causes the incurable chronic fatigue syndrome and bacillus anthracis which could kill hundreds of thousands of victims. Hussein fired at least six SCUD missiles (and probably up to twenty-four) which showered the Desert Storm forces with brucella melitensis. He was poised to fire more armed with anthrax when after 100 hours of battle, George Bush stopped the war and began an immediate withdrawal.

Over the following weeks troops exposed to brucella melitensis began to manifest symptoms of chronic fatigue syndrome, labeled in their case, Gulf War Illnesses. The Pentagon, like the Centers for Disease Control and the National Institutes of Health before them, could only respond by declaring that the veterans were not ill. However, the disease is significantly contagious and family members, fellow employees, and other service personnel are going to be manifesting symptoms for several years.

Endnotes

[1].Peter Grose, *Gentleman Spy* (Boston, New York: Houghton Mifflin Company, 1994) p.76

[2].*Ibid*, p.76

[3].Pierre Salinger and Eric Laurent, *Secret Dossier* (New York: Penguin Books, 1991) p.211

[4].Peter Dale Scott, *Deep Politics and the Death of JFK* (Berkeley and Los Angeles: University of California Press, Ltd., 1993) p.60

[5].*Ibid*, p.101

[6].James F. Dunnigan and Austin Bay, *From Shield to Storm.* (New York: William Morrow and Company, Inc., 1992) p.401

[7].Salinger and Laurent, *Ibid*, pp.239-241

[8].Joel Bainerman, *The Crimes of a President* (New York: Shapolsky Publishers, Inc., 1992) p.21

[9].Grose, *Ibid*, p.87

[10].Davis Crystal, *The Cambridge Factfinder* pages 259 and 269 respectively.

[11].Jimmy Carter, *Keeping Faith* (London: Collins, 1982) p.559

[12].Howard Teicher and Gayle Radley Teicher, *Twin Pillars to Desert Storm* (New York: William Morrow and Company Inc., 1993) p.207

[13].Senate Committee on Banking, Housing, and Urban Affairs. *Report on U.S. Exports of Biological Materials to Iraq.* pp. 36 to 50

[14].Salinger and Laurent, *Ibid*, p.9

[15].*Ibid*, p.4

[16].*Ibid*, p.20

[17].*Ibid*, p.21

[18].*Ibid*, p.23

[19].Timmerman, *Ibid*, p.381

[20].Salinger and Laurent, *Ibid*, p.25

[21].*Ibid*, pp.57,58

[22].Joel Bainerman, *Ibid*

[23].*Ibid*, p.69

[24].Rick Atkinson, *Crusade* (Boston* New York: Houghton Mifflin Company, 1993) p.497

[25].Larry Wayne Harris, *Bacteriological Warfare: A Major Threat to North America*

[26].Timmerman, *Ibid*, p.20

[27].*Ibid*, p.35

[28].Dunnigan and Bay, *Ibid*, p.185

[29].Bainerman, *Ibid*, p.211

[30]. Stephen G. Baum, M.D., "Atypical Pneumonia" in : Rex B. Conn, M.D. Editor *Current Diagnosis 8* (Philadelphia; W.B. Saunders Company, 1966) p.373

[31]. Gail H. Cassell, M.S., PhD, and Barry C. Cole, PhD "Mycoplasmas as Agents of Human Disease". *The New England Journal of Medicine*, Vol. 304. (Jan. 8,1981) pp.80-89

[32]. "Severe Mycoplasma Disease - Rare or Undiagnosed?" *West. J. Med.* Vol. 162(2), (Feb.1995) pp.172-5

[33]. An example of this can be seen in a Memorandum dated 'Aug 98' from Major T. Cook, M.D. FRCPC, Head Medical Services, Can. Armed Forces, to the Chief of the Defence Staff, General J.M.G. Baril. In this Memo, Maj. Cook stated "These organisms were first identified and classified in the 1960's" (page 1). Actually, the term 'mycoplasma' was first used by B. Frank in 1889, and there was a period of time when the organisms were "...referred to as pleuropneumonia-like organisms (PPLO)." In 1967 the reference to PPLO gave way to Mollicutes which were further categorized into three families (i. Mycoplasmataceae; ii. Acholeplasmataceae; and, Spiroplasmataceae)

[34]. August 1998 Memorandum of Major T. Cook to General J.M.G. Baril, p.2

[35]. In such a complex area as evaluating the degree of expertise one possesses in any particular field of science, there is always room for disagreement. However, since Dr. Shyh-Ching Lo was the applicant of record for United States Patent Number 5,242,820 on September 7,1993, and since this was a patent for *"pathogenic mycoplasma"*, we think that our categorization of Dr. Lo is reasonable.

[36]. Dr. Shyh-Ching Lo; "Pathogenic Mycoplasma". United States Patent Number 5,242,820. Sept. 7, 1993 p.43

[37]. Wesley A. Volk and Jay C. Brown: *Basic Microbiology* (Addison Wesley, Longman, Inc., 1997) p.17

[38]. Lo, *Ibid*, p.2

[39].Lo, *Ibid*, p.18

[40]. Wm. B. Coleman & Gregory J. Tsongalis, Eds.,: *Molecular Diagnostics* (Totowa, New Jersey; Humana Press, 1997) p.347

[41]. Lo *Ibid*, p.20

[42]. Hillary Johnson: *Osler's Web* (New York: Crown Publishers, Inc., 1996) p.95

[43]. Peter Morgan, M.D.:Home Medical Encyclopaedia (Montreal; Reader's Digest, 1992) p.1075

[44]. Conn *Ibid*, p.1144

[45]. Conn *Ibid*, p.382

[46]. The broad range of body systems affected by

the various mycoplasmas can be seen in the title of an article in the Canadian Medical Association Journal of October, 1968: "The Protean Manifestations of Mycoplasma Infections in Childhood" by Turner, et al. But an even more compelling case for the protean range of the disease can be seen in the article by Cassell and Cole, referenced in endnote #2 above.

[47]. Peter Morgan, M.D. *Ibid*, p.867

[48]. David S. Goodsell: *Our Molecular Nature* (New York; Copernicus, 1996) p.94

[49]. Peter Morgan, M.D. *Ibid*, p.286

[50]. Lo *Ibid*, p.44

[51]. Joseph B. Martin, M.D., PhD: *Molecular Neurology* (New York: Scientific American, Inc. 1998) p. 206

[52]. Robert Gallo, *Virus Hunting* (A New Republic Book, 1991) p.45

[53]. Conn *Ibid*, p.373

[54]. Gail H. Cassell, M.S., PhD and Barry C. Cole, PhD *Ibid*, p.81

[55]. Conn *Ibid*, p. 542

[56]. Patricia Barnes-Svarney: *Science Desk Reference* (New York; Macmillan, USA, 1995) p.191

[57]. Adapted from Wayne M. Becker and David W. Deamer: *The World of the Cell* (The Benjamin/ Cummings Publishing Company, Inc.1991) p. 459

[58]. Simpson, L.O., Shand, B.I., Olds, R.J.:"Blood rheology and myalgic encephalomyelitis: A pilot study" *Pathology* Vol. 18. (1986) pp.190-92

[59]. Fujii, T., Takashi, S., Tamura, A., Wakatsuki, M., Kanaho,Y: "Shape changes of human erythrocytes induced by various amphipathic drugs acting on the membrane of the intact cells." Biochemical Pharmacology, Vol. 28. (1979) pp.613-20

[60]. Goodsell, *Ibid* p.12

[61]. Becker and Deamer, *Ibid* p.10

[62]. *Ibid*, p.297

[63]. Charles H. Graham, Jennifer Forsdike, Carolyn Fitzgerald, and Shannyn MacDonald-Goodfellow: "Hypoxia-mediated stimulation of carcinoma cell invasiveness via upregulation of urokinase receptor expression". *International Journal of Cancer*, Vol.80. (1999) pp. 617-23

[64]. Lo, *Ibid*, p.14

[65]. David S. Prince, M.D. and James E. Fish, M.D.: "Asthma in Aduklts" Conn: *Ibid*, pp.353-359

[66]. Joanne E. Embree, M.Sc., Juan A. Embil, M.D., PhD, FRCP[C]: "Mycoplasmas in diseases of humans" *CMA Journal*, Vol.123. (July 1980) p.105

[67]. Lo, *Ibid*, p.20

[68]. Peter Morgan, M.D. *Ibid*, p.88

[69]. To note just two:

Gnarpe, H. and Friberg, J.: "Mycoplasma and human reproductive failure" *American Journal of Obstetrics and Gynaecology*, Vol.114, (1972) p.727

and

Schoub B.D., Jacobs, Y.R., Hylen, E., et al. "The role of mycoplasma in human infertility." *South African Medical Journal*, Vol. 50 (1976) p.445

[70]. Embree, et al, *Ibid*, p.107

COMMENTARY

Despite the fact that we had cited the most recent authorities on the mycoplasma and human diseases and had clearly linked these to Lt. Richard's medical situation, the Veterans and Pension Review Committee denied her application. This despite the further fact that according to veterans administration policy in any case where a doubt existed, the benefit of the doubt was to be given to the veteran.

Lt. Richard was not given the benefit of the doubt and like so many of her comrades in arms was denied treatment.

CHAPTER ELEVEN

The Battle of Tahoe-Truckee High School

Casualties of an undeclared war of a government against its citizens.

ABSTRACT: Beginning in the mid-1930's as we have seen, and following a hiatus during the World War Two years, a number of 'mystery epidemics' occurred in the United States, Switzerland and England. In 1946 the hiatus ended with an epidemic in Iceland, followed by several in the USA, Canada, Great Britain, Denmark, Australia and South Africa. Although the epidemics presented with diseases that varied to a minor degree, as a group they 'share a great number of common features and, both clinically and epidemiologically, present a unique and distinctive appearance.' [1] A secret Congressional document dated June 9, 1969 and subsequent investigation into wartime and post-war research, make it evident that the testing of laboratory-developed biological weapons based principally upon brucellosis and visna/maedi antecedents is the probable cause of the mystery epidemics. The documentation also reveals that the biowar researchers had a dual-purpose agenda. The goal was to achieve a 'disabling' disease and a 'lethal' disease. The disabling disease agent, now known to be Mycoplasma fermentans, was based upon the brucellosis toxin{1} isolated in a crystalline form and diffused by aerosol, insect vector and in food/water sources, while the lethal disease agent was based upon the visna/maedi sheep virus, and is contagious by the exchange of body fluids.

The Mystery of Mystery Epidemics

There have been mystery diseases and disease epidemics for as long as there have been people concerned with determining why they or others have lost their health. Possible explanations for such loss of health have ranged from the anger of a Lord whose codes had been ignored [I may smite thee and thy people with pestilence—The Book of Exodus, verse 15] to infected needles of 60 intravenous drug users in a recent Scotland, Ireland and England [2] mystery disease outbreak.

Generally speaking, the mystery has gone out of each new disease outbreak as careful, caring persons have collected data, formulated hypotheses, devised tests for their hypotheses, revised their original conclusions and produced answers that could sustain rigorous challenge.

However, in 1934 an epidemic occurred among the personnel of the Los Angeles County General Hospital when 198 adult employees fell ill with a 'mystery disease'. [3]

We could take a long and careful look at all of the known details of that epidemic and the symptoms of its victims. However, that is not the focus of this study. What concerns us at this point in time is something very unusual about the response to the mystery illness by James P. Leake, Medical Director, United States Public Health Service and others at the National Institutes of Health in Washington, D.C.

At the time of the epidemic a young graduate of Johns Hopkins University in Epidemiology, Dr. Alexander G. Gilliam, prepared a 90 page study of what had happened at the Hospital, and submitted it to his boss, Dr. Leake, with the recommendation that it be published.

To Gilliam's surprise, and a source of continuing mystery, Dr. Leake strongly resisted publishing the results of the "…first scientific review of an epidemic of what is known today as ME [myalgic encephalomyelitis] or CFS [chronic fatigue syndrome]."[4] Even when it was finally published four years later Dr. Gilliam reported that he had been "stymied by his superiors from telling the whole story"!

There are a variety of possible reasons for Dr. Leake's resistance to putting the full story of this mystery epidemic before the public. For example, most of the victims had been given a "prophylactic serum" by their employer before they became ill. The serum would have been approved before use by Dr. Leake's Public Health Service. Was Dr. Leake aware of some flaws in the development and testing of the serum which he did not want to share with the public?

However that may be, we still don't know why Dr. Leake and other top public health officials did not want to tell the whole story. We do know that the Agency of the United States government responsible for protecting the health of American citizens, in its first encounter with what has since become a health problem of immense proportions, responded with a cover-up rather than with candour. This stance has characterized the various branches of the United States health services ever since.

From Dr. James Leake in 1934 to Dr. Brian Mahy in 2000, the public health services of the United States have been characterized by a marked lack of such candour, and, at times, by outright dishonesty and evil. Thus, to the mystery of the disease epidemics themselves, key members of the public health services have added the mystery of their response. What have they had to hide?

Abortions and Population Growth

Two important symptoms or co-symptoms of the mystery diseases known as ME/FM/CFIDS in women are endometriosis and hysterectomy. Dr. Man has observed that 20–30 percent of FM patients have [a] history of miscarriage or abortion. [5]

It is interesting to note that the next appearances of ME/FM/CFIDS mystery epidemics occurred in Switzerland in 1937 and 1939 and that many of the symptoms present in Los Angeles were seen again. However, there was an additional symptom of significance. A large number of the female victims presented with accentuated gynecological problems frequently culminating in abortions or requiring surgical interventions. Is this a possible clue that will help us solve the mystery of the mystery diseases?

Later in this study we will have occasion to consider the role of brucellosis in the etiology of ME/FM,[6] but at this time it should be noted that one species of the brucella pathogen is *brucella abortus*. It is so named because its major symptom is the inducement of abortions in cattle and other domestic animals and pets.[7] We will also have occasion to consider enunciated goals for biowar weapons which include pathogens which will reduce the birth rate in target populations. Anything that induces abortions will *ipso facto* reduce the birth rate.

Looking, but Hoping not to Reveal?

One of the medical professionals who studied the Swiss outbreaks was Dr. Gordon Parish of Great Britain, who in the course of his research, contracted ME/FM himself.

Dr. Parish was to experience what Dr. Gilliam had experienced in his dealings with the U.S. Public Health Agencies. There was an evident need on the part of the CDC/NIH to limit the study of the disease. Dr. Alexis Shelokov tells the story of Dr. Parish at an April 27,1987 meeting of the Centers for Disease Control. The meeting had been called to study outbreaks of the mystery diseases, but:

*"...when someone like Gordon Parish- who is truly a world authority, **has** this disease, and really knows what he is talking about—when **he** tried to open his mouth, one of these guys [from the CDC] would look at him and say, 'Yeah? Well that's very interesting. Thank you very much.' I just said, 'Jesus, it's no use wasting my time here.' and that's how Gordon [Parish] felt. But we stayed politely until the thing was over. Afterwards I said, 'Gordon, what do you think?' He said, 'I think they're going off in the wrong direction.'"* [8]

From Dr. Peake's hiding of information about the Los Angeles mystery disease to the CDC's control and (mis)direction of research, the story was the same: keep the truth from the public.

Why would the Public Health Services seek to cloak the mystery epidemics in further mystery?

Akureyri, Iceland

In 1948 Iceland was garrisoned by the United States Military who had taken over from the British in 1942 to prevent Germany from occupying the island.

In November, 1948, there was another epidemic of a 'mystery' disease. This time it was in the most remote area of northwestern Iceland in the towns of Akureyri, Saudakrokur and Isafordur. Unlike the Los Angeles outbreak which had affected vaccinated medical professionals or the Swiss outbreaks which had mainly affected pregnant women, this time the disease hit over 1,100 teenagers who attended local schools, and spread to other members of the communities.

There are three things worthy of special note about the Iceland outbreak.

First, of the 1,100 victims of ME/FM, five developed Parkinson's Disease and later died. Parkinson's at the time was a very rare disease and was largely confined to patients 65 or over. Five teenagers with Parkinson's was most unusual. Thus a mystery disease had become even more of a mystery. There had been no Parkinson's seen in Los Angeles or Switzerland, but it has been linked to both ME/FM and Gulf War Illnesses. [9]

Second, an Icelandic doctor, Bjorn Sigurdsson, became the principal investigator of the epidemic. There is nothing unusual in that, but there are certain elements in Sigurdsson's career that need to be known. Dr. Sigurdsson had been in Denmark when World War Two broke out. After the Germans occupied Denmark, Sigurdsson was able, despite wartime travel problems, to leave Denmark and turn up in Princeton, New Jersey, where he began a study at the Rockefeller Institute in animal and plant virology.[10] Among the animal bacteria that he studied were the brucellosis species and the retroviruses known as visna/maedi and a related progressive pneumonia of sheep.[11]

Following the war, Sigurdsson returned to Iceland as Scientific Director of a new Institute for Experimental Pathology, financed by his Rockefeller mentors and patrons. Thus, by what may have been a happy coincidence, Sigurdsson was on site when the mystery epidemic struck his homeland and he was able to report it fully to his U.S. sponsors: the Rockefellers.

In passing it should be emphasized that of the animal virology that he studied, brucellosis has very marked links to ME/FM and visna/maedi has equally strong links to AIDS.[12] Also, the features of progressive pneumonia are similar to those of Legionnaire's Disease.(See Chapter Five)

Third, a report at the time of the mystery outbreak in Iceland, concluded by stating that, if another outbreak occurred, the Rockefeller Foundation would probably send a medical commission to study it in even greater detail.[13] Another link to the Rockefeller empire!

Thus, as we shall see, in the whole field of mystery diseases and epidemics, the Rockefellers would play a significant and suggestive role, although the links were more often than not out of the public eye.[14]

What Went on in 1953?

In 1953 Nelson Rockefeller was named by President Eisenhower as Undersecretary to Oveta Culp Hobby, Secretary of Health, Education and Welfare (HEW). It was, of course, Secretary Hobby who was responsible for the Public Health Services.

Very few, if any, people had identified Nelson Rockefeller with health, education and welfare concerns, and when he took on this new job he lived up to any lack of expectations. He largely ignored the areas of philosophy and human resource development and concentrated instead upon personnel restructuring within the Agency.

His first undertaking was to establish a "war room" and he worked "...through advisors that were hazy figures on the periphery of the internal administration. They were people who apparently were tied in with numerous Rockefeller interests."[15] Among these numerous interests was population control, and Nelson Rockefeller was in an ideal position to tie the population control concerns of the Rockefeller Foundation to the public health services which would be monitoring any military/CIA biological weapons development tests. The latter, of course, would include abortion-inducing brucella abortus. A disabling but not usually fatal disease which was suspected of being able to 'jump species' and affect women.[16]

Another of the 'Rockefeller interests' was the World Health Organization which we will have occasion to consider later.

Donald Henderson, MD, and Alexis Shelokov, MD

Donald Henderson and Alexis Shelokov belonged to what Hillary Johnson would some 35 years later term "...a kind of secret fraternity".[17]

Drs. Henderson and Shelokov published a landmark summary of mystery diseases in 1959.[18] The two part article is brief, objective and useful. However, it is not the article nor its contents that need comment at this time, but rather, it is the background and activities of its authors that we should note.

Dr. Henderson received his MD. at the University of Rochester. Later, he was appointed Chief Medical Officer, Smallpox Eradication, World Health Organization, Geneva, Switzerland.[19]

Dr. Shelokov received his A.B. and MD. from Stanford University and was later affiliated with the National Institutes of Health. He had affiliations with several organizations, but the one most worthy of note is his membership in the 'Core Group of the Expert Working Group on Biological Toxin Weapons Verification, Federation of American Scientists.'

It is worth emphasizing that Dr. Henderson had been affiliated with the World Health Organization, while Dr. Shelokov had been on a Committee concerned with 'biological toxin weapons'. Their interests were brought together in 1969 when the WHO established a 'Brucellosis Research Laboratory' at the University of Minnesota Medical School.[20] Research with an emphasis on abortions!

It should also be noted that Rochester University was the alma mater not only of Dr. Henderson but also of Dr. D. Carleton Gajdusek and Dr. Daniel Peterson. As it turned out, all three were to be involved in the earliest stages of the AIDS and CFIDS epidemics.

Why these career events are worthy of note will become clear as we continue our study.

Military Secrets and Mystery Epidemics

"Wouldn't it be more effective to disable than to kill troops?"
Representative Daniel J. Flood, Pennsylvania.
June 9, 1969.[21]

In Chapter Four we reviewed the Hearings of June 9, 1969 when a group of Congressmen filed into a 'secure' meeting room in the Capitol Buildings of Washington, D.C. to hear a report from Dr. D.M. MacArthur, Deputy Director (Research and Technology) of the Department of Defense Research and Engineering in the Office of the Secretary of Defense. The report would help the Congressmen determine how much tax-payers' money should be appropriated in the coming fiscal year (1970) to be spent on the research, development, testing and engineering of biological weapons by the United States Military.

A Secret, Silent War

As it was to turn out, that meeting on June 9, 1969, was to be the date when certain elements within the United States Government effectively declared a secret silent war against carefully selected communities of their own nation, and against several 'lesser developed'(to use Henry Kissinger's terminology) foreign nations throughout the world...with an emphasis upon Africa.

The undeclared war was to employ biological weapons developed in government laboratories such as the one in Fort Detrick, Maryland; in selected industrial laboratories including those of Bionetics Research or Litton Industries; and at a range of Universities throughout the land. It was all to be done in the name of 'testing' the new weapons as researched by 'eminent' scientists; developed by the military in co-operation with the CIA; approved by the Congress; and, monitored by the Public Health Agencies including the Centers for Disease Control and the National Institutes of Health.

The weapons were to fall into two categories: one class of weapons would be 'lethal' and would target the people of the lesser developed nations whose natural resources the US coveted; and, one class would be 'disabling' and would especially target women of child-bearing age in the 'civilized' western nations; although both genders were to be vulnerable on a 'female:male' ratio of approximately 6:1.[22]

The New Nazis

Dr. MacArthur of the Pentagon was accompanied to the meeting by four medical and military persons who evidently felt no compunction about undertaking to develop (or as it was to turn out: to continue to develop) [23] new biological organisms which would kill or disable targeted 'enemies', despite the public 1969 proclamations by President Nixon to the effect that the US was unilaterally terminating its biological warfare research.[24]

The group of eleven elected legislators, together with their Chairman George Mahon heard Dr. MacArthur's plan to develop two new pathogens that would kill or disable millions of human beings across their own nation and throughout the rest of the world. When the doctor was finished, the Congressmen voted him the money he had requested: an initial appropriation of $335,000,000 plus another $10,000,000 for a special lethal agent refractory to the human immune system and ideal for strategic warfare against the growing population of third world countries. They also approved his time frame of five to ten years to develop the latter new disease.

Their vote effectively sentenced hundreds of teachers and students of Tahoe-Truckee High School and various of their family members and friends to an ME/FM disability for life. The vote also sentenced millions of other American citizens to ME/FM; first, in epidemics and later as chronic, pervasive, persistent diseases spread throughout America. Millions more of the world's population were doomed by that vote of Congress, to a slow and cruel death by AIDS.

What Dr. MacArthur Promised

Dr. MacArthur warned the Congressmen that "… there are many who believe such research should not be undertaken lest it lead to yet another method of massive killing of large populations". [Hearings, p.129] This warning echoed his earlier mention of a constraint the Pentagon and CIA had placed upon themselves "…to prevent…a worldwide scourge, or a black death type disease that will envelop the world or major geographical areas if some of these materials were to accidentally escape". [Hearings, p.121]

Dr. MacArthur did not mention the possibility of an 'intentional escape' of the pathogen to reduce the rate of population growth in certain lesser developed countries. The latter problem was to be left for Dr. Henry Kissinger to raise three years later in his NSSM 200.[25]

Such moral considerations seem to have been lost in any further discussions that may have ensued, for Congress voted the entire budget request, plus the extra $10,000,000 for the AIDS pathogen. True to his word, within ten years MacArthur and his covert agents of death, Mahon, Sikes, *et al.* began to witness the first victims of a 'gay plague' in America and the beginning of the massive killing of large populations in Africa and other 'lesser developed countries 'from a mystery disease refractory to the human immune system. Just what Dr. MacArthur had described and the world has witnessed since 1981!

However, our focus in this Chapter is upon that other pathogen that the Pentagon/CIA researchers were working upon: "..agents that are not lethal but incapacitate". [Hearings, p.114]

Agents that Incapacitate

The logic of two new pathogens, one lethal and one disabling, is obvious.

The people of the United States and most of the white citizens of the world can today largely ignore the 6,000 people a day dying of AIDS as long as those people are black and living 'uncivilized' lives in the jungle. The prospects of 6,000 whites dying daily…the equivalent of a fully loaded 747 crashing every two hours day-after-day, week-after-week… cannot be envisioned without it being realized that such a scenario would elicit a huge public outcry and draw immense research efforts greater than any ever seen before to bring the carnage to a halt.

Blacks can be killed, but whites can only be disabled. But, just in case a significant portion of the white population should respond strongly to the plight of the Africans dying of AIDS and the ME/FM-disabled white victims, two pre-emptive actions would be necessary.

First, to head off calls for AIDS research, the Pentagon/CIA/CDC/NIH had to co-operate to make AIDS a so-called 'gay plague'. Given the homophobic nature of the 1970-80's America, one way to ensure that only a minimal amount of research would be generated in the crucial opening years of the AIDS epidemic would be to associate it almost entirely with homosexual males. A 'free' hepatitis "B" vaccination program in 1979 might accomplish this goal if it was laced with MacArthur's new 'lethal' AIDS agent, [26] and the resulting epidemic blamed upon a sinful life-style.

Co-incidentally, in 1979, the New York City Blood Center, the pharmaceutical company of Merck, Sharp & Dohme, and the Centers for Disease Control came up with just such a Hepatitis B vaccination Program, and within months many of the gay males who accepted the vaccination began to present with the symptoms of AIDS.

The subsequent dawning AIDS epidemic was firmly established in the minds of most middle-class Americans as a consequence of an immoral life style and hence drew little or no public demand for research. In fact, it was considered politically astute for the newly elected President Reagan to declare that 'not one cent will be spent on AIDS research' by his administration.

Second, to head off calls for ME/FM research, the same coterie involved above took advantage of the pathogenic requirement of a certain level of pathogen concentration in the blood being necessary before the process of disease could be triggered to label it a 'psychosomatic' disease, principally of women who, it was claimed, could not cope with the stress of the modern world. [See Endnote 2]

In both cases the perpetrators of these great crimes against humanity could call upon their media assets to advance such covering myths. AIDS would dismissively become 'the gay plague' and ME/FM would become 'the yuppie flu'. *The New York Times* and *Time* magazine would warp the reality of the diseases by picking up the NIH themes and passing them along to the world at large. Strange academics from Harvard and Princeton such as Edward Shorter and Elaine Showalter wrote and lectured in a new jargon, psychobabble, to the effect that victims of ME/FM were just escaping the stress of their world by imagining they had an illness that did not exist.

Shorter would "aim at middle-aged women with an imaginary disease"[27] in a scholarly rant while Elaine Showalter would suggest that persons ill with ME/FM might be cured if they 'swam with dolphins.'[28]

Two obscene new pathogens: one that was lethal and one that was disabling, had both been promised by Dr. Donald MacArthur at that June 9, 1969 meeting, and both burst upon the world in the late 1970's and early 1980's. And both were misrepresented to the world in their critical early years by rogues and charlatans in the CDC/NIH and the media.

Back to the Mystery Epidemics

However, none of the Congressmen on hand asked MacArthur how he could be so sure of himself as to be able to set a time limit for success. Had they asked, MacArthur would have had to admit that the plans for both the lethal and disabling weapons were already well under way. Tests had been done on someone somewhere. Could such tests have been the cause of the mystery disease epidemics that we have been examining? Undoubtedly yes.

The Need to Tell the Truth

Of the $335 million Defense Budget approved by Congress in 1969 for the Budget Year 1970, $18 million was for 'Test and evaluation'. [Hearings p.138] To appreciate how the spending of that money and the subsequent monies over the next ten years would impact upon the citizens of the United States and the world in general and of Tahoe-Truckee High School in particular, it is necessary that the program of biological warfare weapons development now be re-considered and certain factors be taken into full account. Only when the truth is told will the secret Battle of Tahoe-Truckee be revealed and the thousands of casualties be seen as the victims they are.

Let's go back and Start with 1942

There are various critical dates in any study of biological warfare. These range from the days of Moses when there was "...a very grievous murrain" that

killed off much of the Egyptians' livestock and contributed to the Pharaoh's decision to allow the Israelites to leave Egypt[29]. A more recent date could be that of the skyburst SCUD missiles, which, in all likelihood, were armed with a cocktail of biological disease agents, that were fired at Israel and Allied forces by Saddam Hussein in 1991.[30] The latter attacks probably contributed to the George Bush decision to call off the Desert Storm attack after just 100 triumphant hours, in case a further volley of anthrax-armed SCUDS should follow.

President Bush would not have had to guess what was going on. Not only had he been President Reagan's Vice-President when the U.S. sold some brucella biological weapons components to Iraq,[31] but a way back in 1975 Bush had been appointed by Gerald Ford to replace William Colby as Director of the CIA...and the CIA at that time was busily engaged in the development of the weapons promised by MacArthur. We will return to President Bush and his Secretary of Defence, Richard Cheney, later. We will also discover who George Bush had selected as his "Associate Director for Life Sciences". 'Life sciences' study is frequently a euphemism for people engaged in biowar activities. Dr. Donald MacArthur in charge of biological weapons development for the Pentagon had once been Manager of the Life Sciences Research Center of Westinghouse.

Tahoe-Truckee High School

The Battle of Tahoe-Truckee had its genesis in 1942, when the United States, Great Britain and Canada entered into an agreement to co-operate fully in the development of biological weapons. Canada and Great Britain were already well underway in such activities as were the enemy nations of Germany and Japan, with the latter engaged in what was probably the most intensive of the programs of weapons development.

When the war ended in 1945, two important things happened. First, the three Allies decided that even though the Axis powers had been defeated, an Allied program of bioweapons development should continue in the face of the perceived Soviet threat. Second, the United States unilaterally engaged in an extensive program to recruit German and Japanese biological warfare researchers who would be spared the prospect of war crimes trials if they shared their secrets with the U.S.

Most of the Japanese criminals who had used Allied prisoners-of-war as guinea pigs to test their new weapons were happy to exchange their information for a full time United States Government job. Under the program labelled Operation Paperclip[32], various Nazi criminals were brought to work in the U.S. Another way to learn the enemies' secrets was to send U.S. scientists to Japan to work with General Ishii Shiro who had headed the Japanese biowar program. Under the latter program people such as Dr. Edwin V. Hill of Fort Detrick travelled to Japan to learn about "...botulim, *brucellosis,* gas gangrene, glanders, influenza, meningococcus, plague, smallpox, tetanus, and tularaemia."[33]

The latter information, plus the as yet unrevealed details about the Japanese biological test site in New Guinea, are of critical importance to this study. It is now evident that the brucellosis bacteria (mutated, as we shall see, by viral DNA) is the antecedent to the pathogen that caused the ME/FM outbreak in Tahoe-Truckee High School, while the New Guinea test site data was the probable basis for the development of the AIDS virus from its visna/maedi antecedent.

BACK TO GEORGE MERCK

On January 3, 1946, George W. Merck,(whose pharmaceutical firm we noted above in the 'free' Hepatitis B vaccination of gay males) the Special Consultant for Biological Warfare to the Secretary of Defense, submitted a Report to his boss.[34] This Report helps place the outbreaks of mystery diseases, the Congressional Hearings of June 9, 1969 and the Battle of Tahoe-Truckee in historic and scientific perspective. The critical points of Merck's report should be summarized here as a necessary foundation for understanding what followed.

First, it is important to note that Merck made the point that "...the U.S. Public Health Service" was involved in the biowar activities from the beginning. [Senate Hearings, p.66] As will be seen, this involvement began as a monitoring of military tests of biological agents developed in military-operated or controlled laboratories and evolved into a more participatory role under Nelson Rockefeller as Undersecretary of HEW in 1953 until, under Henry Kissinger in the Nixon/Ford presidencies, the public health services were literally transformed into full biowar weapons development partners with the military and the CIA.

In effect, a significant part of HEW (later the Department of Health & Human Services) was to become an adjunct of the Department of Defense in the latter's quest for biological warfare weapons development...but more of that later.[35]

The partnership that we have already noted of the U.S., Britain and Canada in biological warfare research was also acknowledged by Merck, and, he reported, "...was continued and provision was made for the interchange of biological warfare personnel between the three countries." It was under this agreement that the City of Winnipeg was to be attacked by U.S. military aircraft spraying a carcinogenic agent in 1953,[36] and with later Canadian tests involving the mosquito vector in the St. Lawrence Seaway Valley and tests at a Montreal Hospital involving contaminated vaccines to follow in 1984.

Another important comment must be noted. Merck reported that: "...the problems of offense and defense were closely interlinked in all the investigations conducted." In 1969 when Nixon made his unilateral declaration that the U.S. was pulling out of all 'offensive' biowar research, he was engaging in insidious double speak. One cannot research defensive biowar without at the same time researching offensive biowar. Just part of the word games associated with the whole subject.

However, it was on page A-7 of his Report [page 70 of the Senate's 1977 release] that George Merck made known some of the most critical 'accomplishments' of his research team's efforts. The first seven of his eleven 'accomplishments' are worth reproducing in full.

"1. Development of methods and facilities for the mass production of microorganisms and their products.

"2. Development of methods for rapid and accurate detection of minute quantities of disease-producing agents.

"3. Significant contributions to knowledge of the control of airborne disease-producing agents.

"4. Production and isolation, for the first time, of **a crystalline bacterial toxin,** *which has opened the way for the preparation of a more highly purified immunizing toxoid.*

"5. Development and production of an effective toxoid in sufficient quantities to protect large scale operations should this be necessary.

"6. Significant contributions to knowledge concerning the development of immunity in human beings and animals against certain infectious diseases.

"7. Important advances in the treatment of certain infectious diseases of human beings and animals, and in the development of effective protective clothing and equipment."

Of these seven accomplishments, the following points merit emphasis:

(1) The earliest efforts to utilize disease microorganisms as biowar weapons involved the production, isolation and diffusion of those organisms. It is important to note that Merck has added an important factor: the 'products' of such microorganisms. This will be better understood after we consider the fourth accomplishment below, when we ask what it is that microorganisms can 'produce'.

(2) The rapid and accurate detection of minute quantities of disease-producing agents will be better appreciated after we consider the events of the 1991 Desert Storm attack on Iraq. [See 'Gulf War Illnesses']

(3) An early problem associated with the airborne diffusion of living biological agents was the latter's tendency to die and to lose virulence. This problem had been largely solved by June 9, 1969, and did not pose a challenge in the Battle of Tahoe-Truckee. The air-conditioning system of Tahoe-Truckee High School was to prove ideal for the diffusion of a new form of bacterial toxin.

(4) *"Production and isolation, for the first time, of a crystalline bacterial toxin"*…This accomplishment is probably the most critical one of all those that Merck lists. It should be noted by every medical practitioner, disease victim and victim's family members in the world who want to understand many of the so-called 'mystery' diseases such as myalgic encephalomyelitis (aka CFIDS) multiple sclerosis, Parkinson's, fibromyalgia, Lyme Disease and other such of which it is said that …there is no known cause; there is no known cure; and whose incidence is increasing dramatically.

Consider carefully what George Merck has written. His researchers had managed 'for the first time' to take various disease-causing bacteria and to have isolated from them the toxin or poisonous protein that does the actual damage to its host. Just what Dr. Shelokov [above] was later to become an expert on. Furthermore, such extracted bacterial toxin had been isolated in a crystalline form. In such a form it could be reduced to an infinitely fine dust and diffused through the air; or, it could be used to contaminate mosquitoes or ticks which would thus become the new vector for spreading the disease agent.

In such crystalline form, the toxin could attack its victim who would present with all of the symptoms of a bacterial disease such as brucellosis, but there would be no sign of the bacteria!

A simple analogy might be helpful

An average rattlesnake cannot seriously hurt anyone. It can wind itself around the arm or leg of a human enemy and squeeze as hard as it is capable of squeezing; but, unlike its cousin the boa constrictor, it can be plucked off and thrown aside without much effort by an average adult. Even if it bites someone, the bite is not apt to be more than an inch across and barely skin deep. Such a wound would scarcely be in need of stitches and would warrant only some iodine and a Band-aid ®. It is not the rattlesnake that causes humans serious harm, it is the toxin that it delivers into the flesh of its victim when it bites that does the harm.

If one were to extract the toxin and then put it into a victim by hypodermic needle, the victim could die of a rattlesnake bite without ever having been near a rattlesnake.

Such, in a simplified form, is what George Merck and his researchers had achieved by 1946 in their search for ways and means to use bacterial toxins as biological weapons to maim and kill perceived enemies. To find out if it would work it would have to be tested on someone.

Just what this crystalline toxin isolated from various bacteria was is still subject to speculation, since the Pentagon has been very circumspect about it.[37] However, the evidence is becoming more compelling that MacArthur was talking about what has come to be known as the 'mycoplasma', a sterol-dependent cell wall-less microorganism originally reported in 1898 by Nocard and Roux.[38]

In turn this microorganism appears to be a particle of the bacterial DNA and has been labelled a 'virus', a designation that may not be accurate, except in-so-far as it may be isolated in crystalline form.[39] Any relationship that the laboratory 'mycoplasma' may have to the microorganism reported in 1898 is not clear.

The Pentagon/CIA/CDC/NIH appears to prefer ambiguity, quite likely to make any effort to track their research more difficult.[40] Despite their efforts at obfuscation, the truth keeps bubbling to the surface and it is clearly evident that the crystalline microorganism called the 'mycoplasma' was the subject of testing by the above agencies of government. It is also more than likely that, as stated above, the mycoplasma was what Merck's researchers had been working with,[41] although at that point in time they would be referring to it as a 'PPLO' - Pleural pneumonia-like organism'.

5) *"Development and production of an effective toxoid".* This 'accomplishment' says more by what it doesn't say than what it does say. An 'effective toxoid' is an inactivated bacterial toxin which can stimulate antibody production by the immune system. However, there is no 'magic bullet' toxin where one form protects against all bacterial disease. It needs to be known which toxoid Merck was alluding to. If it was one which was effective against brucellosis bacterial toxin, it might prove to be helpful in the treatment of the casualties of the Battle of Tahoe-Truckee. But more of that later.

(6) Most living organisms, including human beings, have developed over time "immunological and therapeutic processes upon which..." they depend to maintain their relative freedom from infectious disease.[Quoting from Dr. MacArthur's June 9, 1969 meeting with the Congressmen-Hearings, p.129] That George Merck's researchers were already studying the human immune system in relation to their biological warfare weapons programs is an ominous hint of things that were to come.

George Merck ends his January 3, 1946 Report with a ringing declaration:

"Work in this field, born of the necessity of war, cannot be ignored in time of peace; it must be continued on a sufficient scale to provide an adequate defense."

We are moving towards June 9, 1969, and a union of the mystery diseases and biological weapons testing, but first we must pause to make a special note of the disease called brucellosis.

Brucellosis

Brucellosis is an ancient disease. Animal bones from the time of our caveman ancestors suggest that this disease took its toll of humans and other animals[42] as far back as prehistoric times.

*"From the medical, production, and dissemination standpoints, then, **Brucella** made a fine weapon",* or so says Ed Regis.[43] In fact, the brucellosis species were among the earliest agents experimented with during World War Two by the Allies, and there is considerable evidence that the United

States used their brucella-armed weapons in Korea between 1949 and 1954.[44]

Although lethal in rare instances, brucellosis is largely regarded as disabling and for that reason it has fitted in well with Pentagon/CIA planning.[45]

The most important feature of the various brucella species, however, from a biowar point-of-view, is the fact that brucellosis, like ME/FM, can affect every body system of its victims. As with myalgic encephalomyelitis brucellosis can present as damage to the muscular/skeletal systems; the reproductive system; the respiratory system; the endocrine system; the digestive system; the urinary system; the blood and cardiovascular systems; and, the brain and nervous system.[46]

Brucellosis was one of the first naturally occuring diseases to be studied intensively by Allied biowar researchers. Even the 'school song' of Allied trainees featured a reference to the disease:

"Brucellosis, Psittacosis,
Vee! You! Bah!
Antibodies, Antitoxin,
Rah! Rah! Rah!." [47]

After 1946, when the biowar scientists could isolate and produce its disease-causing toxin in crystalline form, brucellosis was ready for a new lease on life as a disabling weapon.[48] It remained as we shall see for the researchers to enhance it by mutating its bacterial base with a viral agent to make it more virulent and contagious.

Back to June 9, 1969

Congressman George H. Mahon of Texas got the secret meeting of June 9,1969 under way with an important introductory remark:

"This subcommittee and the Congress has, over a period of years, supported the appropriations of funds for chemical and biological warfare" [Hearings, p.105]

The budget in each of those years contained money for testing the new weapons and weapon components developed by the military and its collaborators. Some of the tests could be conducted upon animals, but when the final product was deemed ready to kill or disable people, the researchers had to make sure it would perform up to expectations by actually testing it upon people. That is where the 500,000 human guinea pigs of 1940 to 1974 admitted to by the General Accounting Office had played their unwitting role. These victims sitting in an office building or a hotel[49] or a place of work or riding the New York subway[50] had received a pathogenic substance administered or ordered by their own government and had then been observed for their reaction.

It is the pathogenic substances thus visited upon a huge number of innocent citizens by order of their government that is the focus of our present study. This class of victim is to be seen as distinct from other victims who were regarded by the military/CIA as enemies and were targeted for assassination.[51]

After acknowledging that Congress had been spending money for years to test new and improved biological pathogens upon some of their unwitting constituents, Mahon and his colleagues heard something else from Dr. MacArthur:

"Every attempt is made to use discretion in selection of contractors, and not to ask institutions to do work which might be contrary to their policies and purposes" [Hearings p.108]

In other words, there were some institutions whose administrators might not like the idea that biological weapons to disable and kill were being developed by their government and tested upon the citizens of their own country. This may be seen as pertinent later in this study when we consider the role of the recent Clinton administration Secretary of Health & Human Services, Donna E. Shalala, who accepted with remarkable aplomb the news that one of her employees (Brian Mahy) had engaged in the fraudulent misappropriation of ME/FM research money.

Before accepting her job as Secretary of Health & Human Services, Dr. Shalala had been the Chancellor of the University of Wisconsin which, in turn, was distinguished as one of the major contractors to the military in developing biological weapons. Between May 1950 and October 1969, the University of Wisconsin had 21 such contracts while Yale, for example, had only 2. [Senate Hearings: March 8 and May 23, 1977. pp.99 and 100][52]

Further along, Dr. MacArthur sheds more light on the people involved without actually naming them. Speaking about the 'incapacitants' his researchers were working on he says:

*"Before an agent can be classified as an incapacitant we feel that the mortality must be very low. Therefore, the ratio of the lethal dose to the incapacitating dose has to be very high. Now this is a very difficult technical job. We have had some of the **top scientists** in the country working for years on how to get more effective incapacitating agents. It is not easy".*

Top Scientists

Just who those 'top scientists' were is still classified in the interests of national security! However, one can piece together evidence from a variety of sources. For example, from one source we learn that Dr. Ira Baldwin of the University of Wisconsin [See Shalala reference above] was one 'of the principles [sic] of the biological laboratories from World War ll to early 1960's'[53], and that a colleague was Dr. Edwin V. Hill. From another source we learn that Dr. Hill in October 1947, had been one of the American scientists who de-briefed the Japanese biological weapons researchers such as Dr. Ishii Shiro. Dr. Hill interviewed and collected much data from Masahiko Takahashi about "...the aerosol delivery of infectious agents, a topic of surpassing interest at Camp Detrick."[54]

Thus, when Dr. MacArthur briefs the Congressmen on 'aerosol' diffusion of infectious agents [Hearings p.120] there is a clear trail from MacArthur back through Edwin Hill to Ira Baldwin to Masahiko Takahashi to Ishii Shiro.

Before leaving this point, it needs to be noted that Dr. Hill received 15,000 specimen slides from his Japanese informants. These slides were from the dead bodies of Allied prisoners-of-war killed by Japanese experiments or murdered afterwards. And it should be noted that Dr. Baldwin "...resigned his post as the scientific director at [then] Camp Detrick and returned to the University of Wisconsin."[55]

Finally, in respect to top scientists, both American and Japanese, it should be remarked that among the slides collected by top scientist Dr. Hill were ones detailing damage by brucellosis.[56] And both brucellosis and aerosol diffusion will figure in the Battle of Tahoe-Truckee High School.

Strategic Rather than Tactical

On page 121 of the Congressional Hearings of June 9, 1969, Dr. MacArthur makes an important distinction. He tells the Congressmen that "...the biological weapons are considered strategic rather than tactical." Tactical weapons have to do with the winning of battles in the field. Strategic weapons have to do with the provision of advantage in the field by what takes place away from the actual place of fighting.

A mustard gas bomb that asphyxiates enemy soldiers on the battle field is a tactical weapon. A brucellosis bomb that disables workers in munitions plants and on transport trains is a strategic weapon. And a deadly disease agent (such as AIDS) which reduces the populations of third world countries and so enhances American access to supply sources is a strategic weapon.

Apparently Dr. MacArthur and his fellow researchers had learned something else from Dr. Ishii Shiro. Shiro had written a "treatise on the whole subject", including his ideas about the strategical and tactical use of BW weapons, how these weapons should be used in various geographical areas."[57]

MUTATED TO NEW FORMS

If the Congressmen would approve his budget requests, MacArthur promised another area of research that his key scientists would be seeking to solve: "... whether viruses and bacteria can be mutated to new forms resistant to vaccines" [Hearings, p.144]

On this note, the Hearings of June 9,1969 were ended and the military/CIA went back to their labours, armed with the money they had requested to advance with a 5 to 10 year program their plans to develop two new biological weapons: one which was lethal and one which was disabling.

The plan was to get under way in 1970, which it did, and by 1981, after a few sporadic cases of AIDS, a new 'worldwide scourge, or a black death type disease' as anticipated by MacArthur and approved by the Congress was beginning to ravage the population of certain 'strategic' countries selected by Henry Kissinger. And, by 1983 a new 'mystery' disease was to hit the staff and students of Tahoe-Truckee High School in California. This disease was not the only mystery disease between June 9,1969 and 1983.

There had been a mystery disease that hit the Lackland Airforce base in Texas in 1970. And in 1975 200 hospital staff in Sacramento,[58] California, fell ill and spread their illness to many of the children of the hospital staff and from there to the children's teachers. In 1976 even Ireland was not spared when an 'mystery' epidemic hit that country.

All of these diseases and some twelve other epidemic diseases over the same time frame in the U.S., Canada, Great Britain and Australia had minor points of difference; however, they had much more in common. In fact, besides being largely similar to chronic brucellosis, a fact that for some reason went largely overlooked and unremarked, the disease

symptoms also resembled those of the epidemic that had occurred in Iceland in 1946-47 and 1948-49 which came to be known as Akureyri Disease or Icelandic Disease.

The Icelandic Disease had many features in common with the Tahoe-Truckee epidemic some 35 years later. Both diseases seemed to have as their epicenter, a large school. Both failed to present any known pathogen such as herpes simplex, coxsackie, influenza, etc. Both were largely disabling but in both cases the disability was to persist for many years after on-set. In neither case was the brucellosis bacteria looked for.[59] Both major epidemics had been preceded by a few isolated cases of the mystery disease, and after having peaked, new cases presented in a lower incidence, but continuing in presence.

There was, however, something very unusual about the disabling disease of Akureyri: as noted above, out of the more than one thousand mostly teen-age victims, five developed Parkinson's disease and eventually died. This would not fit Dr. MacArthur's template for a disabling disease...the mortality rate would have been too high. And, one is left to ponder the question whether there is any linkage between the increasing incidence of myalgic encephalomyelitis and the increasing incidence (and younger age of on-set) of Parkinson's Disease? But more of this later.

AT THE END OF A DECADE

Ten years after Congress had voted Dr. MacArthur his budget request to develop two new pathogens, one lethal and one disabling, the world could report that such diseases existed under the acronyms AIDS and ME/FM.

Were AIDS and ME/FM the product of the military/CIA biological weapons testing that had of necessity to follow the research? Had the wartime work of American, Canadian and British researchers extended into peacetime and, augmented by the secrets of the German and Japanese researchers, achieved what Dr. Donald MacArthur had promised twelve Congressmen on June 9,1969?

We will not attempt to answer this question at this point, but will, instead, take a closer look at the challenge of testing deadly and disabling pathogens developed in military, commercial and university laboratories and relate what we learn to Tahoe-Truckee High School and the epidemic that hit teachers, students and staff in 1984.

The AIDS epidemic bears a striking resemblance to the 'worldwide scourge, or a black death type disease'[Hearings p. 121] that Dr. MacArthur described to the twelve Congressmen on that fateful day in June, 1969. Its most dramatic distinguishing characteristic of being 'refractory to the immunological and therapeutic processes' [Hearings, p.129] of human beings is the major characteristic of AIDS. And, Dr. MacArthur had promised that such a lethal pathogen could be produced within 5 to 10 years and the record shows that the first 'official' case of AIDS was discovered in 1981.[60]

CRITICAL TEST CRITERIA FOR A BIOWAR PATHOGEN

If one has developed a pathogen which it is theorized will disable 3 or 5 or other percentage of targeted victims, the test must be carried out on a sufficiently large sample to be statistically valid. A small sample may give a warped result which will not reflect the reality of the pathogen being tested. An example, using a disabling pathogen, of such a small sample warping the results can be seen in what happened in 1946 in Suffield, Canada. Thirty-five hogs had been exposed to a heavy cloud of brucella suis for the theoretically correct period of time. Later the hogs were tested with the expectation that a significant percentage would test positive for the disease.

As it turned out, not a single hog possessed the bacteria nor presented with the symptoms of the disease[61] after the test!

Test rule-of-thumb (i): The sample in any test must be large enough for the results to be statistically valid.

However, before a large target group is exposed to a theoretically disabling disease pathogen it must be determined that the pathogen is not lethal. Therefore, under the same test conditions that will prevail in the large-scale test, a sample must demonstrate that, as MacArthur had said, "The ratio of the lethal dose to the incapacitating dose has to be very high." [Hearings, p. 117] To ensure that the pathogen is not lethal, a small, trial run is made. If the latter demonstrates no lethality, the major test can proceed.

An example of the application of this criterion appears to have occurred in Punta Gorda, Florida, in 1956. An infestation of mosquitoes was associated with a major outbreak of ME/FM [62] in that year. In the two weeks before the major outbreak one or

two people had become mildly ill but were not noted until after the major outbreak drew attention to them. Then, one morning there was a huge influx of mosquitoes, large enough to merit many comments by the Punta Gorda populace. The following week the epidemic began and lasted several weeks.

Taken in conjunction with the fact that the Government of Canada had been breeding one hundred million mosquitoes a month at the Dominion Parasite Laboratory in Belleville, Canada, and had been delivering these to the U.S. and Canadian military, it is reasonable to speculate that infected mosquitoes were the disease vector. However, the largest release would only occur when it had been demonstrated that the pathogen was not lethal.

Test rule-of-thumb (ii): Any major test of a disabling pathogen should not take place until a small trial run has been made to ensure that it is disabling but not lethal.

When the United States detonated its first hydrogen bomb in 1952 the event was witnessed by thousands of service and scientific personnel. The latter were present for a very obvious reason: if one is to make a test of a weapon, someone qualified to evaluate the results must witness what happens.

In 1953 when the U.S. sprayed an attenuated carcinogenic pathogen over the City of Winnipeg, Canada, there were American observers all over the City to evaluate the consequences. How many people presented with coughs, sniffles, runny eyes? From these and similar observed results the researchers could extrapolate a consequence had the pathogen been full strength. Learning what has happened is the essence of testing.

Test rule-of-thumb (iii): The results of any test protocol must be observed and evaluated by the researchers or their agents.

Whenever a test which involves a significant number of people is carried out, there must be a pre-determined spin which can be placed upon what has happened. Such a spin must appear to be logical and to provide an explanation for all aspects of the covert activity.

In the 1953 above-mentioned tests of an attenuated carcinogenic pathogen over Winnipeg, such a spin was ready, should it be needed. As it turned out it was needed.

The Mayor of the City took a very paternal, hands-on interest in all things affecting his City. When he observed that what appeared to be an American military aircraft was flying back and forth over Winnipeg with a vague hint of something coming from it, he phoned the Department of Defense in Ottawa. The people in Ottawa referred him to the Headquarters of the North American Air Defense System, where he spoke with a prepared public relations officer. The explanation he received boggles the mind.

The Mayor of Winnipeg, Canada, was told by NORAD staffers that the plane was spraying out a harmless mist that would obscure Winnipeg on any radar screens. If it should happen that the Russians at the height of the Cold War should launch a surprise inter-continental ballistic missile attack on the West, no missile guidance system would be able to locate Winnipeg and so the City would be free from nuclear devastation! It was essential, the Mayor was told, that this secret defense system be kept absolutely secret or the Russians might find a way to circumvent it.

The Mayor bought the story. After all, there was a Cold War reported daily in the media. Propaganda stories led many people to believe the Soviet Union would stoop to any depth of depravity in pursuit of world domination. There had been reports about radar bafflers before, usually involving metal foil paper. There was a U.S. military aircraft flying back and forth over the City spraying something out as it flew. It all seemed to add up.

The story stayed secret as we noted above, until the middle of May, 1997, when the Pentagon finally confessed what they had been doing.

Test rule-of-thumb (iv): Alternative spin stories must be in place to account for any test data that might emerge from its covert shadows.

For several years after the attack on the City of Winnipeg and the obfuscation story to cover it, bits and pieces of the truth emerged in unexpected ways and places. However, when such occurred it was found to be helpful that major media were cultivated to ignore the truth as being simply more of those 'conspiracy' theories so enjoyed by leftist and liberal agitators.

An excellent example of this cultivation of the media is to be seen in a Memo issued by the CIA as a four-page document Number 1035-960, dated 'Sept 1976' and titled "Countering Criticism of the Warren Report". It provides several suggestions to 'liaison and friendly elite contacts (especially politicians and editors)' as well as 'propaganda assets to answer and refute the attacks of the critics.' Led by influential but insidious media such as *The New York Times* and *Time* magazine, the Memo's key points have become a part of American folk lore and

the dishonest Warren Report continues to hide the truth.[63]

Test rule-of-thumb (v): It is essential that 'propaganda assets' be cultivated to maintain any alternative spin put upon facts and consequences.

Finally, the test site itself must be carefully chosen. An ideal site is an island, since it already has a water barrier around it to limit interlopers bungling into the midst of a critical test.

The Japanese apparently chose to test their visna/maedi sheep inoculant which is the source of human Creutzfeldt-Jakob disease on the Fore tribe of the Island of New Guinea in 1942. The Americans apparently tested their new brucellosis derivative agent on the Island of Iceland in 1946 & 48.

If an island surrounded by water is not conveniently available, then a site surrounded by mountains, accessed by few roads would be a reasonable alternative. Tahoe-Truckee High School was such a site.

Test rule-of-thumb (vi): Most test sites must have a sufficient level of natural barriers as is necessary to ensure a degree of innocuous security.

Planning the Battle of Tahoe-Truckee High School

On June 9, 1969, a very minor disagreement had developed between Dr. MacArthur and Representative Flood of Pennsylvania. Dr. MacArthur had just finished telling the Congressmen that "...agents that we would try to develop would be noncontagious; that is, that it could not be passed on directly from individual to individual."

Mr. Flood responded: "Would they be effective if not contagious?"

Dr. MacArthur: "They could be infectious from the standpoint that they would be used as primary aerosol and infect people inhaling it. After that they could be carried from me to you, say, by an insect vector-a mosquito, for example."

Mr. Flood persists: "Could they be effective and contagious?"

Dr. MacArthur: "No".

Mr. Flood: "I doubt that. I doubt that."

Just what was this all about?

Dr. MacArthur claimed to believe that if a targeted victim was directly exposed by a disabling pathogen in sufficient quantity, then the victim would be infected with the anticipated disease. Once such a disease was in the body of the victim, the theory was that he would not be able to relay the infection by breathing out any of the pathogen. He would be effectively ill, but would not communicate that illness to others by 'secondary aerosol'. That was what Dr. MacArthur believed, but as we shall see, he was to be proven terribly wrong…and Mr. Flood was intuitively correct.

The virulence of the pathogens that MacArthur had in mind must be remarked upon. If a victim were infected by primary aerosol, his blood would carry the disease and even the minute amount taken by a mosquito which subsequently bites another victim would pass the disease to the latter! This level of virulence by insect vector suggests that if the pathogen is proven to be infectious by secondary aerosol, the results could be catastrophic. Only a test would tell whether secondary aerosol could be a consequence.

The need to prove the theory that persons made ill by primary aerosol would not infect others by secondary aerosol was probably one of the main questions that led to the Battle of Tahoe-Truckee High School.

It is evident that disease agents developed in the years between 1970 and 1980 (MacArthur's ten year window) would still be governed by the policy enunciated by MacArthur: they must be infectious but not contagious. It is also evident that a wide variety of naturally occurring biological agents were being experimented with, including the incapacitants: rickettsia causing Q-fever; Rift Valley fever; Chikungunyn disease; and Venezuelan equine encephalitis; as well as lethal agents yellow fever; rabbit fever; anthrax; Psittacosis and the Plague. [Hearings, p.121]

It is to be noted that the above list of agents provided by MacArthur to the Congressmen does not include brucellosis, despite the fact that the latter was and had been the focus of research since the beginning. Why the oversight?

Dr. Peter Dale Scott's negative template hypothesis has provided a likely answer. There is much evidence that the Pentagon/CIA was never fully candid and complete in their dealings with Congress and this is a likely example of that tendency. It is also to be noted that MacArthur did not mention at any time the accomplishment reported in 1946 by George Merck: that the biowar researchers could isolate the bacterial toxin in crystalline form from its source. Certain details were evidently just too critical to publicize, even to Congress.

Thus, by the year 1980, it is reasonable to conclude from all of the hard, confirmed sources of data, that the Pentagon had a disabling weapon based upon a mutated form of the brucellosis bacteria. Distinguishing this pathogen from the brucellosis weapons that the Pentagon had already placed in inventory,[64] was the fact that rather than being based upon the whole bacteria, the 'new synthetic organism' was in crystalline form which, when reduced to an infinitely fine dust and combined with a simulant to provide more efficient diffusion, could infect its victims while leaving no hint as to the disease source.

Bacterial disease without the bacteria!

The victim of the bacterial disease would reveal no trace of the bacteria and hence could be told: 'Your sickness is all in your head.'

Whether this new agent would infect by primary aerosol but not be contagious by secondary aerosol remained to be determined. As Ed Regis has written in another context: "Naturally, it would have to be field tested".[65]

The Field Test

1980

How the military had gone about selecting sites for field testing new biological/chemical weapons on the 500,000 human guinea pigs that they have already admitted to we do not know. Nor can we know what brought them to the Tahoe-Truckee High School in 1984. We can, of course, deduce the broad general principles which would have guided them: a sufficient degree of isolation from major population areas (See above, Point vi) while retaining reasonable access to the site.

The High School, situated to serve Truckee, California, on interstate Highway 80 and Tahoe City on the north shore of Lake Tahoe met both criteria. The school in 1984 served some 600 students and had 35 teachers plus administrative staff. About 500 miles east along Highway 80 was Dugway Proving grounds in Utah which was the major biowar test site in North America, if not the world. This military installation would be a convenient logistical headquarters for activities for any biowar testing that might be conducted in Tahoe-Truckee.

1984

In the summer of 1984, as we have earlier noted,

a construction crew arrived at the high school and installed a new air conditioning/heating system. The new system had an unusual feature: each room was individually serviced by individual intake and exhaust ducts. This meant that the air in a room could be drawn to the air conditioner/furnace, cooled or heated, and then returned to the same room from which it had been drawn! In addition, the windows were all sealed shut and the staff was forbidden from opening them to get any fresh air! An arrangement such as this made it possible to feed a pathogen by primary aerosol directly to the occupants of a specific room, while the occupants of all the other rooms would be spared primary aerosol but would be subject to secondary aerosol.

Someone to Watch Over Me

The Tahoe-Truckee area had access to a number of doctors, but two in particular are important to our study: Dr. Dan Peterson and Dr. Paul Cheney who in 1984 were partners in a clinic in Incline Village, Nevada, a few miles east of the California/Nevada border on the north shore of Lake Tahoe.

Both doctors had received financial assistance

from the U.S. Government in their years of medical education, and both apparently owed a period of time equivalent to their years of training to the Government. That is to say, if the government had need of their services in some particular area for whatever reasonable purpose, both Peterson and Cheney were bound to accept the assignment.

Peterson, in what according to Hillary Johnson had been a 'gamble'[66] had settled in Incline Village in 1981. In 1983 he invited Cheney to join him. Thus, by 1984, just as Tahoe-Truckee High School was being re-equipt with an unusual heating system, two new doctors, both indebted to the U.S. Government, were on site in case some business should come their way, such as an outbreak of a mystery disease.

1985

When Tahoe-Truckee High School had re-opened in the Fall of 1984, eight teachers had found themselves assigned to a separate staff room. In this room, with its windows bolted shut and its air constantly recycled from the newly installed air conditioning/

1-2 PUNCH

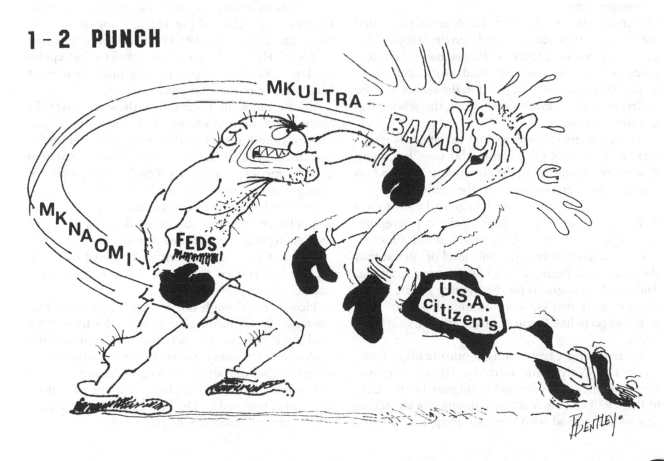

heating system, the teachers became aware of a distressing quality to the air. One of the teachers assigned to this staffroom decided that he would not use his workplace and parked a camper trailer a short distance from the school. Here he ate his lunches, marked his papers, prepared his lessons and took his coffee breaks.

At the end of the school year, seven of the teachers assigned to the small staffroom were ill with a 'mystery' disease which came to be known as CFIDS. Only one of the eight escaped: the teacher who had chosen to keep clear of the room.[67]

Was Flood or MacArthur Right?

MacArthur had stated his belief that only targets exposed to primary aerosol would become ill.

Congressman Flood had expressed doubt.

Congressman Flood was right! Even students who never entered the small staffroom became ill over the course of the school year. The pathogen was contagious by secondary aerosol...far more contagious than anyone had ever dreamed.

The Pentagon/CIA had let loose a new contagious plague: myalgic encephalomyelitis.

Consequences

The illness did not stop at the door to the sealed staffroom. Other teachers and certain students began to present with fever, weakness, nausea, fatigue, aches and pains, cognitive and emotional problems...although the focal point in the school was the staffroom under review, no one in the school was safe from illness.

There was also a growing number of family members of the school population who were becoming ill, and even members of the community who had no obvious link with anyone from the school.

The victims sought medical help, and many found their way to the Peterson-Cheney clinic. It is reported that persons attending the offices of other doctors in the area did not find the same level of interest that the patients of Peterson and Cheney were receiving. And slowly a diagnosis for the mystery disease began to emerge: it was chronic mononucleosis [68], or so the experts like Stephen Straus from CDC/NIH said.

Peterson and Cheney sought outside help...turning to Drs. Werner and Gertrude Henle, a German husband-wife team who had immigrated to the U.S. in the 1930's. This team was among the top scientists of the period who were studying the Epstein-Barr virus[69] which was implicated in Burkitt's lymphoma and mononucleosis. And, it is interesting to note, both Werner and Gertrude Henle had been members of the Kissinger-Nixon 'Great War of Cancer' under which so much biowar research had gone on. But no answers emerged. All of those concerned studied the symptoms which resembled those of chronic brucellosis, but none seemed to link that ancient disease with the new epidemic. Instead, most of the doctors continued their focus upon chronic mononucleosis...and that is passing strange.

What the Good Doctors Seemed to have Overlooked

In the July 27, 1944 issue of *The New England Journal of Medicine* there had appeared an editorial titled "Infectious Mononucleosis versus Brucellosis". The key sentence in the editorial read: "Because of the similarity in the clinical manifestations of undulant fever [another name for brucellosis-Ed.] and infectious mononucleosis, one may easily be confused with the other."

Despite the fact that the two diseases could present in almost exactly the same way, neither Peterson, Cheney, nor either of the Henle's appear to have asked themselves whether brucellosis might be the problem! How did two of the world's top epidemiology specialists happen to miss one of the most likely sources of the epidemic?

In the index to *Osler's Web* there are over 34 citations for mononucleosis, but not a single citation for brucellosis! How does it happen that one of two diseases, so similar as to warrant an editorial in one of America's leading medical journals, does not even get considered when the Tahoe-Truckee High School was hit by all of the common symptoms? How does it happen that the one disease fingered by people such as Stephen Straus turned out to be wrong?

Was it a case of not wanting to find brucellosis because it had been the subject of so much biowar research? Perhaps.

However, although not included as an *index* citation, a careful reading of *Osler's Web* turns up a significant reference to brucellosis. When another epidemic of a mystery disease bearing startling similarities to that of Tahoe-Truckee broke out in 1985 in Lyndonville, New York, the possibility of brucellosis was considered by Dr. Karen Bell, but, "Brucellosis tests were uniformly negative."[70]

Despite the fact that standard tests for brucellosis were negative,[71] Dr. David Bell (then husband of Karen) responded to the illness with treatment by doxycycline, a standard brucellosis remedy, and apparently experienced a good level of success.[72]

Thus, by the end of 1985 one of the major and most logical interpretations of the symptoms seen in Tahoe-Truckee patients, that the illness was somehow linked to chronic brucellosis, had never been investigated. The other interpretation (that the disease was infectious mononucleosis caused by the Epstein-Barr virus) before it gave way to more detailed study and " was finally put to rest"[73] in 1987 led most doctors away from brucellosis as a possible etiologic factor. The spin doctors, led by senior people in the Centers for Disease Control and National Institutes of Health, began their part in the Battle of Tahoe-Truckee High School: hiding the truth.

In the Beginning was Stephen Straus

Science, a weekly magazine published by the American Association for the Advancement of Science, presents its readers with a broad range of subjects as befits its title. After all, " science is that branch of knowledge or study dealing with a body of facts or truths systematically arranged and showing the operation of general laws".[74]

The technical articles appearing in *Science* appear to meet this criterion, but only very well-informed professionals can pass such judgement.

However, *Science* has another area of concern which one must broadly lable as 'editorial': "an article or statement in a newspaper or other medium presenting the opinion of the publisher, editor, or owner." [75] [See Chapter Seven]

Editorially, *Science* is one of the voices of the 'establishment'. This bias shows when it departs from science and wanders off into the realm of politics and power. Consider, for example, its treatment of Stephen Straus,[76] written by Eric Stokstad.

Stokstad's piece begins with the question "Why in the world would a respected researcher like Stephen Straus leave a topflight lab at the National Institutes of Health to run NIH's new National Center for Complementary and Alternative Medicine (NC-CAM)?

To begin a piece in a scientific journal with a rhetorical question is inappropriate since a rhetorical question is "...asked solely to produce an effect and not elicit a reply." [77] If Stokstad were worthy of publication in a journal titled *Science* and if he felt compelled to grab his readers' attention by opening with a question then he should have written: " Why has Stephen Straus accepted the job as Director of the National Center for Complementary and Alternative Medicine? " Expressions such as 'why in the world'; 'respected' ; 'topflight' are also rhetorical and reflect the writer's and his editor's desire to persuade readers of something and only introduce facts incidentally.

In a word, the piece under review reflects the fact that *Science* has a political agenda and Stokstad writes down to that level.

Stephen Straus may well be respected by someone, but to incorporate the adjective so blatantly belies the fact that Stephen Straus is held in very low regard by many who have had occasion to know his work reasonably well. He has proven himself to be unscientific (See definition above), dishonest, inconsistent, mean-spirited, and conceited.

Medical History According to Straus

In 1991, Straus, who was then with the Medical Virology Section, National Institutes of Allergy and Infectious Diseases, National Institutes of Health, released an article titled " History of Chronic Fatigue Syndrome."[78] He introduces his 'history' with an abstract:

"Chronic fatigue syndrome is not a new medical condition. For centuries its confusing array of features has been attributed to numerous environmental, metabolic, infectious, immunologic, and psychiatric disturbances. This is a review and critique of many of these alternative diagnoses, sufficient to provide a historical background for current thinking about the disorder."

Scientist Straus was moved to try his hand at history in response to the mystery disease that had hit so many staff and students at Tahoe-Truckee High School and their community, as well as thousands of citizens in other places such as Lyndonville, New York; the St. Lawrence Seaway Valley, Canada; Chapel Hill, North Carolina; and even as far away as West Otago, New Zealand.

At the time these and other places were hit by their particular epidemic, the disease was labelled a 'mystery'. However, by 1986 the Centers for Disease Control and the National Institutes of Health were working upon a 'case definition' that would de-mystify it. The best way to de-mystify the mystery was to deny it was new. Another way was to make it out to be something related to the victims' inability to cope with the ordinary stresses of life. Straus was an active participant in these efforts,[79] but one would never know it from his 'History'.

Despite the fact (which should according to the definition of 'science' be accorded pride of place) that the victims of the various epidemics presented with a protean range of symptoms just as brucellosis presents with such a range, Straus and his collaborators came up with a case definition and a name which was based solely upon one aspect of the disease: fatigue. This is extremely misleading and fails that other quality of 'science' in that it is not the truth. The disease was labelled by the dismissive title: Chronic Fatigue Syndrome.

An analogy will illustrate the insidious dishonesty of such a label: "Christopher Columbus was an explorer who discovered Watling's Island". Yes, Columbus did indeed discover Watling's Island, but he also discovered Antigua, Barbuda, the Bahamas, San Salvador, Costa Rica...in a word America. Lies are told by telling less than what is true as much as telling more than what is true, and Stephen Straus is insidiously adept at both extremes.

It is to be emphasized that fatigue is a symptom of a wide range of diseases: lupus, sarcoidosis, Lyme's , multiple sclerosis and many others. When Straus picks this one characteristic of the epidemics of the 1980's, and treats it as if it were the only characteristic the victims were suffering from, he is insidiously dishonest. He emphasizes his distortion by the use of definite articles and demonstrative pronouns such as 'its' and 'it' and 'the' and 'this'.

Then Straus introduces another of his insidious themes: 'Mannington noted...the (!) syndrome [was] most prevalent among women of wealthy families and those who are sedentary and studious'. He repeats the theme further along in reference to 'DaCosta's Syndrome' which he has identified as another earlier diagnosis of 'the' syndrome. He writes :"...there was a twofold to threefold preponderance of women and a preponderance among those engaged in light work rather than in the manual trades."

One cannot require 'historian' Straus to be aware of the fact that certain serological diseases only present when a critical concentration of a pathogen is achieved;[80] and, since women have about 20 percent less blood per pound of weight than men

and since they also have 20-25 percent less haemoglobin than men the critical level of concentration will be achieved about 4 to 6 times faster than men. An 'historian' cannot be expected to know that, but certainly a 'scientist' can be expected to know it. Especially a scientist who is Head of Medical Virology.

Again, Straus is being a liar. He knows full well why women become ill from certain diseases faster than men from the same diseases, but it helps him achieve his rhetorical point to let on that this syndrome is not a real illness, it is simply a manifestation of the 'weaker sex' being unable to cope with the harsh realities of life.

Back to Brucellosis

Straus' next heading: "Chronic Brucellosis" is almost startling. Straus, as a senior member of the administration of the National Institutes of Health that had co-operated for several years with the military/CIA researchers into biological warfare weapons development undoubtedly knew that brucellosis had been one of the two first disease pathogens weaponized by the Army. He would also know that as early as 1946 the researchers had learned how to isolate the toxin from that bacteria in a crystalline form. Straus would also be in the loop when it came time to test a crystalline brucella toxin to learn whether it could be targeted at a small group of a larger whole to determine whether it was contagious by secondary aerosol, as well as by primary aerosol.

So, when Straus starts a section of his 'history' with 'Chronic Brucellosis' one must for a wild, unreasoning moment wonder: Is he going to tell the world the truth at last?

Such was not to be. In his account he doesn't appear to remember that brucellosis had been the earliest disease of choice by the biowar researchers; he does not appear to remember that it was one of the first disease agents weaponized; his memory also fails him when he entirely overlooks the fact that several laboratory workers had become ill with the disease, even though they had been vaccinated and wore protective clothes and goggles and worked behind airproof screens. None of these facts, which scientist Straus was used to working with, is noted by historian Straus.

Instead, Straus refers to several early researchers into the subject of brucellosis and he almost gets some of their work correctly reported. Until, that is, he refers to a study at Johns Hopkins whose researchers had studied several persons ill with acute brucella infections and had concluded that those who had developed 'chronic' brucellosis did so because they were not quite well in the head.

When Straus reports this startling phenomenon recognized by the Johns Hopkins researchers, he (typically) neglects to mention that: (i) Johns Hopkins had had twelve contracts to help develop biowar weapons between 1951 and 1970[81]

(ii) Johns Hopkins had had three major contracts in the Special Virus Cancer Program or Nixon's 'war on cancer' which is now seen by many researchers as having been the cover under which the AIDS and ME/FM pathogens were developed

(iii) Straus neglects to mention that the chronically ill victims were all laboratory workers at Fort Detrick, Frederick, MD who had been working on developing brucellosis as a biological weapon

(iv) Straus also neglects to mention that the Johns Hopkins research was paid under the Defense Appropriations Budget, just like the Budget approved on June 9, 1969. The contract number was DA 18- 064- 404- CML-100.

One can scarcely expect a cohort in a crime to come up with an investigative report that implicates the criminals. The Johns Hopkins research team on behalf of themselves and the CDC/NIH monitors of biowar weapons research testing by the military/CIA were brushing away their own footprints in the snow. For Straus to cite their 'research' as proof that such epidemics were 'no more prevalent now' than they ever had been is another insidious distortion of the facts.

Obviously, Straus was as good an historian as he had proven himself to be as a scientist when he was supposed to be researching Tahoe-Truckee High School and other such epidemics.

Straus the Scientist

Writer Eric Stokstad of Science, who believes Straus is 'respected' but doesn't say by whom, also believes that:

"Straus, 53, has the kind of training necessary to get answers. During his 23 years at the National Institute of Allergy and Infectious diseases (NIAID) - including 8 years as chief of the Laboratory of Clinical Investigation - Straus has investigated a range of diseases, a track record that earned him the respect of NIH institute [sic] directors, Varmus says."[82]

Question: Does 'investigating' a range of diseases establish a track record, or does finding answers for the problems investigated establish a track record?

Stokstad may have some list of Straus investigative successes which are not available to the public for reasons of national security, for there is little that the average researcher can find of the 'track record' that has earned him the respect of NIH directors.

Straus was one of the key investigators of the epidemics of ME/FM and in 20 years he can show nothing for his efforts. (This may well answer Stokstad's opening question...See above.) He did come up with the Epstein-Barr hypothesis which had soon fallen apart. Thereafter, he concentrated his skills upon two key points: He claimed:(1) there is really no disease at all; and,(2) what disease there is derives from stress felt by middle aged women who are under-achieving in their professional careers.

In fact, unless (apparently) one is an NIH director, an objective observer might be justified in concluding that Straus is a very poor scientist. Byron Hyde was sitting next to Straus at a 1987 meeting when a paper demonstrating some of the flaws in Straus' theory of EBV etiology for ME/FM was handed out. Hyde describes it this way:

"Straus began talking to himself out loud as the scientific purport of the paper sank in... He held a monologue that lasted at least two minutes...I thought he was having a nervous breakdown. He kept saying, 'They've ruined me. What will my colleagues think? These goddamn patients!' He seemed to be taking it personally, and talked as if the patients had banded together to destroy him."[83]

Conflicts Of Interest

Dr. Donald MacArthur of the Pentagon had made it very clear to the twelve Congressmen whom he had briefed on June 9,1969 about the military/CIA plans to develop two new pathogens: one to disable (ME/FM) and one to kill (AIDS), that any tests would be monitored by the public health agencies: the Centers for Disease Control and the National Institutes of Health.[84]

Stephen Straus worked for the latter.

As a consequence, the government agency that should investigate any mystery epidemic would be aware of any links that epidemic might have with tests conducted by the military/CIA.

A clear and totally unprincipled conflict of interest.

A Trashy Soap Opera

There are other examples in the literature of Stephen Straus playing on both sides of the net at the same time. One such example can be found in his work to solve the mystery of AIDS in which he has as poor an achievement record as he has in his study of ME/FM.

In 1986 the Burroughs Wellcome Pharmaceutical firm had come up with a drug which they claimed would arrest the development of the disease in AIDS-infected people. In their research they had employed Straus on a part-time basis, and then after some near-catastrophic tests they applied to have it approved by the FDA's Anti-Infective Drugs Advisory Committee on January 16, 1987.

On that critical morning, Burroughs Wellcome turned up to present their case to the Committee and lo and behold...sitting there in judgement of a drug he had been paid to help develop was none other than Dr. Stephen Straus! As Bruce Nussbaum was later to put it:

> *"All this was very strange. In the world of Big Science, one of the major rules was that a scientist who had received money from a drug company to run tests on its drugs would generally not be permitted to sit on a committee reviewing that company."[85]*

But that didn't keep Straus from supporting the application. Apparently at this stage of his career, he had not yet developed the 'scientific principles' which, according to Eric Stokstad, had gained him 'credibility and stature'.[86] Others saw it in a different light. One scientist deeply involved in AIDS research, would call what happened on that January morning evidence that 'science really is nothing but a trashy soap opera.'[87]

Another scientist, Michael Lange, declared that "AIDS was the most politicized disease " he had ever seen."[88]

Politicized!

Which brings us back to ME/FM which had also been a subject of Straus's peculiar kind of science. Quoting from Hillary Johnson's magnificent *Osler's Web:*

> *"Some suspected that there were darker reasons for Straus's shift, having to do with the government's need to soft-pedal the disease...Commented one [ME/FM] sufferer who was among Straus's tiny patient cohort in Bethesda: 'This is exactly what happened to AIDS patients. It becomes necessary to psychologize this disease to make us an 'other'.*

> *This is not a medical event; this is a political event.'"[89]*

How marvellously intuitive!

A patient, looking desperately for help with his disease, had fallen into Straus's web, and had come to perceive all the essentials of what was going on: the linkage between ME/FM and AIDS as revealed in Dr. MacArthur's June 9,1969 briefing of the Congressmen; the government's efforts to 'soft-pedal' [ie cover-up] the truth about the tests that they would have to do; and, Straus's insidious political role that removed the latter's efforts from the realm of medicine to the realm of political propaganda.

Straus the Accountant

In 1991, Congress had voted six million dollars to investigate chronic fatigue syndrome.[90] Of this amount $946,225 was being orchestrated by principal investigator Straus. Investigations at the time revealed that approximately two million dollars of the money voted by Congress was missing!

Apparently Straus was as skilled an accountant as he was a scientist and historian. Neither he nor anyone else at CDC/NIH could say where one third of their budget had gone.

As if that were not bad enough, of the money that was accounted for, most of it went to a psychiatric study designed to prove that ME/FM victims were mentally not physically ill:

> *"It is of interest that, in the recent $6,000,000 NIH funding to ME/CFIDS research, not one penny was allotted to an investigation of the retroviral theory. Curiously, one of the three grants went to a specialist in stress."[91]*

Enter Brian Mahy, or "Who stole the tarts"

> *"As Alice said this, she looked up, and there was the Cat again, sitting on a branch of a tree.*
> *"Did you say 'pig' or 'fig'?" said the Cat.*
> *"I said 'pig'," replied Alice; "and I wish you wouldn't keep appearing and vanishing so suddenly: you make one quite giddy!"*
> *"All right, "said the Cat; and this time it vanished quite slowly, beginning with the end of the tail, and ending with the grin, which remained some time after the rest of it had gone."[92]*

There is an Alice in Wonderland quality about the CDC/NIH, only instead of the Cheshire-Cat appearing and vanishing it is the money voted by Congress to investigate Chronic Fatigue Syndrome.

As noted above (Straus the Accountant), as far back as 1991 the Centers for Disease Control had problems handling money. In that year, Congress had voted $6,000,000 to study the terrible disease that was taking an increasing toll among American citizens.

Two million of that appropriation vanished without a trace, and of the remaining four million, a major portion was allotted by the CDC to a study of stress in CFIDS patients.

Like the Cheshire-Cat, over the next few years money appeared by vote of Congress to study the disease and then it vanished. In 1996 Hillary Johnson spelled out the reality of CDC dishonesty in careful detail.[93]

Johnson's data became the basis for a letter from Congressman Jerrold Nadler to Secretary of Health and Human Services, Donna E. Shalala. The Congressman focussed upon certain scientific questions rather than financial questions, but the evidence in Osler's Web made it clear that the neglect of actual scientific data was largely due to under-funding of the research.[94] If, as seems likely, Secretary Shalala had neglected to read Johnson's book, one could understand her weak response. However, Shalala's response is a two page re-hash of the CDC/NIH official position with no evidence whatsoever that the Secretary had extended any personal effort to fulfill her official duties and it reeks of dishonesty. For example, Ms. Shalala reports that "CDC has been unable to confirm the occurrence of a cluster of CFS cases"!

Had no one thought to tell her about Los Angeles General Hospital; Tahoe-Truckee High School; Lyndonville, New York and other such clusters?

Apparently giving up on the Secretary of Health and Human Services, Congressman Nadler directed a follow-up request to The General Accounting Office on September 4,1996. The follow-up consisted of nine critical questions concerning the abysmal failure of the Department of Health and Human Services to investigate real scientific evidence about CFIDS which was being neglected by the 'scientists' under Shalala's oversight. To date, the GAO has not provided any reasonable and convincing explanation.

Secretary Shalala, during her tenure, had demonstrated the same level of ineffective control over the likes of Stephen Straus and Brian Mahy as the Queen

of Hearts exercised over the Cheshire-Cat. And the money kept on vanishing...

Until, that is, August 13, 1998, 17:46 EDT

William Reeves is a balding, bearded scientist, who on the above date was and still is, the Director of the Viral Exanthems and Herpesvirus Branch of the Division of Viral and Rickettsial Diseases. As such, Reeves was 'directly responsible for CDC's chronic fatigue syndrome (CFS) research program'.

On the date cited, Reeves addressed a news conference that he had called and, under the protection of the Whistle Blower Act, declared that his boss, Brian Mahy, had improperly misused money that had been voted by Congress to research chronic fatigue syndrome and his successor had lied to Congress to cover up Mahy's actions. Reeves provided all the details necessary to substantiate his charges, and June Gibbs Brown, Inspector General for the Department of Health and Human Services was asked to conduct an audit.

Ms. Gibbs Brown reported on May 10, 1999 that Congress had voted $23,409,000 between 1995 and 1998 to research chronic fatigue syndrome. She also reported that of that amount, $9.8 million (42 percent) was actually spent on what might by rather generous criteria be regarded as 'Acceptable Charges'. However, almost as much, $8.8 million (39 percent) of the expenditures were "Unacceptable" (ie 'misappropriated'). The balance of $4.1 million (18 percent) had simply vanished.[95]

The auditor also determined that Brian Mahy's cohorts and successor had lied to Congress:

"The CDC provided inaccurate and potentially misleading information to Congress concerning the scope and cost of CFS research activities."[96]

Then came the auditor's remarkable finding: the misappropriation of money voted by Congress to look for the cause of and cure for a terrible and tragic disease which has destroyed and continues to destroy the lives of millions of Americans and the cover-up lies that followed the misappropriations were due to..."Ineffective Internal Controls"![97]

Science New-Speak

As we saw above (Straus the Scientist) Science writers and editors have a way with words. Stephen Straus whose research into AIDS had probably done more harm than good, and whose research into ME/FM had gone barking up the Epstein-Barr tree until he was proven wrong and whose foray into history is dishonest, distorted and insidious, was found by writer Erik Stokstad to be "respected", and "receptive to new ideas and scientific rigour"

In January, 2000, Science turned its attention to the Brian Mahy fraud and lies, and writer Martin Enserink makes it all sound, well, almost virtuous. Enserink even quotes a former CDC researcher, Jack Woodall, to the effect that:

> *"Of course you shouldn't break the rules. But I'm sure [Mahy] did what he thought was in the best interest of public health."[98]*

In a letter to the Editor two weeks later, a reader tries to set the record straight. John H. Gagnon, Emeritus Professor of Sociology, State University of New York wrote as follows:

"Misallocation of CDC Funds"

According to the Centers for Disease Control and Prevention (CDC), the reason for the misallocation of $8.8 million (plus another $4.1 million that is impossible to trace) mandated by Congress for the study for chronic fatigue syndrome is because some 'brilliant scientists' are 'not very good managers'. But the use of this 'dizzy scientist' stereotype by the CDC as an explanation seems to be an attempt to conceal what is a more serious problem - a government scientist apparently arrogating to himself the choice of what is to be studied after Congress decided otherwise. That the acting director of the CDC provided Congress, in the words of the inspector general of the Department of Health and Human Services, with 'inaccurate and potentially misleading' information supports this view. The fundamental problem is the tension between 'experts' and elected officials, and the publics they represent, about what is or is not an important health problem.

"What makes this report more troubling is that William Reeves, the whistle-blower, is the one who appears to be in trouble with the CDC, rather than the administrator-scientist who misallocated the funds to the acting director who misled Congress or its representatives. Perhaps the scientific community could hear more about what administrative and personnel actions the CDC and other federal health agencies are taking to clarify the difference between the authority to select appropriate scientific problems and the authority to select appropriate scientific procedures to study those problems."[99]

Professor Gagnon has made a couple of valid points, but has missed some others. First, when he speaks of 'experts' and elected officials and the 'publics' they represent, he is putting the personnel of the CDC on the same footing as the Congress. This is wrong. The 'experts' are employees of the government which derives its authority from the one and only 'public' which chooses its representatives in duly authorized elections. It is the very essence of democracy.

When the duly elected representatives of the public direct how the public money is to be spent, the hired employees are bound to spend it according to the directions they receive.

Furthermore, Professor Gagnon failed to comment upon the editorializing such as that in a "News" column by the writer of the piece and the editors of *Science*. For example: "Indeed, some researchers both within and outside CDC say that there may well have been sound scientific reasons to emphasize diseases known to be infectious rather than something as elusive as CFS." This specious argument is not news, it is a rationalization of a dishonest action, and ranks with comments such as "He may well have had a good reason to beat his wife." And, if something is 'elusive', it merits more attention, not less.

But the fundamental problem is this: the public health services of the United States are a power unto themselves, and do not see themselves as serving the people of the United States, but serving 'some darker reasons...having to do with the government's need to soft-pedal the disease.' And, it is the responsibility of journals such as *Science* to employ 'a prose of reportorial calm' such as that employed by Hillary Johnson when she reported upon her nine year study of CFIDS, rather than serve as a propaganda asset for the powers of darkness.

Chronological Summary Of The United States Biowar Research

1942: Canada, Great Britain and the United States enter into a tripartite agreement to research, develop and test biological weapons. Their principal bacterial agents of choice were the species of brucellosis bacteria.

1945: At the end of World War Two the three Allies agreed to continue their secret biowar research.

The United States secretly reached a deal with

Japanese war criminals who had used Allied prisoners-of-war as guinea pigs to test bio weapons. The criminals would be spared a war crimes trial in return for their sharing what they had learned about biological warfare with the United States.

1946: George Merck, head of biowar research in the U.S. reported to the Secretary of Defense that U.S. researchers had managed to isolate the bacterial disease toxin in crystalline form. In effect, the disease could be isolated like a teaspoon of salt while the rest of the bacteria could be discarded. A person could be infected with brucellosis without ever encountering a brucella bacteria.

With the new pathogen isolated from its bacterial antecedent new delivery systems could be developed such as aerosol diffusion, introduction into food supplies such as goat's milk; contaminated insect vectors; and others.

Testing of the new pathogens was undertaken in various sites, including Akureyri, Iceland; Lakeland, Florida; Chestnut Lodge Hospital, Rockville, Maryland; and Seward, Alaska.

Bjorn Sigurdsson, a Rockefeller protege, began studies of visna/maedi, a lentivirus antecedent to Creutzfeldt-Jakob/Kuru/and AIDS.

American Biowar researchers de-brief Japanese Biowar researchers. Learn of test-site activities in 1942 in New Guinea. Later an epidemic of Creutzfeldt-Jakob ravaged the isolated Fore tribe in the region. The Fore tribe called the disease 'kuru'.[100]

1957: D. Carleton Gajdusek, a graduate of Rochester School of Medicine whose education had been paid for by the U.S. military and who had agreed to serve equivalent time on 'military assignment', turned up in New Guinea where he studied the outbreak of Creutzfeldt-Jakob disease among the Fore tribe. Found 'scrapie-like' features.

1965: Dharam Ablashi, a veterinarian, later an expert on ME/FM, and Paul Levine, another future ME/FM expert, turn up in Africa, trying to infect chimpanzees with a variety of human diseases including herpes saimiri, Burkitt's lymphoma and sarcoma. The program continued for three years under the supervision of Robert Gallo who would later 'discover' the AIDS virus. Before the program ended, it also involved Carleton Gajdusek

who tried to infect chimpanzees with Creutzfeldt-Jakob disease. It is not clear what all of this very unusual activity meant but by...

1968: Dr. Donald A. Henderson agreed to serve the World Health Organization (WHO) in a vaccination campaign to eradicate smallpox. Millions of Black Africans (among others) were inoculated. Five years later the first cases of AIDS had begun to appear on a sporadic basis.

1969: Dr. Donald MacArthur reported to Congress that the military/CIA researchers were ready to move to a more dramatic level of weapons development. Based upon tests which had been conducted in as yet unrevealed locations but which would fit with the locations of the here-to-fore 'mystery diseases' locations, two new pathogens could be developed: one to disable and one to kill...a division which corresponds to the ME/FM and AIDS outbreaks. Of course MacArthur did not explain how the researchers knew what they knew (from testing and their activities in Africa inoculating chimpanzees) and the Congressmen did not ask. Evidence is suggestive that the Pentagon/CIA were simply bringing the Congress into the 'loop'; that the AIDS pathogen was already a reality needing only an official blessing, and the ME/FM pathogen was being fine-tuned to be disabling but not lethal. According to MacArthur, the latter task 'was not easy.'

Congress voted the budget requests and the development of the ME/FM pathogen and the AIDS pathogen continued.

1971: Nixon 'declared war on cancer'. Established the 'Special Virus Cancer Program'. Now seen as the 'cover story' under which the continuation of research into ME/FM and AIDS could be carried out. Major work done by Werner and Gertrude Henle, Robert Gallo, Dharam Ablashi, L. Dmochowski, R.V. Gilden, Y.Ito, Paul Levine and others.

1974: Henry Kissinger submitted National Security Study Memorandum 200 to President Nixon and Joint Chiefs of Staff. Made population growth rate a matter of national security. Urged action to address the 'population problem'.

1977: Test on Stock Island, Florida of ME/FM pathogen; however, a large number of victims presented with multiple sclerosis and the pathogen was deemed too lethal to serve as a 'disabling' biological weapon.

1978: Four year hiatus during Carter Administration when activities were somewhat curtailed, but not totally abandoned. SVCP cancelled.(It appears that Republican administrations [Nixon, Ford, Reagan, Bush] are more inclined to such covert biowar enterprises, although individual Senators and Congressmen cannot be so categorized. Senator Reigle of Michigan, a Republican, was one of the best friends the Gulf War Veterans had. Congressman Robert Filner of California, a Democrat, is one of the most committed supporters of justice for CFIDS/GWI victims.)

1980: Program of bio-weapons development re-invigorated with election of Ronald Reagan. Vice-President Bush and CIA Director William Casey 'in the loop' and supporting the program.

1981: Dr. Daniel Peterson took a 'gamble' and established a medical practice in Incline Village, near Tahoe-Truckee High School.

1983: Dr. Peterson recruited Dr. Paul Cheney to come to Incline Village, continuing 'gamble' that business would pick up. Both Dr. Peterson and Dr. Cheney had their medical education paid by the U.S. government and had agreed to serve an equivalent time where ever they were assigned on government duty. Cheney still had three and one half years on his contract with the military. Cheney stayed in Incline Village for three and one half years!

1984: Test at Tahoe-Truckee for primary aerosol diffusion of ME/FM pathogen. Among first persons consulted by Drs. Peterson and Cheney were some from the Nixon SVCP, especially the Henles, Dharam Ablashi and Paul Levine.

Test at Lyndonville, New York, for goat milk vector.

Test in St. Lawrence Seaway area, Ontario, Canada for mosquito vector, with co-operation of Canadian Military elements.

1985: Stephen Straus publishes E-B/psychosomatic dis-information.

1986: First shipments of brucella bioweapon components sold to Iraq by the U.S. Also shipped West Nile Fever virus.[101]

1987: Dr. Paul Cheney relocated from Incline Village to North Carolina. Strongly suggestive that he was in Incline Village as a military monitor of the Tahoe-Truckee High School tests that went dreadfully wrong.

1991: Iraq employed brucella-derived mycoplasma in SCUD-missile attack. Forced a halt to Desert Storm attack.

Gulf War Veterans begin to present with ME/FM now labelled "Gulf War Syndrome". U.S./British/Canadian military begin cover-up by claiming symptoms were "all in the head".

1992: Propaganda asset, Edward Shorter, published From Paralysis to Fatigue, continuing and embellishing Straus dis-information.

1993: Professor Garth Nicolson and Professor Nancy Nicolson of the University of Texas in Houston and of the M.D. Anderson Cancer Center began study of bacterial particle mycoplasma in Gulf War Veterans.

1994: Senator Reigle released his 'Report' which revealed sales of brucella components to Iraq. Links brucella to ME/FM with following quotation from the Report: "Brucella Melitensis: a bacteria which can cause chronic fatigue, loss of appetite, profuse sweating when at rest, pain in joints and muscles, insomnia, nausea, and damage to major organs." [Page 266] Note dramatic similarity to the 'mystery epidemics', ME/FM and GWI!

Professor Garth Nicolson fired from M.D. Anderson Center for publishing evidence of mycoplasma infection in Gulf War Veterans and Chronic Fatigue Syndrome victims.

1995: Congress votes $22.7 million for CFIDS research. Brian Mahy head of the Division of Viral and Rickettsial Diseases fraudulently diverts large part of these funds for other purposes. Transactions kept secret.

1998: William Reeves of the CDC reveals under Whistle Blower Act protection Brain Mahy's fraud.

1999: Pentagon forced to initiate mycoplasma test

protocol treatment of Gulf War Veterans, using Garth and Nancy Nicolson protocols.

2000: Dr. Charles Engel, head of Gulf War Veterans mycoplasma study suggests that "...mycoplasmas are the probable cause of Chronic Fatigue Syndrome and Fibromyalgia."[102]

SUMMARY

Within the daunting constraints imposed by the fact that so much of the material dealt with in this study has been zealously hidden from public view by the military/CIA/and the public health services of the United States, we have attempted to discover and report the salient facts about the advent of ME/FM and AIDS, with an emphasis on the former.

In addition to attempts to hide the facts of what has been going on since (and undoubtedly prior to) 1934 when Dr. James P. Leake of the United States Public Health Service wanted to keep the facts about the 1934 Los Angeles County Hospital Epidemic secret, until 1995 when Dr. Brian Mahy diverted research money away from solving the mystery of CFIDS, the CDC/NIH and the U.S./Canadian military have engaged in a planned and persistent program of dis-information through their media assets.

Despite these constraints, and by virtue of seven years of almost single-minded research, we have managed to draw together from several sources the data we cite herein.

We have made as much effort as our limited research resources would permit to ensure that the data are correct. We have interviewed Dr. Gajdusek and Dr. Shorter. We attempted to interview Dr. Showalter but were rudely hung-up on. We have written and faxed Drs. Peterson and Cheney but have received no replies.

From the data that we have located, we have drawn the following inferences which we state in as straight-forward a manner as we can:

1. The so-called mystery disease epidemics since 1934 were to a very large extent if not entirely, the consequences of tests being conducted by (first) private, wealthy interests epitomized by the Rockefeller empire; (second) by wartime generated research for biological weapons development drawing upon much of the earlier, private research; (third) by peacetime continued co-operation between the United States, Great Britain and Canada.

2. The program of biological weapons development (with the testing which that carried with it) had been secretly supported for many years by Congressional funds with certain key persons intimately involved. However, it was not until the election in 1968 of Richard Nixon and his appointment of Henry Kissinger as head of the National Security Council that the use of new pathogens developed by the military/CIA with constant monitoring by the public health services, that ME/FM and AIDS were officially integrated into National Security efforts. AIDS was to be used as a strategic weapon in 'lesser developed countries' while ME/FM *may* have become epidemic in error (which we doubt). Dr. MacArthur had assured twelve Congressmen in 1969 that such a disabling weapon would be 'infective by primary aerosol but not contagious by secondary aerosol.' Perhaps he knew better, but didn't want to alarm the Congressmen.

3. Testing was a necessary part of the development of the CFIDS pathogen and we infer from our studies that Tahoe-Truckee High School was one test site and that Drs. Peterson and Cheney were military/CIA monitors put on site to evaluate the consequences.[103]

4. Because of their role in monitoring and later in active research into the CFIDS pathogen certain key personnel in the Health and Human Services Department have wittingly participated in covering up the reality of the disease. This includes Dr. Brian Mahy and helps explain why he diverted money voted by Congress from the study of Chronic Fatigue Syndrome. He and others cannot afford to have the truth discovered.

5. Because of their role in supplying Iraq with both the disabling weapons components and also many lethal biological agents such as anthrax, the military and President George Bush, Sr. and his Secretary of Defense, Richard Cheney, had to participate in the cover-up of the Gulf War Illnesses reality.

6. Because of their role in developing and testing of the ME/FM pathogen, the public health services of the United States, especially the CDC and the NIH have had to mask the reality of the initial epidemics and then of the on-going spread of the disease throughout North America and other parts of the world. Their first line of defense was to be the 'its all in their head' thesis. This myth could be maintained for several years because the crystalline bacterial toxin could infect a victim without leaving any evidence of the bacterial source.

7. Today the CDC estimates that approximately 800,000 Americans are ill with CFIDS. From our research we infer that this figure is too low. By personal observation and research, we suggest that at least one percent of the American public suffers from ME/FM. This means about 2,560,000 are disabled to some degree. The disability can range from mild to severe. Among the tasks assigned by Congress to Brian Mahy was that of determining the full extent of the disaster. To date the CDC has defied the direction from Congress, quite likely because of a desire to keep the full extent of the disaster hidden.

8. Although ME/FM is the principal form, numbers wise, in which the disease presents, we infer, based upon seven years of study, that other neuro/systemic degenerative diseases such as multiple sclerosis, Crohn's-colitis, Parkinson's, Alzheimer's and bi-polar depression are caused by the same pathogen. The disease presents differently in different victims due to varying patterns of genetic pre-disposition. We are constantly amazed to find a family where, for example, the mother will have CFIDS, the father Parkinson's and the daughter multiple sclerosis.

The pathogen has been present for centuries as the bacterial toxin of the various species of brucellosis, and the diseases have also been present. For example, neurobrucellosis in the lateral ventricles appears to share so many characteristics that it may well be a variant of or even the fore-runner of multiple sclerosis. At this point in our research, we theorized that the human immune system had evolved to cope with such challenges. Then, when the bacterial toxin was isolated in a crystalline form and diffused by aerosol or other more concentrated routes, we concluded that the immune system could not cope to the same extent that it had coped with the bacteria. Further, we believed, when the bacteria was mutated with the visna/maedi virus a greater range of brain damage ensued, presenting as cognitive dysfunction and emotional lability.

We were wrong! As we will demonstrate in Chapter Fifteen, long hidden information became available to us which demonstrated the truth.

9. From the family constellations of disease that we have studied, we infer that all of these disease presentations are contagious. However, one will not necessarily become ill unless one has a genetic pre-disposition; one's immune system is compromised; and, (usually) one experiences a trauma. Because so many people are initially infected by secondary aerosol, the lungs are a focal point and present with respiratory distress syndrome, sarcoidosis, atypical pneumonia, Wegener's disease, atypical asthma, etc.

Also involved in the initial stages of illness are the nasal passages and the salivary, submandibular, parotid and sublingual glands. In a word, the nasopharynx area. There is also compelling evidence that the pathogen plays a role in causing cancer.[104]

Following the initial infection which is usually improperly responded to, secondary and tertiary levels of damage occur, which must be addressed independently. If, in its earliest stages, the disease is responded to with vigour and a minocycline protocol, it may well be stopped at that first stage.

10.Finally, we infer that if our principal hypothesis in correct, then the illnesses can best be responded to by seeking to contain the inciting pathogen, rather than by responding to the symptoms. And, if the pathogen is indeed derived from the bacterial disease toxin it can hopefully be limited by certain antibiotics such as the minocycline/doxycycline protocols noted above.

Credo

We believe that the human family has endured a grievous assault from powerful people utilizing scientific knowledge to achieve misguided and illicit ends: more power and control even of the growth of the world's population.

The leadership in this great crime against humanity has derived from those who control the wealth of the western world and all which follows that state: the control of the media; the control of the political leaders; the control of the governmental bureaucracies; and the control of the military/CIA.

We believe that only if the full story of what has gone on in the name of 'national security' and 'population growth rate control' is told, it will be extremely difficult if not impossible to find the answers needed to stop the ravages of ME/FM and AIDS and the related epidemics of multiple sclerosis, Parkinson's, etc.

Further, we believe that since the crimes have been so horrid and the consequences so tragic and the effects so wide spread, only a full disclosure through the medium of an undertaking along the lines of the South African Truth and Reconciliation Commission will ever allow humanity to recover from the effects of these terrible seven decades.

Such a Commission will allow those who have

committed these great crimes to share all of their secrets with us, and so allow our scientists, liberated from the tyranny of evil money controlled by the tyranny of evil bureaucrats, to follow up on the answers to ME/FM and AIDS which we reveal in Chapter Fifteen, and so allow each human being to enjoy a greater level of health than he or she might otherwise be able to achieve.

Then, more of our human genius and our human energy and our human love can be directed towards attaining a garden for human growth here on earth.

But it must all start with facing up to reality and requiring that the truth be told.

Please do not say 'I believe that this is indeed what has happened' or 'I do not believe that this is what happened.'

It is not a matter of faith, but a matter of evidence. Until all evidence has been fully presented and carefully evaluated, please suspend your decision.

Footnotes

{1} When the authors began their search for answers to Diane Martel's 'mystery' illness, we early concluded that it was somehow related to the ancient disease, brucella melitensis. However, this conclusion had been a working hypothesis. At the time of the present writing, we have now the advantage of genomic probe sequencing, and our hypothesis is confirmed. "It would appear that the specific probe for M.fermentans also reacts with Brucella melitensis..." redflagsweekly.com 3/18/02 p.4.

Endnotes

[1]. Henderson, Donald A., M.D. and Alexis Shelokov, M.D."Epidemic Neuromyasthenia- Clinical Syndrome? [conclusion]. Re-printed in : Byron Hyde, (Editor) (Ottawa, The Nightingale Foundation: *The Clinical and Scientific Basis of Myalgic Encephalomyelitis/Chronic Fatigue Syndrome,* 1992) p.173

[2]. "Mystery illness kills intravenous drug users". *The Toronto Star* (Friday, June 9,2000)

[3]. For an overview of the Los Angeles epidemic you are referred to a review chapter written by Dr. Byron Hyde of the Nightingale Foundation in The Clinical and Scientific Basis of Myalgic Encephalomyelitis (Editor Dr. Hyde and published in Ottawa by the Nightingale Foundation, 1992) pp.119-128

[4]. Hyde, *Ibid,* p.120

[5]. S.C. Man, MD. *Fibromyalgia* (Winnipeg; Henderson Books, 1998) p.37

[6]. Because of the protean range of symptoms in the mystery disease, finding a satisfying name for the illness has posed a challenge for many years. Indeed, it has been called 'the disease of a thousand names'. It is now generally accepted that the name 'chronic fatigue syndrome' was conjured up by the CDC/NIH and their cohorts as a 'put-down' name to discourage a sympathetic response to the ill victims. In Canada and Great Britain the terms 'myalgic encephalomyelitis' and 'fibromyalgia' have gained favour as being more scientific and less dismissive than chronic fatigue syndrome.

[7]. L.Garry Adams; *Advances in Brucellosis Research.* (College Station, Texas: Texas A & M University Press, 1990) pp.470-495

[8]. Johnson; *Ibid,* p.206

[9]. John Hanchette (Gannett New Service) "Gulf vets, Parkinson's linked". Rochester; *Democrat and Chronicle* (Sept. 17, 2000)

[10]. Hyde, *Ibid,* p.704

[11]. Carleton Gajdusek; Nobel Lecture, December 13, 1976 Bethesda, MD., National Institutes of Health

[12]. "Animal virus is linked to origin of AIDS" Associated Press *Herald* (Jan.4, 1985)

[13]. "A Polio-like Epidemic in Iceland" British Medical Journal (April, 1951) pp.934-5

[14]. Some of the links may be completely innocent and of a purely coincidental nature. For example, Fort Detrick, Maryland, the principal location of U.S. biowar installations after 1943, was named after Major Frederick L. Detrick who graduated as a medical doctor from none other than the Rockefeller Institute, New York City. See: Norman M. Covert, *The Cutting Edge* (Maryland: Fort Detrick 1997) p.9

[15]. Collier, Peter and David Horowitz; *The Rockefellers.* (New York: New American Library, 1976) p.271

[16]. Although known to be able to jump species from cattle to humans, there is little published literature on the incidence of abortion in female victims. However, there are some studies showing that such risk occurs. See, for example,

the abstract by E.J. Young: *Brucella Antibodies in Veterinarians Exposed to Strain 19.* p.465: L.Garry Adams, (Editor); *Advances in Brucellosis.* (College Station, TX. Texas A. & M. University Press, 1990)

[17]. Johnson, *Ibid,* p.196

[18]. Henderson, Donald A. and Alexis Shelokov: "Epidemic Neuromyasthenia- Clinical Syndrome?" *The New England Journal of Medicine,* (Vol. 26, No.'s 15 & 16, April 9 and 16,1959)

[19]. Donald A. Henderson; "Smallpox- Epitaph for a Killer?" (Washington, D.C.: *National Geographic.* Vol.154, No.6. December, 1978) pp.796-805

[20]. *The Lancet,* November 8, 1969. p.1000

[21]. Hearings before a Subcommittee of the Committee on Appropriations; House of Representatives, Ninety-first Congress. "Chemical and Biological Warfare". Monday, June 9, 1969. p.114. Hereafter, reference to these Hearings will cite just the page number in the body of the text.

[22]. The gender differential is due to the fact that the disabling pathogen is only triggered when an appropriate level of concentration in the blood has been attained, similar to that identified by Carleton Gajdusek in his Chapter 91 of *Fields Virology,* Third Edition. Philadelphia: Lippincott-Raven Publishers (1996) p. 2853. Since women have approximately 25 percent less blood than men and since the blood of a woman has approximately 20 percent less haemoglobin than that of men, the critical level of pathogen concentration is achieved in women about six times as frequently as that of men.

[23]. Although officially Dr. MacArthur is asking permission at this meeting to do certain things in the realm of biological weapons development, there are hints all the way through the record of the Hearings that much of the work was already under way. For example, on page 117 MacArthur tells the Congressmen:" We have had some of the top scientists in the world working for years on how to get more effective incapacitating agents. It is not easy."
There are other sources which also reflect the fact that with or without the approval of the elected representatives of the people, the military/CIA/industrial complex follows its own agenda. For example, although Richard Nixon did not declare his 'war on cancer' until 1971, the record of that 'war' contains several references to activities later

included under its rubric, even though they occurred five or more years earlier. The Progress Report # 8 of the Special Virus Cancer Program (ie 'The War on Cancer') dated July, 1971, describes research that took place as early as 1962 [p.286]

[24]. Norman M. Covert: *Cutting Edge* A history of Fort Detrick, Maryland. Headquarters, U.S. Army Garrison, Fort Detrick, Maryland. (Second Edition ; September, 1994) p.51

[25]. Henry Kissinger: National Security Study Memorandum 200. National Security Council, Washington, D.C. (April 24, 1974)."Subject: Implications of Worldwide Population Growth for U.S. Security and Overseas Interests." Although purportedly created in response to a request from Nixon, this Memorandum more than likely reflects the influence of Kissinger's sponsors, the Rockefeller family. It should be noted that, in keeping with the strategic war paradigm of the Pentagon's interest in world population control, Kissinger provided copies of NSSM 200 to the 'Chairman, Joint Chiefs of Staff.'

[26]. Leonard Horowitz: *Emerging Viruses: Aids & Ebola* (Rockport, MA. Tetrahedron, Inc. 1997) p.245

[27]. Scott, Donald W. and William L.C. Scott: *The Brucellosis Triangle.* (Sudbury; The Chelmsford Publishers, 1998) pp.87-96

[28]. Elaine Showalter

[29]. *The Holy Bible;* Exodus 9:3. (Cleveland, Ohio. The World Publishing Company) p.86

[30]. Mark Perry: *Eclipse.* (New York: William Morrow and Company, Inc. 1992) p.393

[31]. Hearing before the Committee on Banking, Housing, and Urban Affairs; United States Senate. "United States dual-use exports to Iraq and their impact on the health of the Persian Gulf War Veterans" (The Riegle Report).Washington, D.C.; U.S. Government Printing Office. May 25, 1994

[32]. See, for example, Horowitz '*Emerging Viruses*' page 331 where he draws upon the research of Peter Dale Scott.

[33]. Endicott, Stephen and Edward Hagerman: *The United States and Biological Warfare.* (Indianapolis: Indiana University Press. 1998) p.41

[34]. The Report in an abbreviated and carefully edited version is reproduced in the Senate Hearings of March 8 and May 23, 1977.

[35]. It is probably more than chance that has led to the phenomenon noted by Hillary Johnson in

her magnificent study: *Osler's Web*. On page 43 Johnson writes: "The disease detectives at the Centers for Disease Control are often described in military terms. The nation's 'shock troops' against epidemic diseases and the 'front line' in public health emergencies are two metaphors that have found their way into print in recent years."

[36]. "Germ Warfare Tests Were Safe-Pentagon". *Toronto Star*. May 15, 1997.

[37]. It is to be noted that in the June 9, 1969 Hearings Dr. MacArthur still spoke about the limited 'shelf life' of biological weapons as if he had never heard of the crystalline form of the disease toxins. This is just another example of the Pentagon's failure to be fully forthcoming with Congress.

[38]. Shmuel Razim: "Mycoplasma Taxonomy and Ecology". Jack Maniloff(Editor): *Mycoplasmas*. (Washington, D.C. American Society for Microbiology, 1992) p.3

[39]. The term 'virus' is sometimes thought of as a minute life-form, but this is far too simplistic.

[40]. An example of this deliberate ambiguity can be found in the inter-change of terms. The 'amyloid' written about by Carleton Gajdusek is the same microorganism as the 'prion' written about by Prusiner. Also, according to Gajdusek, this 'embraces viroids, virioids, virinos, nucleating agents of industrial infections, infectious amyloids, and computer viruses.' See. chapter 91 of *Fields Virology, p.2862*

[41]. We have in our files several supporting documents. For example we have a photocopy of a classified ad in a Maryland newspaper from the mid-1970's. It reads:
"Research Volunteers needed for 30 day in-patient vaccine safety test. Very pleasant environment. $20. per day. Call University of Maryland Hospital Mon. 9 - 3 P.M. at 528-6624 or 528-6621, ask for Tina or Sylvia."
The ad was responded to by our informant who saw it as a kind of 'job'. Later she ascertained that the vaccines employed contained mycoplasmas and that the test protocol was under contract to the "Division of Microbiology and Infectious Diseases, National Institute of Allergy and Infectious Diseases, NIH, Bethesda, Maryland 20892. Some time later our informant developed sarcoidosis. Please see our JODD, Vol. 2, #1. (July 2000) pp. 57-60

[42]. Arno Karlen: *Men and Microbes*. (New York: Touchstone, 1995) p.19

[43]. Ed Regis: *The Biology of Doom*. (New York: Henry Holt and Company, 1999) p.139

[44]. Endicott, Stephen and Edward Hagerman: *The United States and Biological Warfare*. (Indianapolis: Indiana University Press, 1998)

[45]. Scott, Donald W. and William L.C. Scott: *The Brucellosis Triangle*. (Sudbury: The Chelmsford Publishers, 1998)

[46]. See Colmenero, et al: "Complications associated with *Brucella melitensis* infection; A study of 530 cases." *Medicine*, Vol.75, No.4

[47]. John Bryden: *Deadly Allies*. (Toronto: McClelland & Stewart, 1989) p. 200

[48]. There is evidence that the canine-feline disease referred to as 'parvo-virus B-19' is actually caused by a bacterial DNA particle from *Brucella-Abortus*, Strain 19. It may well be that the world-wide epidemic among dogs in the late 1970's was initiated in American/British laboratories and the pathogen got out of control. The researchers were able to develop an effective toxoid in record-breaking time and is now used universally. Arno Karlen comments as follows about the so-called 'parvovirus': "Equally disturbing is the fact that often we do not know just how some microbes speed around the globe. In recent decades, several new types of cat and dog infections (feline and canine parvoviruses) have spread worldwide within a few years." *Man and Microbes*, p.223

[49]. There is compelling evidence that the outbreak of Legionnaire's Disease in the Bellevue Stratford Hotel in Philadelphia in 1976 was a consequence of biological weapons testing by the Military/CIA. See Chapter 5 above.

[50]. See pages 20-21 of the March 8 and May 23, 1977 Senate Hearings.

[51]. Hearings before the Subcommittee on Health and Scientific Research of the Committee on Human Resources; United States Senate. (March 8 and May 23,1977) page 244. The evidence revealed in this source demonstrates that assassination of perceived enemies was provided for under CIA project MK-NAOMI, the records of which were largely destroyed during and after the Watergate investigations. However, enough remains to make it clear that Gerald Ford, George W. Bush Sr., Henry Kissinger, Alexander Haig and Richard Cheney among others were in the 'assassination loop'. The same group also provided the key political direction for the biological warfare program.

[52]. It may, of course, be just a coincidence, but a mystery illness hit LaCrosse, Wisconsin, in 1963. Like many other mystery epidemics of the time, it was characterized by headaches, fever, disorientation, seizures and stomach problems. Also of interest is the fact that mosquitoes were identified as the vector. See: J.J.Stambaugh: "7 cases of La-Crosse virus reported". *The Knoxville News-Sentinel.* (Sept. 9, 2000) p.A6

[53]. Norman Covert: *Cutting Edge* (Maryland: Fort Detrick 1994) Photograph on page 59. In the same photograph is Dr. Edwin V. Hill of Fort Detrick.

[54]. Regis, supra, p.126

[55]. Regis, *Ibid*, p.114

[56]. Regis, *Ibid*, p.128

[57]. Regis, *Ibid*, p.111

[58]. It may be relevant that Sacramento is just 110 miles southwest of Tahoe-Truckee.

[59]. For a summary of these and other 'mystery' epidemics of the same period, see: Sir Ernest Donald Acheson "The Clinical Syndrome Variously Called Benign Myalgic Encephalomyelitis, Iceland Disease and Epidemic Neuromyasthenia." Byron Hyde (Ed.) : The Clinical and Scientific Basis of Myalgic Encephalomyelitis Chronic Fatigue Syndrome. (Ottawa; The Nightingale Foundation, 1992) pp.129- 175

[60]. David Crystal (Ed.) *The Cambridge Factfinder,* 1993) p.161

[61]. Regis, *Ibid*, p.139

[62]. Poskanzer, *et al.* NEJM 1957; 257: 356-64

[63]. Robert J. Groden: *The Killing of a President.* (New York; Penguin Books, 1993) p.144

[64]. Regis, *Ibid*, p.210

[65]. *Ibid*, p.139

[66]. Johnson, *Osler's Web.* (New York; Crown Publishers, 1996) p.20

[67]. Johnson, *Ibid*, p.28

[68]. Johnson, *Ibid*, p.27; 29; 31; 33...

[69]. See, for example, the report on the Henle's and their work with Epstein-Barr: *JAMA,* Vol. 210, # 3. (1969) p.438. Also see page 1451 of *JAMA,* June 1, 1970. Vol.212, No 9 "E-B virus related to Hodgkin's disease".

[70]. Johnson, *Ibid*, p.62

[71]. Even under the best of circumstances the brucella bacteria species are extremely hard to locate. With the bacterial toxin removed in a crystalline form, the presence of the pathogen is almost beyond discovery. So Karen Bell's failure to find the bacteria is to be expected, and is, of course, what the biowar researchers knew.

[72]. This information was passed to us by a colleague of Dr. Bell who does not wish to be identified.

[73]. Byron Hyde" The Search for a Retrovirus in ME/CFS, A Review". Byron Hyde (Ed.) *supra,* p.333

[74]. Jess Stein, Editor in Chief: *The Random House Dictionary,* (New York; Ballantine Books, 1980) p.785

[75]. *Ibid*, p.277

[76]. Erik Stokstad, "Stephen Straus's Impossible Job." *Science* Vol. 288, # 5471;(2 June 2000) pp.1568-1570

[77]. Jess Stein: *supra,* p.757

[78]. Reviews of Infectious Diseases 1991; p.13 (Suppl 1):S2-7 Bethesda, Maryland; NIH

[79]. Johnson, *Ibid*, p.175

[80]. Carleton Gajdusek" Infectious Amyloids". *Fields Virology,* (Philadelphia; Lippincott-Raven Publishers, 1996) p. 2853. Gajdusek is referring to amyloids, but the principle is the key point.

[81]. Senate Hearings; March 8 and May 23, 1977. p.89

[82]. Stokstad, *Ibid*, pp.1568-9

[83]. Quoted in: Johnson, *Ibid*, p.321

[84]. Hearings, June 9,1969: *supra*, p.110

[85]. Bruce Nussbaum: *Good Intentions* (New York: The Atlantic Monthly Press, 1990) p.162

[86]. Stokstad, *Ibid*, p.1569

[87]. Nussbaum, *Ibid*, p.162

[88]. *Ibid*, p.162

[89]. Johnson, *Ibid*, p.321

[90]. Johnson, *Ibid*, p.587

[91]. Hyde, *Ibid*, p.335

[92]. Lewis Carroll: *Alice in Wonderland.* (Newmarket, England: Brimax Books, 1988) pp.56-7

[93]. Johnson, *Ibid*, pp. 370-71; 448; 454; 477; 554; 642

[94]. Nadler's letter of April 11, 1996 and Shalala's reply of June 25, 1996 are in the author's files.

[95]. June Gibbs Brown: "Audit of Costs Charged to the Chronic Fatigue Syndrome Program at the Centers for Disease Control and Prevention." Washington; Department of Health and Human Services. (May, 1999) p.7

[96]. *Ibid*, p.12

[97]. *Ibid*, p.10

[98]. Martin Enserik: "CDC Struggles to Recover From Debacle Over Earmark. *Science,* Vol. 287, #

5450. (7 January 2000) p.22

[99]. John H. Gagnon. *Science,* Vol. 287 #5452. (21 January, 2000) p.427

[100]. The first western contact with the Fore tribe was in 1932 when Ted Eubanks, a gold prospector, encountered them. Then, in 1949 a Lutheran Mission was set up in the area. Our research has failed to locate any references from Eubanks or the Mission that kuru was present in the period of 1932 to 1949. However, on Sunday, December 6, 1953 an Australian Patrol Officer named J.R. MacArthur reported the first known western encounter with a kuru victim.

In 1957 when D. Carleton Gajdusek arrived to study the disease, he stated in a letter to Joseph E. Smadel, a biowar weapons researcher at the Walter Reed Institute of Research, that kuru was the 'major disease problem of the region...for the past five years'! ie since 1952!

The most likely scenario: the Japanese had inoculated a certain number of the Fore tribe in 1942. In 1945 Ishii Shiro shared this information with the American researchers from Fort Detrick. In 1954 Patrol Officer MacArthur told District Medical Officer, Dr. V. Zigas of his encounter with a case of kuru. In 1956 brain samples were sent to Walter and Eliza Hall of Melbourne, Australia where Gajdusek had arrived a few months before. Gajdusek travelled to Fore country and began his study of kuru which earned him a Nobel Prize.

Since kuru is derived from a lentivirus which can take from 5 to 20 years to present with symptoms, it is reasonable to assume that the Fore tribe had indeed been the test victims of Japanese biological warfare weapons development in 1942 and that the disease had begun to show in the early 1950's.

Carleton Gajdusek is likely to be the greatest fraud in medical research and the Nobel Committee should re-examine his entitlement to the prize he accepted for his work.

[101]. "United States Dual-Use Exports to Iraq and their Impact on the Health of Gulf War Veterans" (The "Riegle Report) Washington, D.C. The U.S. Government Printing Office. May 25, 1994. pp.36-51

[102]. Sean and Leslee Dudley; "Mycoplasma Registry Report". *The Journal of Degenerative Diseases.* Vol. 2, #1. (July, 2000) pp. 41-50

[103]. It is of interest that a patient of Dr. Peterson ordered three copies of the original edition of *The Extremely Unfortunate Skull Valley Incident* in 1997. She stated on a note with her order that Dr. Peterson had suggested the book to her. How one should interpret this cannot be ventured. We have attempted to involve Dr. Peterson in our research but he has refused to reply to faxes and an Express Mail ® letter we sent him.

[104]. "Study Links Epstein-Barr Virus to Nasopharyngeal Carcinoma"; *JAMA,* Oct.20, 1969. Vol. 210, No. 3. P.438. Also, see the *JODD,* Vol.1, # 3-4. "Cancer and the Mycoplasma" (March, 2000) p.58

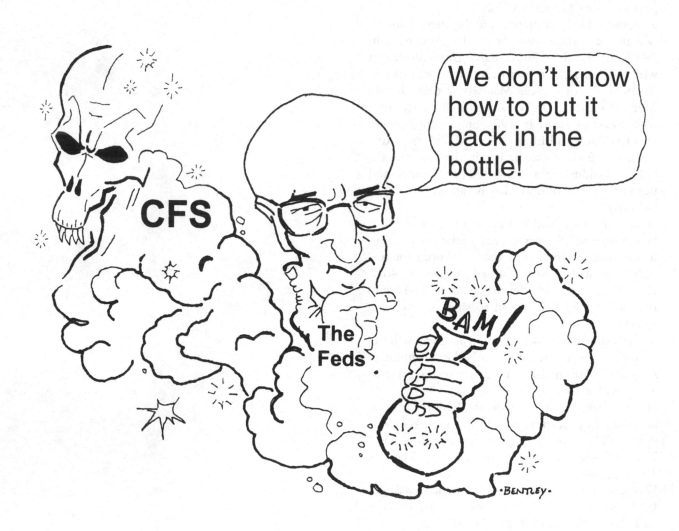

CHAPTER TWELVE

THE CHRONOLOGY OF AIDS...

A population Growth Rate Control Strategy
The Rockefellers had a Dream

Holistic Evil

It is much more satisfying psychologically to think of our society with its manifold social, political, financial, religious, medical, educational, business and media institutions as inter-related but independent of each other and as being basically good with occasional lapses into evil by 'misfits' than it is to contemplate a profound and powerful core of evil that dominates our world through control of these very institutions.

For example, even though there is not a single iota of sustainable evidence that Lee Harvey Oswald murdered President John F. Kennedy or that he even knew the President was being targeted, most writers, commentators, historians, researchers and others when they talk about the November 22, 1963 coup d'etat often or indeed usually, refer to "assassin Lee Harvey Oswald." Even our esteemed colleague in research, Dr. Leonard Horowitz, wrote in a recent communication to us "Following the assassination of John F. Kennedy by Lee Harvey Oswald..."

We immediately responded: "Please, please, please...do not..."refer to the "assassination...by Lee Harvey Oswald." Then we cited the key evidence which makes it most unlikely that CIA agent Lee Harvey Oswald was anything other than a 'patsy' to draw attention away from the real assassins.

Even when someone advances a theory that others were involved in the crime, there is a tendency to keep Mr. Oswald in the scenario:

"In a peer-reviewed paper published in the British Forensic Science Society's journal Science and Justice, scientist D.B. Thomas adds weight to the 'grassy knoll' theory that a second gunman shot at the president at almost exactly the same moment as Oswald fired his three shots." [National Post; March 27, 2001, with files from Reuters]

How satisfying! Into the midst of our bliss-blessed goodness there suddenly appears someone evil [Lee Harvey Oswald] who commits a terrible crime and then gets what he deserves at the hands of a perverse and insidious Mafia hit-man [Jack Ruby] who is saddened by the thought of a suffering widow having to return to Dallas to testify at a trial.

And in regard to another great crime [AIDS] it is so satisfying to accept the quaint myth that a Canadian airline steward once had a sexual encounter in Paris with a woman who in turn had had a liaison with a black man from Africa and whose previous encounter in Africa had been with a black woman who had been bitten and infected by a green monkey which had a dysfunctional immune system and so this steward became the first carrier of a human immunodeficiency virus...AIDS.

My oh my! Talk about fairy tales.

However, this modern myth further claims that the steward (who was celibate in his home town of Montreal, heterosexual in Paris and homosexual in New York, Los Angeles and San Francisco) had carried that green monkey virus to all his 2500 gay sexual partners in the next five years. At which point he died of AIDS, or extreme exhaustion.

A wonderfully complete explanation. It explains how the virus got from the green monkey to humanity. It explains how it got from the black population of Africa to the gay white population of the United States. Even the steward's airline pass explains how he could get from coast-to-coast so easily. And the happy fact that he was Canadian put the steward beyond the reach of U.S.health authorities and enquiries, so they were spared the task of exploring the mystery of the AIDS epidemic in America.

It is a stupid, preposterous idea yet it has been accepted in whole or in part by eminent scientists such as Robert Gallo and Stephen Straus; by acclaimed medical writers for the *New York Times;* and, by beloved politicians such as Ronald Reagan. And it has been accepted, again in whole or in part, by the majority of persons who have heard it. It has entered into our folk lore: AIDS came from monkeys; AIDS came from Africa; AIDS is a disease of homosexuals, a 'gay plague'.

The *New York Times* purports to believe and persistently disseminates both these and many other myths that fit the template of a single evil misfit who does immeasurable harm in and to an otherwise good society. In fact, it was the *New York Times* that first referred to the accused Lee Harvey Oswald as "the President's assassin" even before Oswald had been charged or tried for the crime. And, when the *Times* says it's so, the rest of the world's media can take up the myth as fact without having to support their position with evidence…they just have to quote the *New York Times*. Then, also, history professors can cite the *Times* as their authority for advancing the myth to their students; thus it begins its insidious passage into folk lore which eliminates the need for thinking and questioning and so preserves a flawed self-image: America is a nation of laws democratically enacted, not a nation of men having their undemocratic way.

The same 'lone misfit' social myth was recognized by the great Harold Weisberg in his study of the official government position that the purported assassin of Dr. Martin Luther King, James Earl Ray, had acted alone:

"With the truth so unpleasant [ie. that Dr. King had actually been executed by the U.S. Military/ CIA/ FBI] was it not better to rescript the King assassination, to make it seem detached from life, an odd and unexpected, isolated crime by a single, unassociated man, it and he removed from connection with anyone and anything?" [Weisberg: Frame-Up, p.411]

But, is the lone misfit theory of social evil really true?

The evidence suggests that it is not.

There are, of course, lone persons who do evil deeds. However, are many or even most of the great tragedies of our times random acts of evil done by such lunatic loners?

We strongly suggest that they are not random; and, we suggest that the perpetrators have a unity and cohesion beyond our wildest imaginings.

It is time that the thesis be clearly put forth that most of the great crimes and tragedies of the last six decades, including the murders of John F. Kennedy, Robert Kennedy, and Martin Luther King, Jr. and the epidemics of AIDS and CFIDS, as well as the Vietnam War and the Gulf War, although superficially disparate entities, actually reflect the reality of a holistic evil at the very core of society.

It is time to put the case that the middle-aged woman disabled by what she has been told is 'chronic fatigue syndrome'; or the Kenyan child, orphaned by the AIDS virus; or Lee Harvey Oswald, murdered by Jack Ruby; or the black tennis player, dead from

an infusion of AIDS-infected blood; or even the President of the United States who is shot dead in Dealey Plaza, Dallas at high noon are all victims of an evil at the core.

An evil core that puts forth its criminal tentacles through the very institutions of society that are believed to stand for goodness and law and health and human fulfilment. Tentacles which present in an example as small as a Supreme Court Justice whose petty immature sexuality is seen in an office light switch plate (given to him by his wife) shaped as a naked man whose penis is the switch toggle. Or as significant as the Supreme Court Chief Justice who is so oblivious to the true nature of majority rule in a democracy that he votes to effectively establish the loser of an election (by one and a half million votes) as the President of the United States.

An evil so profound that twelve elected Congressmen can approve a request in 1969 from a Pentagon biological warfare researcher for ten million dollars to develop a "new microorganism…for which no natural immunity could have been acquired". That is AIDS !

An evil hinted at in linkages such as that between Dr. Jose Rivera and Dr. Brian Mahy, former Director of the Centers for Disease Control who has been transferred to another post within the CDC because he misspent $8 million voted by Congress to study 'CFIDS' and who 'lost' another $4 million voted for the same purpose.

Earlier in his career Dr. Mahy had worked with Dr. Jose Rivera and through Mahy's influence, had Rivera appointed to Dr. Hilary Kowproski's Wistar Institute to work with Dr. Elaine DeFreitas when she was researching CFIDS.

Was Dr. Mahy totally oblivious to the fact that Dr. Jose Rivera was by some strange route, linked to none other than Lee Harvey Oswald…several months before the murder of Mr. Kennedy? [Dr. Rivera had given a colleague Lee Harvey Oswald's new telephone number in New Orleans even before Oswald had moved to that address!]

Then there is the link between Oswald and David Ferrie of New Orleans. Ferrie had links with Oswald dating back as far as the latter's New Orleans high school days, and both had attended parties hosted by Clay Shaw. However, it was only after his death that it was learned that Ferrie had been studying methods of transferring certain monkey viruses (recall the so-called monkey origin of the AIDS virus) to mice. Furthermore, Ferrie was apparently closely linked to

Dr. Mary Sherman of Tulane University who was also engaged in mysterious research until she, like Ferrie, was murdered by someone who has never been identified. It was to another Tulane University researcher that Dr. Rivera passed Oswald's phone number five months before the assassination of Mr. Kennedy.

Without attempting at this point to draw any firm conclusions about what these and several other startling linkages portend until they have been carefully and completely studied, one must initially wonder at those linkages: from Mahy (who attempted to sabotage the Congressional efforts to study CFIDS); to Jose Rivera who knew Lee Harvey Oswald and who may have sabotaged certain Wistar Institute research into CFIDS; to David Ferrie who was studying in an area closely linked to Mahy's early work [such as his 1965 investigation with K.E.K. Rowsen and M.H. Salaman of lactic dehydrogenase elevating virus's effects on the reticuloendothelial system in conjunction with T-lymphocytes and macrophages involved in cell-mediated immunity]. These studies can be closely linked to certain AIDS factors.

There are those in various positions to influence the common view of things who will explain these links as 'coincidences'. 'Coincidence buffs' such as the editors of *Time* and *The Readers Digest* will also make it a point to disparage the 'conspiracy buffs' who think that such linkages don't just happen but are planned by someone and are purposeful, not random, in effect.

Is it just a coincidence that there is a linkage from CFIDS to Mahy and from Mahy to Rivera? And is it just another unbelievable coincidence that Rivera had links with Lee Harvey Oswald who, in turn, had strong links to David Ferrie? Is it a coincidence that Ferrie had been studying how to transfer monkey viruses to mice when the folk myth now tells us that AIDS comes from a monkey virus? Is it a coincidence that David Ferrie had links to an eminent cancer researcher, Mary Sherman, and is it a further dramatic coincidence that Oswald, Ferrie and Sherman were all to die under very strange circumstances?

And, to bring the coincidental wheel full circle, is it a coincidence that Brian Mahy's early research has identifiable links to the disease mechanics of AIDS and that AIDS has been called a mirror image of CFIDS? Could that be the reason why Mahy, as Director of the CDC misspent and/or lost $12 million assigned by Congress to study CFIDS? Could it be that if he spent that money honestly on honest and

honourable men doing unpoliticized science, the truth would come out?

Enough already!

The Mahy; Rivera; Oswald; Ferrie; Sherman linkage is just one out of several such coincidences that we could cite.

But, we won't cite those here. Rather, we will state our firm position that there are no coincidences in the whole sorry mess of AIDS and CFIDS and the warped and evil financial, political, military, medical, educational, pharmaceutical and media power core that makes and breaks (or if necessary murders) political leaders; develops biological weapons to disable or to kill; recruits former Nazi and Japanese war criminals; turns AIDS loose among the people of 'lesser developed countries' and CFIDS loose among the people of the 'civilized, developed' nations.

No, there are no coincidences in all of this. There is a holistic core of evil that links military with medical; medical with media; media with educational; educational with politicians; politicians with wealthy patrons; wealthy patrons with population control fanatics; and population control fanatics with biological warfare weapons research and testing and deployment.

You'll find representatives of all of these in the chronology to follow.

The focus of this chapter is on the AIDS epidemic and its links to the holistic core of evil. However, one cannot separate just the AIDS threads from the whole cloth. All have links to the others. We begin with an overview of the years from 1942 until the present. And woven through those years are the elements that have made the AIDS epidemic a reality.

These elements can be categorized as the scientific, the financial, the political and the tactical. Under the 'scientific' we must look for clues as to which microbiologists, medical doctors, veterinarians, and others did the actual work in the laboratories (military, industrial, university and commercial) to isolate the disease agents, modify these as required, stabilize and standardize, etc. In this effort we must try to determine which were witting participants and which were unwitting. Under the latter category will be those scientists whose work provided a necessary detail, but who had no idea about the covert activities they were unwittingly serving.

Under the financial we must try to trace the money flow. Basically, of course, it came from government, but a considerable amount appears to have come from private money such as that provided by the Rockefellers through the Foundation of that name to institutions such as Cold Spring Harbor Laboratory in New York. That part of the money that came from government had (and apparently still has) three parts: *i.* that which is voted in the budget to various branches and departments and is more or less wittingly employed for covert research; *ii.* that which is part of the 'black currency' such as the Nazi gold stolen from Europe at the war's end and placed in the U.S. Treasury under John W. Snyder. The gold was stolen by Allen Dulles, transported by the U.S. Navy under orders from James Forrestal and supervised by Navy Lieutenant C. Douglas Dillon; *iii.* that which is strictly criminal money such as that made from the CIA running drugs between Columbia and the U.S. through Panama. George W. Bush, Sr., was intimately involved in this operation.

Under the political we must look for the role played by John F. Kennedy who basically opposed anything to do with population control strategies and whose administration paid very little towards such. Then we must look at his successor, Lyndon Johnson, who did not try to hide his sympathy with the whole concept of population control efforts, and who said so and openly asked Congress for money to finance such efforts. Then we must search out the devious political financial support as developed by the likes of Richard Nixon and Gerald Ford. Nixon hid his efforts under the guise of waging a war on cancer, and Ford continued this and other projects through his special assistant, Richard Cheney (now vice-president under George Bush, Jr.)

Finally, under tactical, we must look for those who did the necessary organizing and leg work to move the created pathogens from the laboratories to the test sites, and from the test sites to inventory and then deployment.

Who selected Tahoe-Truckee High School as a test site for the 1984 'CFIDS' pathogen tested upon eight teachers in a separate staff room? Who ordered the renovation of the air conditioning/heating system? Who monitored the results? How were those involved paid for their efforts? Who brought Dr. Tom Merigan of Stanford University into the picture? Who was Dr. Evelyn Lennette, and who brought her in? Did her work with the Special Virus Cancer Project provide her with insights into the disease affecting the students and staff of Incline Village? What was the significance of her work with Huebener and Oshiro and Riggs ...all of whom played a role with the *SVCP* when they did research

to isolate a syncytium-forming agent from domestic cats?

Such work tied in with the work of others on simian foamy viruses and the maedi-visna virus, and the latter was the probable source of the kuru infection of New Guinea tribesmen. How does Evelyne Lennette, a self-styled 'child of the Henles' come to be involved with the victims of Tahoe-Truckee High School? And just who were the Henles' who with Huebener emerge as among the most significant SVCP researchers?

It is an intricate and complicated web of questions, but we must make an effort to follow some of the strands if we are to understand where AIDS and its mirror-image CFIDS came from. We must know where both came from if we are to ever get a handle on how to stop these twin plagues.

Special Acknowledgement
We want to acknowledge with sincere thanks, the great work of Robert E. Lee, M.S., M.S.W., of Black Hawk College, Kewanee, Illinois. Mr. Lee permitted me to read his manuscript in progress: "AIDS: An Explosion of the Biological Timebomb?" The book is a goldmine of information.

Thesis
The thesis of this chapter is that all the objective evidence that we have been able to access and study carefully makes it clear that the AIDS-inducing pathogen was researched, developed, tested and deployed by the United States Government.

Biological Warfare Weapons Development and Testing and the Deployment of the AIDS and 'CFIDS' Pathogens as Agents for World Population Growth Rate Control: A Chronology and Commentary.

Silently slaying the peoples of the 'Lesser Developed Countries' while disabling the women of the 'civilized' world.

THE SECRET WAR

"Men like John J. McCloy, C. Douglas Dillon, James Forrestal, Robert Patterson, Robert A. Lovett, the Dulles brothers, and Winthrop Aldrich were never elected to office, but wielded a power that was in many ways greater and more sustained than that of the elected officials they served." [Peter Collier and David Horowitz in The Rockefellers : An American Dynasty p.276]

Some months ago Mr. Robert E. Lee of Kewanee, Illinois, drew our attention to a dramatic statement made in 1946 by Perry Githens, the editor of Popular Science. Mr. Githens' thesis was that by the use of biological weapons, one nation could destroy another nation without the latter even knowing that it was under attack.

We will paraphrase Githens' comments to better illustrate that thesis which needs to be emphasized when one studies the great tragedy of the dual plagues of AIDS and 'CFIDS'. [We reluctantly use the latter acronym to accommodate those readers who have not yet learned the true nature of the disease so labelled: new variant brucellosis]

> *"Now suppose a few men in one [country] decide that [an] other nation must be 'removed', that it must be wiped out by a war without warfare. Supposing they plan a war without the formalities of overt acts, a kind of global sabotage aimed not at capture but at destruction, a truly 'preventive war'. In this creeping war there would be no blitzkrieg, no declaration, no massing of forces. The weapons for secret warfare exist...In a secret war the countr[ies] under attack might wither as nation[s], without even knowing [they] had even been sick..."*

Perry Githens' terrible scenario has come to pass.

The United States of America (with some help from France and certain covert allies in Britain, Canada and Australia) has embarked upon an undeclared war against several 'lesser developed countries' as identified in Henry Kissinger's NSSM 200 to Richard Nixon, using the AIDS pathogen, and against the general population of the 'civilized' industrial nations, including the population of the United

States itself, using a biologically engineered variant of brucellosis and presenting as 'CFIDS'.

The concept of a lethal biological weapon and a disabling biological weapon was presented by a Pentagon researcher in the early days of Richard Nixon's presidency.

The evidence is now compelling that AIDS is the 'lethal' weapon referred to on June 9, 1969 by Dr. Donald MacArthur of the Pentagon's bioweapons research section secretly reporting to twelve Congressmen, and CFIDS [new variant brucellosis] is the 'disabling' weapon he promised at that same meeting.[See Chronology below: 1969]

The post-war population control cabal which had grown out of the ranks of the 'nouveau riche' in the first two decades of the twentieth century among the U.S. Eastern elite and which consisted of the likes of John David Rockefeller lll, General Richard Draper, and Senator Prescott Bush of Connecticut took advantage of the wartime biowar research to lay the foundation for an all out assault on world population growth rate.

Therefore, although the eugenics movement had existed throughout the early 1900's , I begin this chronology in 1942. It was only during and immediately after the Second World War that the plans of the elite to reduce the numbers of lesser mortals could get seriously under way by incorporating the wealth of the Rockefellers, the Fords, the Morgans and others, with the power of the Government of the United States through its Department of Defense, the soon to be created Central Intelligence Agency, and later the Centers for Disease Control and the National Institutes of Health.

An Overview of Biological Warfare Weapons Development and its Links with other Elements of the Holistic Core of Evil: A Chronology

1942: Canada entered into a secret agreement with Britain and the United States to participate in a program to develop biological weapons for possible use against Germany, Italy and Japan. The principal diseases used as starting points in their research included anthrax (as a lethal weapon) and brucellosis (as a disabling weapon).

In that same year Japan which had also been developing a range of bioweapons, had occupied most of the island of New Guinea. The Japanese Military expected to control New Guinea for the foreseeable future and one of the first things they did under the direction of their biological weapons development commander, Dr/General Ishii Shiro, was to establish a 'biological test site' in the remote interior of that island. At this test site we can now conclude that they inoculated several members of the Fore Indian tribe with a visna virus-derived inoculant. Visna in sheep is an antecedent to bovine spongiform encephalopathy ('mad-cow disease') in cattle and Creutzfeldt-Jakob in humans.

Japanese plans to study the long-term effects of their inoculation program were cut short by the Australian / American counter attack over the Owen Stanley Mountain range, and the infected members of the Fore tribe were left to their deadly fate. A fate that would not become apparent until the lentivirus which can take up to twenty years to present as disease, had begun to show its effects.

1942: Dr. Bjorn Sigurdsson of Iceland had made his way from Nazi-occupied Denmark to the United States where he joined the Rockefeller Foundation. Although a medical doctor, his studies focussed upon visna, maedi and rida (a chronic encephalitis in sheep). Visna, which causes sheep to scrape their itching bodies against trees and posts (hence the word 'scrapie') has a genomic sequence almost indistinguishable from the AIDS virus, HIV.

1943: The United States designated "Camp Detrick" at Frederick, Maryland, as the control center for their biological weapons research and development. The Camp was named after Frederick Louis Detrick, a medical graduate from the Rockefeller Institute and a staff/faculty member of the Johns Hopkins University Hospital. Detrick was also an officer in the Maryland National Guard. [Thus, appropriately, Dr. Detrick incorporated within himself, the Rockfeller/ Johns Hopkins/ Military biological warfare research co-operation that was to lead to both AIDS and CFIDS]

1943: Dr. Ira L. Baldwin, professor of bacteriology at the University of Wisconsin, was named first scientific director at Camp (later 'Fort') Detrick. Baldwin

represented the first of a long list of U. of Wisconsin faculty involved in biowar research. It may be relevant that before her appointment as Secretary of Health and Human Services by President Clinton, Donna Shalala had been Chancellor of the U. of Wisconsin. Furthermore, the U. of Wisconsin had enjoyed the benefits of at least 21 Department of Defense biowar research contracts up to 1961. Contracts after the latter date have not been made public, but it is clear that the U. of Wisconsin ranks very high in the bioweapons development program. (Other universities with a very significant bio-weapons role include the University of Rochester, probably one of the most insidious, and Johns Hopkins University)

1944: O.T. Avery *et al.* published "Studies on chemical nature of substance inducing transformation of pneumococcal types: induction of transformation by deoxyribonucleic acid fraction isolated from pneumococcus type lll". This line of investigation can be traced through the later work of researchers such as Steven Rosenberg [See–1992: Rosenberg] and [1987: Lennette]. As well as the research of Don Francis, Max Essex [See-1983, Essex] Robert Gallo, and others.

1945: Dr. Ishii Shiro was spared prosecution and execution as a war criminal for his use of Allied prisoners of war in lethal biological weapons tests in exchange for his agreement to tell his United States captors all that he had been doing. He also turned over all documents, autopsy slides, laboratory specimens (ie: the hearts, brains, etc in formaldehyde of murdered American, Chinese and British prisoners) eye-witness descriptions of dying victims' symptoms, etc. Included in his revelations was the fact that the Japanese Army had established the biological weapons test site in New Guinea in 1942 referred to above.

Camp (now re-named 'Fort') Detrick sent Dr. Norbert Fell and Lt. Col. Arvo Thompson to Japan to de-brief Ishii Shiro about the New Guinea test site and the (now) infamous "Water Purification Unit 731" near Harbin, China, where the Allied prisoners of war had been used as guinea pigs. The reward in death to these Allied martyrs was to be betrayed by their commanders who included General Douglas MacArthur and his staff members, Generals Willoughby and Fox, and Colonel Alexander Haig, the latter's son-in-law. [Such high level military betrayal of killed and injured service men and women continues to the present. Disabled veterans of the Gulf

War such as Canadian Lt. Louise Richard, have been betrayed by their Commanders and their military medical doctors. Of this more later].

1945: At the end of the war the 1942 Tripartite U.S., Canadian, British Agreement was continued into peacetime due to a perceived Communist threat.

1945: Leon Jaworski was named to the war crimes trial section of the Judge Advocate General's office to prosecute selected Nazi war criminals. He was accompanied to Europe by a medical doctor who would later turn up as a strong defender of the Warren Commission. [Of this, more later] Certain Nazi scientists and doctors were excused the ordeal of a trial at Nuremberg, as was SS officer Otto von Bolschwing who was known as the 'Butcher of Bucharest' for his particularly cruel murder of Jews in that city. von Bolschwing was not only spared trial, he was hired first by the U.S. Army CIC and later he was transferred to the CIA. He was brought to the U.S. in 1954.

1945: On July 6, the American Joint Chiefs of Staff authorized Project Overcast under which 350 German and Austrian scientists and medical researchers were secretly brought to the United States. Although the Nazis had lost the war, their leading theorists and thinkers became an integral part of the American holistic core of evil.

1946: With the 350 former enemy scientists brought to the U.S. under Project Overcast securely ensconced in America, the Pentagon's Joint Intelligence Objectives Agency identified another 1000 former Nazi scientists and medical researchers to be brought to the United States. In September President Truman accepted the idea and under the code name 'Paperclip' they too were given jobs in the U.S. Thus was a significant part of the defeated Nazi brain trust woven into the American holistic core of evil.

1946: Unit 406 of the U.S. Army's Far East Medical Section was established at Yokohama. Its first commander was Lt.Col. W.D. Tigertt, MD. who had done extensive work on insect vectors relating to the diffusion of Japanese B encephalitis. [See also-1956: Fort Detrick]

1946: Dr. George Merck head of biological research in the U.S. reported in a secret memo to the Secretary of Defence that his researchers had managed to extract the disease toxin from various bacteria in a crystalline form. Thus, a disabling bacterial disease such as brucellosis could be isolated in a crystalline form and diffused by aerosol, insect vector or in the food chain. The victims would be sick with the protean range of the disabling brucellosis infection, but no trace of the bacteria would be found. [See below-1987: Lennette]

1946–49: The first major tests of this disabling agent were conducted by the U.S. Army with the co-operation of the Rockefeller Foundation and Dr. Bjorn Sigurdsson in Akureyri, Iceland. It proved to be unsatisfactory as a 'disabling' disease because five of the targetted test children in the local school who presented with a major epidemic of 'CFIDS' developed Parkinson's Disease and died.

1947: On May 15 *The New England Journal of Medicine* published an article by Lieutenant Calderon Howe of the U.S. Navy, et al titled "Acute Brucellosis among Laboratory Workers". The laboratory workers were employed at Camp Detrick, Frederick, Maryland. Their symptoms were almost totally compatible with the symptoms to be presented later in the emerging new entity: Chronic Fatigue Syndrome. [See-1958: Brucellosis]

1947: Dr. Kurt Blome who had been a leader of Nazi biological warfare research which included experimentation on prisoners in concentration camps, was acquitted by the Jaworski Nuremberg International War Crimes Tribunal. Dr. Blome was then hired by the U.S. Army Chemical Corps to conduct a new round of biological weapons research.

1948: Allen Dulles and Frank Wisner achieved a secret agreement with the top U.S. media bosses including DeWitt Wallace of *Reader's Digest* and Henry Luce of *Time-Life,* and the editor-in-chief of *Fortune,* C.D. Jackson, wherein critical news concerning the CIA projects would 'never be mentioned' in the press.

1949: Defence Secretary James Forrestal proposed in March that a "medical intelligence unit" be established within the CIA. This proposal was taken up by private citizen and former OSS Director, Wm. (Wild Bill) Donovan who, with William Colby, conducted their own study and reported to Forrestal that such a task should be undertaken.

1949: Components for a wide range of biological weapons were tested at the Dugway Proving Grounds in Utah for possible use against North Korea and their Chinese Allies, and one weapon based upon brucellosis was actually taken into the arms inventory of the U.S. Military.

1951–53: Brucella-armed biological weapons were deployed by the U.S. in Korea. Evidence also suggests that a pathogen presenting as haemorrhagic fever was deployed along the Hantaan River, but it 'blew back' over American troops, killing several hundred. Thus (in 1951) Seoul hantavirus was introduced into the human family. Dr. D. Carleton Gajdusek was sent by the Pentagon to help contain the damage.

1953: Allen Dulles appointed Director of the CIA immediately embarked upon a program of 'medical' intelligence in a major way.

1954: U.S. military personnel who had handled brucellosis-armed weapons in Korea were given a document upon discharge which told them: *"If within two years of discharge you develop multiple sclerosis (a kind of creeping paralysis) it will be deemed to be due to the nature of the work you were performing."*

1950s: Canada agreed to breed one hundred million mosquitoes a month at the Dominion Parasite Laboratory in Belleville, Ontario. The mosquitoes were to be contaminated with bacterial crystalline agents at Queen's University, Kingston, under the direction of Biology Head, Dr. Guilford B. Reed and then tested by the U.S. and Canadian military in various Canadian and American communities.

1952: The 8003 Far East Medical Research Laboratory founded by the U.S. Military in Tokyo on March 10. This new unit was in addition to the already extant biowar unit 406, and was specially created so that it could recruit former Japanese biowar researchers into its ranks.

1952: The CIA launched a covert war against China with "Operation TROPIC" which included the use of biological weapons against Chinese civilians. On November 29 a CIA plane was shot down by the Chinese, killing Robert Snoddy and Norman Schwartz and leading to the capture of John T. Downey and Richard Fecteau. It was assumed by the U.S. officials that Downey and Fecteau would reveal the truth of their activities to the Chinese, but publicly, American spokes-persons vigorously denied the story. Later, E. Howard Hunt [See 1960: Bay of Pigs; 1963: Dealey Plaza; 1972: Watergate] who had served with the North Asia Command in 1955, admitted that Downey and Fecteau had indeed revealed the truth about the U.S. use of biological weapons. [See 1971: Fecteau and 1973: Downey] Meanwhile, journals such as the *New York Times, Time* and *The Readers' Digest* vigorously denounced the Chinese claims of American use of biological weapons.

1953: A CIA memo dated April 11 to the Chief of CIA's plans and Preparations revealed that the U.S. had used biological weapons in Korea and that UN Ambassador Henry Cabot Lodge had been so briefed. Lodge had protested that he didn't want to hear of such distasteful things, especially since his job required him to deny in the UN chambers that the U.S. had used biological weapons. Here he took a page from Eisenhower's book. The latter had told Allen Dulles that he wouldn't order such immoral things as assassinations to stop; however, he didn't want to be told about them because he would find it hard to lie about them later.

Despite the discomfort the briefing caused Lodge, the CIA report continues that he was briefed anyway and, among other things was told that one of the biological ' bugs' came"...from a very hardy strain and had exhibited appalling vitality." This latter allusion probably referred to the U.S. diffusion attempts on the Hantaan River in Korea when the virus 'blewback' over the U.S. units. Several thousand fell ill and 400 died. It is important to note that it was this catastrophe that led to Dr. Carleton Gajdusek being rushed out from the U.S. to help in the damage control. [See also-1957: Gajdusek / New Guinea / kuru]

1953: December 6, Australian Patrol Officer J.R. MacArthur recorded the first ever case of 'kuru' or Creutzfeldt-Jakob among the Fore tribe of New Guinea to be seen (or at least recorded) by non-native travellers. The eleven year span from the Japanese occupation in 1942 would be compatible with the 'lentivirus' characteristics of the AIDS-related visna virus being studied by Dr. Sigurdsson in Iceland. Dr. Sigurdsson's Icelandic laboratory was principally funded by the Rockefeller Foundation.

1953: President Eisenhower named Nelson Rockefeller his Undersecretary in the Department of Health, Education and Welfare. The first thing Nelson Rockefeller did in his new 'social/ humanitarian' post was to establish a 'war room'. Then he began converting the public health agencies into adjunct agencies of death by replacing the strictly medical/researcher type of top leadership with politically trustworthy Rockefeller Institute alumni.[The transformation was not completely traumatic since the United States Public Health Services had participated in such immoral projects as far back as 1932 when in the Tuskegee Syphilis Study, 400 black males had been used as unwitting guinea pigs. However, Nelson Rockefeller's work left the CDC and NIH as essentially Military minions, a role they continue to play.]

1954: Nelson Rockefeller left HEW to become President Eisenhower's Special Assistant for Cold War Strategy, succeeding C.D. Jackson. [See-1963: *Life* magazine] As such, Rockefeller was the President's coordinator for the CIA. In this role Rockefeller worked with Allen Dulles in an invigorated biological warfare research program.

1956: Colonel W.D. Tigertt was named Commander of the Medical Unit at Fort Detrick, and held this office until 1961. He maintained his interest in the use of insect vectors as a method to diffuse various biological pathogens. [See-1946: Unit 406 above and 1959: Q Fever below]

1956: An outbreak of 'CFIDS' occurred in Punta Gorda, Florida, after an unusual infestation of mosquitoes [See above: 1950's]. Government entomologists suggested that the mosquitoes were uncharacteristically 'fleeing' a forest fire in the Everglades some 30 miles away. Five days after the mosquito infestation, the first residents of Punta Gorda became ill with a 'mystery' disease, now labelled 'CFIDS' or 'CFS'. Donald Henderson, the chief of the Epidemic Intelligence Service of the Communicable Disease Center [now the Centers for Disease Control] conducted the investigation. It is important to note that the CDC was one of the U.S. Public Health agencies that were charged with the monitoring of biological warfare weapons testing. [Also, see below -1976: Smallpox Eradication Program]

1956: Dr. Robert Huebner, together with researchers from the Naval Medical Research Unit published "A Study of the role of Adenoviruses in Acute Respiratory Infections in a Navy Recruit Population." *American Journal of Hygiene* Vol. 64, pp.211-219. (1956) Evidence suggests that Huebner, et al who were studying the "adenoid degeneration agents" were actually pioneering what was to become known as PPLO's (pleural pneumonia like organisms), and at one time referred to as the 'Eaton' Agent. These names were to be re-placed in May, 1963 with the term 'mycoplasma'.

1957: Dr. V. Zigas, the District Medical Officer in Goroka, New Guinea, sent blood and brain specimens from Kuru victims to Walter and Eliza Hall at their Institute of Medical Research in Melbourne Australia. By an unusual coincidence the U.S. military-trained Dr. Carleton Gajdusek happened to be there at the time and was able to get an introduction to the disease characteristics.

1957: Carleton Gajdusek turned up in the remote New Guinea highlands where hundreds of the Fore tribe were suffering from a visna-like (scrapie) version of Creutzfeldt-Jakob disease which the Fore people termed 'kuru'. On March 15 he wrote his first letter since arriving in New Guinea. It was to his mentor, Dr. Joseph E. Smadel, Chief of Microbiology at the Walter Reed Army Institute of Research, Washington, D.C. It was Joseph Smadel who in 1942, had been experimenting with the West Nile fever virus and who later had sent Gajdusck to Korea to help control the haemorrhagic fever outbreak.

1958: A child born at the University of Wisconsin [See-1943: University of Wisconsin and Donna Shalala] Hospital was infected with Serratia marcescens. Investigations revealed that the organism was being used at the time by the university's biochemistry laboratory under Defense Department contract in a study of aerosol diffusion of disease agents. In an adjoining laboratory genetic studies for the D. of D. were also being conducted. [See 1969: June 9-'aerosol' diffusion of biowar agents]

1958: The *A.M.A. Archives of Internal Medicine* published a three-part article: "Brucellosis" by Robert W. Trever, et al. The article deals with sixty cases of acute brucellosis among laboratory workers at Fort Detrick. The article is significant because it illustrates Professor Peter Dale Scott's 'negative template' hypothesis [See: 1993: Peter Dale Scott and 1969: June 9 Hearings]

1959: General William Draper, a great friend of Senator Prescott Bush and of John D. Rockefeller lll, and the head of President Eisenhower's Committee to Study the United States Military Assistance Program incorporated into his report on U.S. military preparedness a statement that world population control had to be made part of the U.S. national security planning. Thus the Rockefeller and Eastern elite private goals of population growth rate control were melded with official U.S. military planning.

1959: Responding to the Draper alarm bells, the Senate Foreign Relations Committee published a report prepared by the Stanford Research Institute which concluded: "some means of controlling population growth are inescapable".[See-1986: Stanford and Thomas Merigan]. The major voice raised against such activities was that of Senator John F. Kennedy who expressed the opinion that the "available resources of the world are increasing as fast as the population" and hence there was no need for population control initiatives by the U.S.

1959: Col. Tigertt published "Studies on Q Fever in Man". Q fever was one of the pathogens being studied and developed as a biological weapon by the U.S. military/ CIA. [See-1969: June 9 Hearings]

1959: On November 27, Senator Kennedy repeated his position to a *New York Times* reporter: "I think it would be a mistake for the United States Government to attempt to advocate the limitation of the population of under-developed countries," he said.

1960: November: John F. Kennedy elected President, defeating Richard M. Nixon. On the eve of the election Kennedy declared: "The kind of society we build, the kind of power we generate, the kind of enthusiasm that we incite, all of this will tell whether, in the long run, *darkness or light overtakes the world.*"

1961: January 20, John F. Kennedy inaugurated as President of the United States.

1961–63: Honouring his pre-election commitments, the new President of the U.S. (JFK) discouraged population control activities by his administration.
1960: President Kennedy allowed a plan to invade Cuba, developed by the CIA in conjunction with former Vice-President Richard Nixon, to proceed. Following the invasion's complete failure, CIA head, Allan Dulles was advised by Kennedy that after a face-saving interval, he would be fired.

1960: One of the key planners in the Allen Dulles/ Richard Nixon/ plans to invade Cuba after the election was E. Howard Hunt [See-1952 : E. Howard Hunt] who was in charge of the 'Miamian Cubans', a loosely run covert group under CIA operative and later President, George W. Bush. Bush, with the logistics help of Col. L. Fletcher Prouty, assisted in securing two re-painted and re-named United States Navy vessels. The new names for the vessels provided by Bush were the 'Barbara' and the 'Houston'. The plan to send in the American military in support of the Cuban exiles failed to develop when Kennedy won an unexpected election victory over Nixon. Both Hunt and George Bush had been brought into the CIA by their mutual friend, Allen Dulles. One of Dulles strongest supporters was Senator Prescott Bush, grandfather of the present president.

1960: Allen Dulles approved a plan by his Deputy, Richard Bissell, to assassinate Patrice Lumumba of the Congo. Bissell delegated the job to CIA operative Justin O'Donnell who protested his orders on moral grounds. Bissell, a former professor of President Kennedy's staff members William and McGeorge Bundy and of Walt Rostow, insisted that his orders be carried out. O'Donnell protested to Inspector -General Lyman Kirkpatrick who supported O'Donnell's position and who then went directly to Allen Dulles to protest. Dulles heard him out, but never-the-less carried on with the planning.

1960: Richard Bissell continued his efforts hatched during the Eisenhower administration, to assassinate Fidel Castro. Bissell enlisted the aid of his science adviser, Sidney Gottlieb, to investigate the use of chemical/ biological agents to kill foreign (and probably domestic) enemies.
1
961: Despite the fact that President Kennedy was on record as opposing any U.S. role in trying to modify the world population growth rate and, by inference, any work on biological weapons to achieve such a goal, Secretary of Defense Robert McNamara in May gave the Joint Chiefs of Staff the go-ahead to "evaluate the potentialities of BW/CW, considering

all possible applications." This McNamara quality of being on both sides of many important questions at the same time was also demonstrated in matters dealing with the Vietnam war when he told Mr. Kennedy one thing about the progress of the struggle and, using information from the Joint Chiefs, told Vice-President Lyndon Johnson another.

1961: The Pentagon biological weapons researchers reported to the Secretary of Defense that "The development of vaccines for Q fever and tularaemia enabled work on Q fever and tularaemia to proceed to standardization as BW (biowar) agents." This important statement suggests that there was (and is?) a policy that production of a biowar agent would not go ahead before an antidote had been developed for that agent. Does this mean that the mass-production of CFIDS-causing brucellosis and AIDS-causing visna did not get fully under way until there was a known antidote?

Is there a known antidote for both AIDS and CFIDS buried somewhere in the archives of the medical component of the 'establishment'?

1962: On Tuesday, October 16, President Kennedy asked Attorney-General Robert Kennedy to come to the White House. "We are facing great trouble" he said. U-2 reconnaissance planes had detected Soviet missiles being installed in Cuba.

Over the next thirteen days President Kennedy negotiated his way towards the withdrawal of the missiles, coping on one hand with the Soviets, divided evidently into two camps of 'hawks' and 'doves' and his own 'Ex-Comm': the Executive Committee of the National Security Council which had its own division of hawks and doves.

President Kennedy was resolved to have the weapons out of Cuba, while at the same time avoiding the risk of a nuclear war with the Soviet Union. At the outset, the majority of the Committee wanted an immediate bombing of the installation. Only the President, his brother Robert and Adlai Stevenson (out of the total group which ranged from 15 to 20 at any one time) opposed immediate military action. Some of the Ex-Comm appeared to Robert Kennedy to 'lose their judgment and stability'. Although he doesn't state such in his account of the crisis, *Thirteen Days,* it is evident that among those who lost his stability was Air Force General, Curtis LeMay. Even

after the Soviets had turned the ships carrying missiles around in mid-ocean and headed for home, LeMay wanted to go ahead and attack Cuba anyway.

The same dichotomy apparently existed in the Soviet Union. During the crisis two messages had arrived from Moscow; the first had personal style features to suggest it was from Khrushchev himself... reasonable, conciliatory and human; the second appeared to have been written by a hardline committee...obdurate, unyielding and militaristic. When Ex-Comm began debating a response to the two letters, especially the second one, Robert Kennedy came up with a stroke of genius. "Let's just reply to the first message from Khrushchev and ignore the second." That's what they did and President John F. Kennedy drafted and sent a wise and temperate reply that led to the achievement of his goals: the missiles were withdrawn, and there was no nuclear war.

With the crisis resolved without resort to arms, and with the world granted a reprieve, and after all of the generals and advisors had gone home, John Kennedy said to Robert Kennedy:"This is the night I should go to the theatre", making reference to Abraham Lincoln. And Robert replied: "If you go, I want to go with you."

In thirteen months John F. Kennedy, like Abraham Lincoln, would be shot dead and within five years Robert Kennedy, too, would be shot dead. The way in each case, was opened for the forces of darkness. John Kennedy's death made it possible for Lyndon Johnson to succeed to the power of the presidency and increased American involvement in Vietnam, while the death of Robert Kennedy opened the way for Richard Nixon and the Congressional Hearings of June 9, 1969; the NSSM 200; and the development and deployment of the AIDS and CFIDS pathogens.

In The Shadows

Although Tuesday, October 16, 1962, is the generally accepted date for the beginning of the 'Cuban Missile Crisis', there were silent, covert moves several weeks before that date.

Cuban refugees in September, 1962, had reported that logistic support equipment for missile launch sites was arriving in Cuba, and one refugee even reported that Fidel Castro's personal pilot had drunkenly referred to a plan to instal missile sites.

Kennedy's National Security Council accepted

these reports with marked concern, but the President played them down, while privately sending his brother, Robert, to meet with Soviet Ambassador Dobrynin. The latter assured the Attorney-General that the rumours of offensive arms build-up in Cuba were false and that Khrushchev would do nothing during the run-up to mid-term elections that would embarrass the President.

To make sure that there was no ambiguity in his position, President Kennedy sent Khrushchev a strongly worded letter warning of the consequences if such offensive weapons were placed in Cuba.

However, these activities were played close to the vest by the President and his closest advisors. He did not want the hawks like LeMay to become too agitated and involving Republican critics in the Congress. Never-the-less, information apparently was passed to the hawks, possibly by McGeorge Bundy, Walt Rostow, Robert McNamara or even Lyndon Johnson. The President's low key response was interpreted as another weakness of will on his part, and the incipient plot to assassinate him was moved ahead another notch. Word was sent to at least three handlers, to put in motion existing plans to begin building easily traced 'patsy' dossiers. One such projected patsy was Lee Harvey Oswald.

Thus it was that on the evening of October 7, 1962, well before any hint of a new Cuban crisis had reached the public, George DeMohrenschildt and his wife called in on Oswald's modest Fort Worth duplex for a surprise visit. While Marina Oswald and baby June chatted with Mrs DeMohrenschildt, George and Lee secluded themselves in another room for a long and secretive chat. At the end of this unusual meeting, Lee emerged to tell his startled wife and the others that he had lost his job as a welder and that the family would be moving to Dallas.

Just as the Cuban Missile crisis sealed the fate of President John F. Kennedy, it also set in motion a new phase of Lee Harvey Oswald's life that would end in his death as well.

1962: Bjorn Sigurdsson, who had studied at the Rockefeller Foundation in 1942 and had been financed upon his return to Iceland in 1946 by the Rockefellers, reported upon the "Pathology of visna. Transmissible demylinating disease in sheep in Iceland." Visna is the starting point for 'mad cow disease' in cattle and Creutzfeldt-Jakob in humans. It was C-JD that the Fore tribe in New Guinea called 'kuru'.

1963: Dr. Leonard Hayflick, together with fourteen colleagues in a letter to *Science,* Vol.140 p.662 (10 May 1963) proposed that the pleural pneumonia like organism, or Eaton Agent be named Mycoplasma pneumoniae.

1963: Dr. Leonard Hayflick of Stanford University was awarded a NIH contract title: Procurement, Processing, Storage, Distribution and Study of Human Tumor Cell Cultures and Operation of a Central Mycoplasma Diagnostic Laboratory. The latter interest in the mycoplasma is not explained in the literature of the day, but obviously it was important to the NIH, Military and CIA biowar researchers. The evidence suggests that initially it was part of a CIA covert program labelled MK-SVLP, which was converted to a mainstream research effort after the election of Nixon. At that point, the 'MK' was dropped and the SVLP (Special Virus Leukemia Program) was changed to SVCP (Special Virus Cancer Program). In other words, the covert activities became part of Nixon's Great War on Cancer. A purely political move to cover the reality.

1963: November 22: John F. Kennedy murdered in Dallas while his Secret Service detail looked on. Secretary of the Treasury, C. Douglas Dillon, who was in charge of the Secret Service was the same Douglas Dillon whose family's financial firm (Dillon, Read and Company) had financed Hitler's rise to power in the 1930's; Dillon had also been seconded in World War Two as a naval lieutenant to Secretary of the Navy, James Forrestal, when the latter arranged with Allen Dulles to transport stolen Nazi gold to the U.S. Treasury. This 'black currency' was given the name 'Economic Stabilization Fund' and was later to be used to finance illegal government activities. The Internal Revenue Service of the U.S. helped 'launder' the wealth as 'Israeli bonds' with the assistance of the fledgling state of Israel and Jewish Mafia leader Meyer Lansky who was Jack Ruby's boss. Thus, in one incredible show of their power, the coalition that killed the President, was combined with the forces who had helped the Nazis rise to power; with those who had stolen the Nazi gold and brought it to the U.S.; with those who controlled the Mafia; and, with the U.S. Military. All met on November 22, 1963 in the seminal act which clearly established who it was that governed the United States of America: the assassination of President John F. Kennedy.

1963: Minutes after the assassination of the President, E. Howard Hunt, [See-1961: Bay of Pigs] dressed as a 'tramp', who had been one of the leaders of the Bay of Pigs invasion, and a key link with several of the Miamian Cubans, was taken into custody by Dallas police. Hunt and his two fellow 'tramps' were led to the Dallas County Criminal Courts building from behind the 'grassy knoll'. They were escorted into the front door and later exited from the rear without being interrogated or finger-printed. It should be noted that the 'Miamian Cubans' were under the overall control of CIA operative, George W. Bush.

1963: On the day after the assassination of President Kennedy, J. Edgar Hoover of the FBI directed Special Agent W.T. Forsyth to visit George Bush of the CIA and brief Mr. Bush on 'potential problems related to the assassination 'and involving the Miamian Cubans. SA Forsyth was accompanied on this mission by Captain William Edwards of the Defense Intelligence Agency.

SPECIAL ATTENTION REQUIRED

1963: Former President, George W.P. Bush has said "I am what I read", a testimony to the fact that human beings only know and hence are what they have learned. They may learn most from parents and the public school system, augmented by their social circle and their church (if they have one). However, in the modern world most of us are molded to an astonishing extent by the print and electronic media. Those who control the media control what people see and read and hence what people believe and thus what people are.

In this context it is important to note that several of the major media flatly lied to the world about what went on in Dealey plaza on November 22, 1963.

One example of lying can be seen in the December 6, 1963 issue of Life magazine. In an article titled "End to nagging rumours: the six critical seconds", written by (or at least attributed to) Paul Mandel, and edited by former Eisenhower CIA intermediary, C.D. Jackson. Jackson was well known for his extreme hatred of John F. Kennedy and he worked closely with Allen Dulles. [See-1954: Jackson/Rockefeller]. The Mandel article contains the following two paragraphs:

"The description of the President's two wounds by a Dallas doctor who tried to save him have added to

the rumors. The doctor said one bullet passed from back to front on the right side of the President's head. But the other, the doctor reported, entered the President's throat from the front and then lodged in his body.

"Since by this time the limousine was 50 yards past Oswald and the President's back was turned almost directly to the sniper, it has been hard to understand how the bullet could enter the front of his throat. Hence the recurring guess that there was a second sniper somewhere else. But the 8mm film shows the President turning his body far around to the right as he waves to someone in the crowd. His throat is exposed-toward the sniper's nest-just before he clutches it."

A blatant and total lie! [See-1964: Warren Report] The Zapruder film shows Mr. Kennedy sitting back in the limousine, looking ahead, when he clutches his throat. Since *Life* had bought the Zapruder film and could prevent their readers from seeing it and hence becoming aware of the lie they had been told, Mandel and Jackson could feel secure in their dishonesty.

Just how blatant this account is can also be seen in the fact that if the first bullet blew off part of the President's head, how could the latter turn far to the right to wave, and so get hit in the throat with a second bullet?

This media misrepresentation can be verified by anyone who accesses the December 6 issue of Life and turns to page 52F. After reading the two paragraphs themselves, they can then rent the video JFK by Oliver Stone. The Zapruder film is in that movie. The lie will be immediately apparent, and the power of the media to mold the unthinking public will be confirmed.

Truly, we are what we read (and/or see), and what we have been told and shown about AIDS and CFIDS by the NIH and the CDC with their media assets Elaine Showalter and Edward Shorter and the New York Times are lies.

1963: November 24. On the day after Mr. Kennedy's death at a 3:00 p.m. meeting with Rusk, McNamara, Ball, McGeorge Bundy, McCone, and Lodge, the new President, Lyndon Baines Johnson made some startling remarks."I am not going to lose Vietnam. I am not going to be the President who saw Southeast Asia go the way that China went." He then told Lodge to "tell those generals in Saigon that Lyndon Johnson intends to stand by our word…I have never been happy with our [ie President Kennedy's] operations in Vietnam."

This hard-nosed tone was to become effective policy immediately, when Johnson altered National Security Action Memorandum 273 that had been prepared on November 21 for President Kennedy's signature. Johnson, largely guided by McGeorge Bundy, altered the Memorandum and reversed Kennedy's decision to withdraw American forces from Vietnam. Instead of getting out of Vietnam as Kennedy wanted to do, Johnson was going to escalate American efforts.

On November 26 Johnson signed the re-written NSAM-273, and the death sentence for nearly 50,000 young Americans was sealed, not to mention the hundreds of thousands of Vietnamese soldiers and civilians who were to be killed over the following decade.

Darkness had overtaken the world.

1963–68: After the November 22, 1963 coup d'etat, Mr. Kennedy's successor, Lyndon Baines Johnson, *reversed* his predecessor's stand on population growth control, just as he reversed Mr. Kennedy's plans to withdraw from Vietnam [see: November 24 and 26, above]; to curb the powers of the Federal Reserve; to break up the CIA and 'throw the pieces to the wind'; to compel Israel to stop production of an atom bomb and to pay displaced Palestinians for confiscated property; and to enter into an arms limitation agreement with the Soviet Union.

It was this combination of Kennedy policies, plus Mr. Kennedy's refusal in October, 1962, to bomb missile sites in Cuba without first making every diplomatic effort to solve the crisis, that led to the final plans by the Rockefeller banking interests, the population control fanatics, certain of the U.S. Military brass such as Generals Lyman Lemnitzer and Curtis Lemay, and certain members of Kennedy's own administration and staff to give the go-ahead for the assassination of Mr. Kennedy and his replacement by Johnson.

Special Attention Required

1964: On September 24 the President's Commission on the Assassination of President Kennedy submitted its Report to President Johnson. Within the first two dozen pages the Report described how an 'eyewitness', Howard L. Brennan told a policeman that "…he had seen a slender man, about 5 feet 10

inches, in his early thirties, take deliberate aim from the sixth-floor corner window and fire a rifle in the direction of the President's car." Within another 50 pages the Commissioners repeated Brennan's story with added details:

"Well, as it appeared to me he was standing up and resting against the left window sill, with the gun shouldered to his right shoulder, holding the gun with his left hand and taking positive aim and fired his last shot. As I calculated a couple of seconds. He drew the gun back from the window as though he was drawing it back to his side and maybe paused for another second as though to assure hisself that he hit his mark, and then he disappeared."

Totally impossible and dishonest. The Commissioners knew it was impossible and they knew it was dishonest, but they chose to print Brennan's fabrication anyway. When they made that decision and then when they signed the covering letter to President Johnson, seven men, Earl Warren, Richard Russell, John Cooper, Hale Boggs, Gerald Ford, Allen Dulles and John J. McCloy, made liars of themselves.

Why was Brennan's story impossible?

The window from which Oswald is purported to have shot has a lower sill 12 inches from the floor. Furthermore, the window (as confirmed by photos taken at the time) was open another 12 inches. If Oswald were "standing" he would have had to be either an 18 inch midget with a 32 inch rifle, or, he would have had to fire through the closed window, shattering the glass. He was neither a midget, nor did he shoot through the glass and Howard Brennan never saw him do such. Brennan never saw what the Commissioners reported.

Later in their Report the seven liars say that Brennan's story was not credible, but the harm had been done. The picture of Oswald taking deliberate aim, firing carefully and then pausing to ascertain the results of his handiwork were part of the public's picture of Dealey Plaza, Dallas at 12:30 noon on November 22, 1963.

A lone gunman had killed the President.

To 'support' their 'findings' the Commission was thorough enough to also publish twenty-six volumes of 'evidence' with no table of contents and no index. Enough evidence to keep even the most conscientious reader busy for several months, until the heat of the moment had cooled.

It was a ploy that McCloy had employed many years before when the Milwaukee and St. Paul Railroad had filed for bankruptcy. To keep the major stockholders from knowing what was going on, Mc-Cloy filed with each stockholder thousands of wordy documents with no table of contents and no index. One of the sentences alone ran to 2250 words. Then the stockholders were given a very short deadline to accept McCloy's proposal or risk losing all hope of a return. The stockholders had to give in by accepting.

Not only were there 26 volumes of Warren Report 'evidence', most of that evidence was useless garbage. For example, in one spot the Commissioners report that Jack Ruby's mother wore false teeth. As Jim Garrison pointed out, this fact would not have been relevant even if Ruby had bitten Oswald to death.

The Warren Report is also deficient in the fact that wherever it suited their purposes, they left out critical details. One such detail was the fact that Dr. Jose Rivera, later a colleague of CDC Director, Brian Mahy, had known Lee Harvey Oswald and had attempted to communicate with the latter some five months before the assassination. Another important omission was all mention of PFC Eugene B. Dinkins a military cryptographer serving in Europe who intercepted a top-secret memorandum from the Army's high command. The Army wanted help from certain French military officers in locating a 'hit man' for a 'wet job' in Texas in November, 1963.

In summary, The Warren Report is a dishonest description of the details of the President's assassination, and is blatantly evil in declaring that Lee Harvey Oswald was a lone assassin. The Report is a further reflection of the power of those people involved in the *coup d'état*.

And, to the point of this chronology, it was John F. Kennedy's death in 1963 that opened the way for Lyndon Baines Johnson and his increased spending on biological warfare agents [See-below], and it was the Commissioners such as Allen Dulles, Gerald Ford and John J. McCloy who were members of the Rockefeller coterie, that lied to the world and to history.

1965: Johnson in his State of the Union message of January, called for the U.S. to "seek new ways to use our knowledge to help deal with the explosion in world population." He was later to boast that "When I entered office we were investing less than $6 million annually for population control. During my last year in the White House [1968] that investment had grown to $115 million." He was also to boast "In the last year of my administration I assembled a committee of men and women who represented a Who's Who in population control." Among his proud recruits to the Committee: John David Rockefeller lll!

The Rockefeller, military, financial, political, population control program had been cranked up a notch.

1966: In April and May Drs. Carleton Gajdusek, C.J. Gibbs, Jr. and M. Alpers reported in the February 19 issue of *Nature* on their joint efforts to transmit a kuru-like [ie Creutzfeldt-Jakob] syndrome to chimpanzees. The Report does not mention that it was related to a 'Special Virus Cancer Program', but it later turned up in Progress Report #8 of that very program! [See below-1971] Gajdusek *et al.* share some dramatic evidence with us that can only be seen in its full import after the AIDS and CFIDS epidemics ravaged millions of victims.

For example:
"In view of the close similarity in the clinical picture and the neuropathological findings of kuru in man with those of scrapie in sheep and mice, the remote possibility of scrapie infection in the affected chimpanzees must be considered, although so far there is no evidence of the scrapie virus producing disease in primates...there is no such syndrome of chimpanzees known to occur spontaneously ..."

In other words, rather than looking for primates that would later be tagged as the source of the AIDS virus, Gajdusek and his SVCP colleagues were trying to pass the disease from man to the primates. And, just as the best evidence clearly suggests that the kuru victims of the Fore tribe in New Guinea had been inoculated with visna/C-JD by the Japanese in 1942, the SVCP researchers were inoculating chimpanzees with kuru/C-JD from humans.

Gajdusek, *et al.* also share this information:
"The diseases under study included kuru, amytrophic lateral sclerosis, parkinsonism, parkinsonism-dementia, sub-acute inclusion encephalitis (Dawson's), myastheniagravis, multiple sclerosis, Schilder's disease, progressive multifocal leucoencephalopathy, and necrotizing encephalitis."

Finally, it should be noted that although reported in 1966, the actual program had begun in late 1963 and into 1964. These dates correspond with Lyndon Johnson's boast that his administration had significantly increased biowar funding. [See-1965 above]

1966: In May, the World Health Organization embarked upon a global smallpox-eradication campaign in conjunction with the U.S. Public Health Service. The latter assigned Donald A. Henderson, MD. to head up the program. [See 'Henderson -1956' above] Over the next decade millions of black Africans were vaccinated and as many as sixty percent, although spared the infection of smallpox, had developed a new disease: AIDS. [See below-1981: First official report of AIDS]

1966: U.S. Army Biological Laboratories, Fort Detrick and the Laboratory of Clinical Investigations, National Institute of Allergy and Infectious Diseases co-operated in testing effectiveness of aerosol transmission of viral infections.

1968: WHO begins a re-newed Smallpox vaccination campaign in certain Third World countries, with an emphasis on South Saharan Africa. They had made initial attempts as early as 1959, but it was only after the election of Richard Nixon and his appointment of Henry Kissinger as his National Security Advisor that the CDC in Atlanta was directed to provide all necessary teams to launch a major campaign under the direction of Donald A. Henderson, MD. There is evidence to suggest that certain of their early programs were represented to be polio vaccination campaigns. The latter campaigns involved Huebner and Hayflick.(See 1956 and 1963 entries respectively)

1968: At approximately 6:00 pm on April 4, The Reverend Doctor Martin Luther King, Jr. was assassinated while standing on the second floor balcony of the Lorraine Motel, Memphis, Tennessee.

The Rev. King had recently become an outspoken critic of President Johnson's/military-industrial war in Vietnam which had been initiated during the Presidency of Dwight Eisenhower by the Rockefeller/Council on Foreign Relations in 1954.

1968: On the evening of June 5, Robert Kennedy, who earlier that day had said that only the President of the United States could mount the necessary effort to solve his brother's murder, was shot dead. Mr. Kennedy's death opened the door for the election later that year of Richard Nixon.

1969: In January Richard Nixon was sworn in as President of the United States. His administration reflected his pre-election deal with the Rockefeller forces: John Mitchell who had assisted Governor Nelson Rockefeller of New York in fraudulently evading state constitutional debt limitations, was appointed Attorney General. In a less public role he was assigned by Nixon to work with the National Security Council and the national intelligence apparatus. In these roles he worked with Henry Alfred Kissinger who was appointed as Special Assistant to the President for National Security Affairs.

1969: The Pentagon's chief researcher asked Congress for ten million dollars to develop a new weapon 'refractory' to the human immune system and 'for which no natural immunity could have been acquired.' ie. An acquired immunity deficiency: AIDS. Dr. MacArthur also promised a new 'disabling' pathogen that would not be fatal.

At the same June 9, 1969 secret Hearings Dr. MacArthur told Congressmen that his researchers were going to 'mutate bacteria with viruses' to create the new microorganism. The brucellosis bacteria mutated with the visna virus would potentially present with all the symptoms now seen in myalgic encephalomyelitis (CFIDS) and Gulf War Illnesses. However, when asked for a list of the lethal and disabling disease agents that his researchers were working on, MacArthur tabled a list that had neither brucellosis nor visna! This despite the fact that brucellosis had been the single most worked with disease agent, and had even been officially taken into inventory as the Pentagon's first biological weapon!

[See-1993: Peter Dale Scott and the 'negative template']. Dr. MacArthur also discussed 'aerosol' and 'mosquito vector' diffusion techniques.

1970: In October Dr. Dharam Ablashi , a veterinarian [See-1986: Gallo collaborator; and,-1984-CFIDS research] reported upon his efforts to inoculate 22 chimpanzees with a *simian* and *human* saimiri inoculant. Rather than monkeys giving viruses to man, man was busy trying give man's viruses to monkeys.

1970: In Mol, Belgium, Robert Gallo spoke to NATO military scientists about the methods and materials used to produce AIDS-like viruses. The very fact that it was a military audience demonstrates the involvement of NATO in biological warfare planning. In essence, Gallo's presentation heralded the dawning age of AIDS. As Dr. Leonard Horowitz has written:

"I sat stunned while reading that Gallo and his coworkers had also published studies identifying (1) the mechanisms responsible for reduced amino acid and protein synthesis by T-lymphocytes required for immune system failure; (2) the specific enzymes required to produce such effects along with a 'base pairswitch mutation' in the genes of WBCs to produce the small DNA changes needed to create extreme immune system failure [See-1987: Lennette]; and (3) the methods by which human WBC 'DNA degradation' and immune system decay may be prompted by the 'pooling' of nucleic acids, purine bases, or the addition of specific chemical reagents." [**Emerging Viruses: AIDS and Ebola;** *Leonard Horowitz, p.72]*

1970: Baylor University School of Medicine in cooperation with the Texas Department of Corrections begins mycoplasmal studies on 46 prison inmates.

1970: On December 28 the Organization of Petroleum Exporting Countries delivered an ultimatum to the oil companies of the western nations: renegotiate the contracts for oil purchases or the OPEC nations would take concerted and simultaneous action. Nixon refused to provide the companies, with their strong Rockefeller components, any show of solid government support. This lack of government [ie. Nixon] support led to large increases in the price of foreign oil and earned Nixon the hatred of the Rockefeller/ McCloy/ oil executive group. When the opportunity permitted (or was created), this group would use that opportunity to bring Nixon back in line. That opportunity would present itself on June 18, 1972 with the help of the 'Miamian Cubans' under the control of George W. Bush.[See -1972: Watergate]

1971: In May the senior staff of the Viral Oncology Area, Etiology, NCI submitted an Annual Report to the National Institutes of Health. It was updated in July for the Annual Joint Working Conference of the Special Virus Cancer Program at the Hershey Medical Center on October 24-27...just five days after President Nixon had declared a 'War on Cancer'. [See next item] The Report is a dramatic albeit convoluted trail through the labyrinth of the AIDS/ CFIDS development programs about which Dr. MacArthur had reported to the twelve Congressmen on June 9, 1969. It brings together as a so-called 'Progress Report #8 of the Special Virus Cancer Pro-

gram' many of the names that were later to become known as 'experts' on AIDS and CFIDS. Among those names: Robert Gallo; Carleton Gajdusek; Paul Levine; Dharam Ablashi; Gertrude and Walter Henle; and D.A. Stevens! It also introduces terms such as Mycoplasma; Burkitt's lymphoma; Simian viruses 5, 20 and 40 which have become the argot of two epidemics: AIDS and CFIDS.

It is also important to note that various strange experiments were going on under this program long before Dr. MacArthur in June, 1969, had briefed the Congressmen on what his researchers 'planned to do.' Actually, the twin programs to limit population growth

[AIDS and CFIDS] were already underway before the elected representatives were told of them.[See-1966: kuru]

SPECIAL ATTENTION REQUIRED

1971: Dr. T.C. Merigan and Dr. D.A. Stevens co-wrote an article titled "Viral infections in man associated with *acquired immunological deficiency states* (AIDS)." The startling fact that the acronym AIDS [for: acquired immunodeficiency syndrome] was not to be officially coined for almost a decade, requires that the research and careers of Drs. Merigan and Stevens be given special attention.

Although immunodeficiency states existed and were the subject of study for several years, the disease now labelled by the acronym AIDS was distinct from the earlier immune system studies because of that key word " acquired."

Dr. Merigan was later to play a significant early role in making money off the as yet non-existent AIDS epidemic. As a 'brilliant' researcher into the emerging science of genetic engineering, Merigan founded the Cetus Corporation to develop and market interferon [See-1980: Cetus]. He was also to play a critical role after the early epidemic outbreaks of CFIDS [See-1984: Tom Merigan] while D.A. Stevens was recruited into Nixon's 'war on cancer'.[See above 1971: *SVCP*, Progress Report #8] Stevens is credited with four research papers, including one with the highly significant title: "Infectious mononucleosis followed by Burkitt's tumor." Another article that he co-authored with none other than Paul Levine [See-1986: "Robert Biggar and Paul Levine"] has the arresting title: "Concurrent infectious mononucleosis and acute leukemia case reports."

Drs. Merigan and Stevens merit this 'special attention' request because they straddle the two catastrophes of modern health: AIDS and CFIDS. Their research as early as 1971, just two years after the June 9, 1969 revelation by Dr. Donald MacArthur that the Pentagon was developing a new lethal pathogen which would be 'refractory' to the human immune system and a disabling pathogen, can be seen as early work on what were to emerge in the 1980's as AIDS and CFIDS. This, plus their associates in the early days of both epidemics, suggest that both were participants in unleashing the two great plagues against which we must now mobilize.

1971: President Nixon arrived at Fort Detrick on October 19 to announce that Fort Detrick was to become the center of a 'War on Cancer'. The Frederick Cancer Research Facility of the National Cancer Institutes would be the leading facility in that war. Later the War on Cancer was expanded to include a War on AIDS. In the latter work it has established strong working links with the Walter Reed Army Institute of Research in efforts to develop a vaccine for AIDS. [It is to be recalled that the latter Institute spawned Dr. Joseph Smadel, the patron of Dr. Carleton Gajdusek who, in turn was the researcher in New Guinea studying 'kuru' or Creutzfeldt-Jakob disease among the Fore tribe.]

1971: China quietly released CIA agent Richard Fecteau from prison as a good will gesture two months before President Nixon's historic visit. [See 1952: Operation TROPIC]

1972: In the early morning hours of June 18 a group of people first identified as Miamian Cubans were arrested in the Democratic Party offices in the Watergate Complex, Washington D.C. Although purportedly working for the re-election of Richard Nixon, the Miamian Cubans and their leader, E. Howard Hunt, had had very strong ties to both Allen Dulles (until his death on January 29, 1969) and former CIA Director, later President, George W.P. Bush. A careful study of the break-in suggests that it was set up and sabotaged, even though it took a heavy toll of loyalists such as E. Howard Hunt and G. Gordon Liddy. Nixon's neurotic, paranoid response to the break-in contributed greatly to his downfall, and gave the 'establishment' a pliant and corrupt Gerald Ford to deal with.

1973: On February 28, President Nixon learned from John Dean that critical intelligence was being passed to Nelson Rockefeller, who then passed it to Henry Kissinger. Nixon began to get the picture as to who was in the center of the web as shown by this conversation from the Watergate tapes:
> *"President: Hoover to Coyne to Nelson Rockefeller to Kissinger. Right?*
> *John Dean: That's right.*
> *President: Why did Coyne tell it to Nelson Rockefeller?"*

1973: On March 13 President Nixon referred for the first time to another force in the shadows. It wasn't the Democrats nor the media nor anyone on his 'enemies' list. It was *'the establishment':*
> *"There is not a Watergate around in this town, not so much our opponents [the Democrats], even the media, but the basic thing is the establishment."*

Here Nixon makes a statement which indicates that he had no idea of just how powerful that 'establishment' was…and still is:

"The establishment is dying, and so they've got to show that despite the successes we have had in foreign policy and in the election, they've got to show that it is just wrong just because of this. They are trying to use this as the whole thing."

Basking in the glow of his huge electoral victory, Nixon believed that he was now free of the establishment [ie. Rockefeller] hold upon him. He had no idea that within 20 months the 'dying' establishment would see their principal representative, Nelson Rockefeller sworn in as vice-president of the United States. Then their full agenda including population control would be back in play.

[At this point it may be appropriate to suggest that it wasn't so much Nixon's major policies that the 'establishment' disliked, it was Nixon as a person. However, that problem could be lived with as long as the President essentially advanced the goals of the powers in the shadows. When he began asserting himself by denying the Rockefeller oil companies special privileges he became marked for removal by the establishment. In this the Rockefeller/ McCloy/ Dulles brothers' response to Naziism is similar. It was not a case of disliking Naziism before the second world war, it was a case of not liking the leadership of Naziism to lie in the hands of men like Adolph Hitler and his cohorts. After the defeat of the German armed forces, the American establishment essentially embarked upon a 'Fourth Reich' by re-building Germany, hiring Nazi scientists and biologists, hiding war criminals like Klaus Barbie, etc. In fact, Germany later made McCloy an "Honourary Citizen of Germany".

Thus it came to be that the United States allowed itself to be transformed into one of the most evil nations in history with its institutions such as the CDC and the NIH participating in the creation of AIDS and CFIDS by the Nazi hierarchy.]

1973: March 30, President Nixon and John Ehrlichman developed a public relations strategy . Nixon tells Ehrlichman: "Get it to Congress...Get it to George Bush". The anticipated help from George Bush never materialized ['Bush resisted Administration pressure to involve the Republican Party in the President's defense'] and so Bush was able to join the forth-coming Gerald Ford administration as Director of the CIA. [See-1976: Bush/CIA], while Richard Cheney would become Ford's 'special assistant'.

1973: In October Vice-President Spiro Agnew pleaded 'nolo contendere' to very flimsy fraud charges, and announced that he would resign as Vice-President. A careful reading of the public data reveals that Agnew was forced out of office by Alexander Haig and certain Rockefeller/ CFR stalwarts. Given the growing likelihood that Nixon would have to resign, it was necessary to have someone more pliable to the 'establishment' in place. With Agnew gone, the way was open for the appointment of Gerald Ford.

1974: Henry Kissinger wrote National Security Secret Memorandum 200 wherein he proposed to President Nixon that the world population growth rate needed to be reduced. Dated December 10, 1974, NSSM 200 was delivered to the President with copies to the Joint Chiefs of Staff. On April 24 Kissinger had sent requests to the Secretary of Defense, the Secretary of Agriculture, the Director of the Central Intelligence Agency, the Deputy Secretary of State, and the Administrator, Agency for International Development, inviting input into the proposed study. Thus, with the December 10, 1974 delivery to the President of NSSM 200, the idea of slowing down the rate of the world's population growth had been officially and definitively incorporated into United States National Security planning and operations.

Thus, on December 10, 1974 the U.S. picked up the Nazi superior race, eugenics, banner from the slime and hoisted it over the White House. Let the killing of blacks and the disabling of whites begin in earnest.

1974: Between the conception of NSSM 200 and its presentation, President Nixon resigned and President Gerald Ford took charge.

1976: U.S. Centers for Disease Control embarked upon a free smallpox vaccination program for designated African and Far East countries. Five years later 60 percent of smallpox vaccine recipients had presented with HIV and many had progressed to full blown AIDS.

Tests were begun in US on gay men. Public antipathy to homosexual life style prevented serious public demand for a proper medical response.

1976: George Bush nominated by Gerald Ford as Director of the CIA, was confirmed by the Senate on January 27.

1976: In September the CIA, which according to its Charter was forbidden to interfere in domestic matters, issued Document Number 1035–960 to "Chiefs, Certain Stations and Bases", which contained instructions on "Countering Criticism of the Warren Report". The instructions included: "...discuss the publicity problem with liaison and friendly contacts (especially politicians and *editors*) [emphasis added]" and suggest that Warren Report critics were "generated by Communist propagandists". Also, "...book reviews and *feature articles* are particularly appropriate."

The Chiefs were also to "...employ propaganda assets" to spread the word that critics of the Warren Report were: i. wedded to theories developed before the evidence was in; ii. politically interested; iii. financially interested; iv. hasty and inaccurate in their research; v. infatuated with their own theories; vi. no new evidence has emerged since the Report.

[For an interesting example of how the CIA suggestions found their way to the medical profession see below: 1992, May 27]

1978: Richard Nixon published his *Memoirs*. Nowhere does he mention population control nor his purported request of Henry Kissinger that the latter prepare National Security Study Memorandum 200: Implications of Worldwide Population Growth for United States Security and Overseas Interests. In NSSM 200 Kissinger was to declare that 'greatly intensified population programs' would be required. [See-1993: Peter Dale Scott and his negative template].

1979: Henry Kissinger published *White House Years* in which he purports to tell the story of his first four years as National Security Adviser to President Nixon. Nowhere in the 1500 pages does Kissinger discuss population growth rate and the crisis it posed for the U.S. Nowhere does he refer to Nixon's and his own concerns about the 'problem' which was to lead to his National Security Study Memorandum 200 of 1974 wherein he predicted dire consequences for the U.S. and the world if the rate of population growth was not reduced by the year 2000. [Again, see-1993: Peter Dale Scott and the negative template] Significantly Kissinger dedicated the book to "Nelson Aldrich Rockefeller", his "ever thoughtful" patron and a avowed eugenics fanatic.

1979: Advertisement placed in New York newspapers to recruit homosexual men into experimental Hepatitis 'B' vaccination program. Over one thousand gay men in New York, San Francisco and Los Angeles took the free shot.

1981: First 'official' report of AIDS, which begins to approach epidemic proportions in the gay male population of New York, San Francisco and Los Angeles. Dr. Stephen C. Joseph [See-1995: mycoplasma fermentans] is New York City Health Commissioner and becomes an expert on the emerging AIDS crisis. Authors a book on the subject: "Dragon Within the Gates: The Once and Future Aids Epidemic."

1981: With less than three months in office, President Reagan was shot on March 30 by a would-be assassin. Had the attempt succeeded it would have placed the George Bush, William Casey, Alexander Haig faction of the Republican Party more solidly in the driver's seat. Even though the George Bush covert cabal had a relatively free hand under the amiable but bumbling Ronald Reagan, their New World Order agenda would have been advanced by eight years had the President died.

1982: Volume Two of Henry Kissinger's service to Richard Nixon, starting with Nixon's visit to China and ending with his August 9, 1974 resignation. As with the first volume *White House Years,* the second volume *Years of Upheaval,* makes no mention of the world population growth rate and the crisis it posed. Again, no mention of NSSM 200. [See-1993: Peter Dale Scott and his negative template]. Kissinger does make one critical point however. After assuring Nixon [in 1974] that his presidency would receive full and proper credit in history, Nixon had said: "It depends upon who writes the history". The latter reality deals with the same idea expressed by President George Bush, Sr. who had once said "I am what I read."

1983: Mathilda Krim, an early activist for research into AIDS and a former member of the Rockefeller Foundation Board, went to Kenneth Warren, the head of the Foundation's health program, for financial help to try to stem the tide of the plague. Warren replied: "This is a small local problem. We deal with big questions." Krim turned to the Ford Foundation and received the same rebuff.

1983: Max Essex contributed "Horizontal and vertical transmission of retroviruses" to E.A. Phillips [Editor] *Viruses Associated with Human Cancer.* Essex drew upon his extensive work with G. Klein who had been cited over 35 times in the *SVCP,* Progress Report #8.

1984: Dr. Robert Gallo officially announced that he had discovered the AIDS virus which, he speculated, came from a green monkey in Africa. The virus had been around for thousands of years, claimed Gallo, but had only managed the species jump in very recent times. One needs to note that Gallo had been the principal researcher at Bionetics Research Laboratories from May, 1962 through June, 1971, when much effort was expended trying to jump human pathogens to monkeys. [See-1971: *SVCP;* Progress Report # 8]

1985–89: U.S. sells enhanced brucellosis pathogens, plus anthrax to Iraq for use against Iran with knowledge and approval of Ronald Reagan and George Bush. On May 21 of 1985 the U.S. also shipped West Nile Fever Virus to Barah, Iraq.

1986: Robert Gallo reported that he and his associates Zaki Salahuddin and Dharam Ablashi had discovered a new human herpes virus which they labelled 'human B-lymphotropic virus' or HBLV. Both Salahuddin and Ablashi had been early consultants on the outbreak of CFIDS.

1987: Evelyne Lennette suggested that the possible viral origin of CFIDS was difficult to detect because "…most of the time they do not exist as virus particles…Part of the viral genome-the only part that is required to propagate-is integrated into the whole cells. So you can't see them." (Was Lennette talking about the crystalline disease agent isolated by George Merck's researchers in 1946? And is the disease agent the asparagine/ glutamine component of the prion and the amyloid?[See below-1998: De-Pace, *et al.*]

1988: In March the *Annals of Internal Medicine* published the dishonest, dismissive, tragically misleading article titled "Chronic Fatigue: A Working Case Definition" by Gary Holms of the Centers for Disease Control and twelve co-authors. This article consolidated the previous efforts by the CDC to mislead the victims and their medical doctors as to the reality of this tragic disease, and added untold suffering to those already ill.

1990: On July 3 the *Journal of the American Medical Association* continued its role as a 'media asset' of the holistic core of evil by publishing an article essentially setting forth the government's purported view that CFS was a psychological, not a physical, disease. In a letter to *JAMA* (never published) Dr. Paul Cheney wrote that the study "had little scientific merit and its appearance in your journal says a great deal more about the biopolitics of *JAMA* editors…than the real scientific concerns about this…issue."

1991: Gulf War Desert Storm Forces hit by Iraq SCUD missiles. Desert Storm attack stopped immediately on order of George Bush. Within hours of the attack by SCUDS many allied and enemy forces began to present with Gulf War Illnesses.

1991: Luc Montagnier, purportedly the co-discoverer (with Robert Gallo) of the AIDS virus, told the San Francisco AIDS Conference that he believed that the mycoplasma [See -1968: Mycoplasma Experiments; -1993: Dr. Shyh-Ching Lo; -1995: Dr. Stephen Joseph.] might be a necessary co-factor for the AIDS virus to become lethal. Robert Gallo repudiated Montagnier's hypothesis.

1992 to present: American and Canadian Military at upper levels agree to cover up record of weapon supply to Iraq and to deny that the 100,000 sick veterans were really ill. Story developed that their illness was imagined due to stress.

1992: Edward Shorter published *From Paralysis to Fatigue,* a 'put-down' of chronic fatigue syndrome, its victims, and those rare medical professionals who treated the victims with respect. Shorter, who had earlier written a National Institutes of Health 'history', *The Health Century* [which had been financed in part by the Blackwell Corporation , a champion of right-wing, Republican Party causes and by the NIH itself] has admitted that in his book he had 'targetted middle aged women with an imaginary disease.' [See-1994: Justice Rawlins].

1992: On May 27, George D. Lundberg, editor of the *Journal of the American Medical Association (JAMA)* published a two part article by Dennis L. Breo titled "JFK's death" which purported to prove that the "…1964 Warren Commission conclusion that Kennedy was killed by a lone assassin, Lee Harvey Oswald" was correct. The article employed almost every guideline established by the CIA for media assets to follow in attacking Warren Report critics. [See 1976, September above] For example, "I can only question the motives of those who propound these ridiculous theories for a price and who have turned the President's death into a profit-making industry" [Commander James Humes; see point iii above under September , 1975] or "…300 people at a convention in Dallas, each hawking a different conspiracy theory".[Humes, point v, above] However, Lundberg and *JAMA* went too far when their article stated that Dr. Charles Crenshaw, MD. was not present at Mr. Kennedy's death in Parkland Hospital. *JAMA* was sued by Crenshaw and had to retract their dishonest claim and pay damages to Dr. Crenshaw.

It may be just a co-incidence, but it should be noted that Dr. Humes received part of his training at the Armed Forces Institute of Pathology in Washington, D.C….the same Institute at which Dr. Shyh-Ching Lo was employed when he patented his infamous "Pathogenic Mycoplasma". [See 1993: September 7, below]

1992: Dr. Steven A. Rosenberg published *The Transformed Cell; Unlocking the Mysteries of Cancer,* wherein he traces his efforts to genetically engineer natural cells by inserting particles of foreign DNA into them. Although he had been included in the

Special Virus Cancer Program, and earlier had participated in MK-NAOMI (the program within the military/CIA to develop biological weapons) he makes no mention of either. It may be significant that in the early 1980's he named his youngest daughter 'Naomi'?

1993: September 7, Dr. Shyh-Ching Lo of the Armed Forces Institute of Pathology is granted Patent Number 5,242,820 for a "Pathogenic Mycoplasma" associated by him with" AIDS or ARC, Cchronic [sic] Fatigue Syndrome, Wegener's Disease, Sarcoidosis, respiratory distress syndrome, Kibuchi's disease, autoimmune diseases such as Collagen Vascular Disease and Lupus and chronic debilitating diseases such as Alzheimer's Disease." [Page 20 of Patent]

1993: Mycoplasma fermentans; despite the fact that Dr. Shyh-Ching Lo had gone to the trouble of patenting a "pathogenic mycoplasma" [See above-September 7] the United States military publicly took the position that the pathogen was not a source of disease in humans. This was a position they held as late as August 28, 1995 [See below-1995: Dr. Stephen C. Joseph]. However, in the 1993-1994 Pathology Student Workbook Syllabus No. VI of the Uniformed Services University of Health Services, the U.S. military state as follows:

"The most serious presentation of M.fermentans (incognitus) infection is that of a fulminant systemic disease that begins as a flu-like illness. Patients rapidly deteriorate developing severe complications including adult respiratory distress syndrome, disseminated intravascular coagulation, and/or multiple organ failure. The organs of patients with fulminant M.fermentans (incognitus) infection exhibit extensive necroses." ['necroses': death of a living tissue]

1993: Alan Cantwell, MD. published *Queer Blood,* a slim but fact-packed expose of the origin and spread of AIDS.

1993: In the journal: *Clinical Infectious Diseases,* Dr. Shyh-Ching Lo co-signed a letter to the editor along with: Dr. Anthony L. Komaroff [who was one of the thirteen signatories to the misleading and blatantly dishonest 1988 "Chronic Fatigue Syndrome: A Working Case Definition"; see 1988: March above]; Dr. David S. Bell [who, with his wife Karen, had

been practising in Lyndonville, N.Y. when the 1985 epidemic of CFIDS hit]; Dr. Paul Cheney [who had been practicing in Incline Village, Nevada, when the same type of epidemic hit in 1984]. Dr. Shyh-Ching Lo [of the Armed Forces Institute of Pathology] was the researcher who had applied for and received a patent on a "Pathogenic Mycoplasma"...now increasingly seen as the etiological factor or co-factor in AIDS and Chronic Fatigue Syndrome. What a strange cluster of bed fellows!

1993: Peter Dale Scott of the University of California published *Deep Politics and the Death of JFK.* Unlike most books dealing with the assassination of President Kennedy, this one fits the Rockefeller family into the total scenario, and it represents the most important and comprehensive study published to date. However, there is a special bonus for the reader: Professor Scott's 'negative template'. Scott noted the fact that when the Justice Department compiled an index of Jack Ruby's acquaintances who had been interviewed by the FBI before February 4, 1964 it had left out over one hundred names. Furthermore, many of those whose names were omitted had played very significant roles in Ruby's life. Scott writes:

"These missing names were recurringly so sensitive that I formed the testable hypothesis...that...the missing ...provided a negative template or clue for further investigation...for a name to be missing from the Justice Department list was itself a lead..." [page 60]

This testable hypothesis is not only extremely valuable in learning what is really critical in anyone's account of an incident or activity, but helps establish hidden relationships vital to a full understanding of events. For example, Scott goes on to say:

"The sanitized index was in short a phenomenon of our deep politics, a symptom that our justice establishment was by no means at arm's length from the criminals it was supposed to prosecute." [page 61]

In other words look for what is left out as a measure of significance. [See-1969: brucellosis and visna]

1994: On June 10, almost 25 years to the day [June 9, 1969] after Dr. MacArthur of the Pentagon had promised twelve Congressmen two new pathogens, one lethal (AIDS) and one disabling (CFIDS), Madam Justice B.L. Rawlins delivered a ruling in the Case of Mackie versus Wolfe wherein she determined that fibromyalgia did not exist as a physical disease. Madam Justice Rawlins arrived at this unusual conclusion after having accepted the testimony of Dr. Keith Pearce, a psychiatrist appearing for the defendant (Wolf). Dr. Pearce supported his testimony by introducing into the evidence the book by Dr. Edward Shorter, *From Paralysis to Fatigue*. In arriving at her peculiar, if not stupid ruling, Madam Rawlins dismissed the evidence of qualified medical doctors and accepted the evidence of a doctor of medical history!

The early position of the culpable NIH/CDC spokespersons such as Paul Levine and of collaborating gangsters such as Tom Merigan had succeeded-even in a court of law!

1994: Richard Preston published *The Hot Zone*. He unwittingly alerts the concerned and thoughtful reader about the trustworthiness of his tome when he acknowledges "...a research grant from the Alfred P. Sloan Foundation." [See-1997: Richard Rhodes and the Sloan Foundation]. The Sloan organization had been an early participant in the research leading to AIDS.

1994: Karen MacPherson of the Scripps Howard News Service reported that the General Accounting Office of the United States had announced that between 1940 and 1972, over 500,000 unwitting American citizens had been used as guinea pigs for Pentagon/CIA radiation, biological and chemical tests. The number of guinea pigs from 1972 to the present is still classified. Just who was being used by whom to test what?

1995: On December 5 Dr. Garth Nicolson was stripped of his chairmanship of the Department of Tumor Biology at the M.D. Anderson Cancer Center in Houston because he insisted upon reporting his scientific findings that Gulf War Illnesses appeared to be caused by the *Mycoplasma fermentans* (incognitus strain). This mycoplasma had been patented by Dr. Shyh-Ching Lo, a United States military researcher on September 7, 1993. [See-1993: Mycoplasma Patent] It is important to note that Dr. Lo had linked this disease agent to both AIDS and CFIDS, as well as a number of other degenerative diseases.

1995: Dr. Stephen C. Joseph, now the [See-1981: AIDS] Assistant Secretary of Defense, wrote a letter to Senator William V. Roth and other legislators to the effect that the Mycoplasma fermentans, incognitus strain, has not been identified as an agent which

can cause disease in man. This despite the fact that the pathogen had been described as extremely dangerous to man by the Uniformed Services University of the Health Sciences just months before. [See-1993: *M.fermentans*]

1996: Hillary Johnson's magnificent history of 'chronic fatigue syndrome' from 1984 to 1994, *Osler's Web*, was published by Crown Publishers, Inc. New York. This great work must be viewed as all the more amazing by virtue of the fact that Ms. Johnson was herself seriously ill with 'CFIDS' when she researched and wrote it. Ms. Johnson in a calm reportorial style tells the story of how one of the epidemics of the decade under study hit its victims; their families and communities; their medical care givers; the media; and, the medical bureaucracy. Although she never allows herself to judge, a sensitive and informed reader recognizes that the story she tells is a story of evil in high places.

The holistic evil core is all there in *Osler's Web*: the military, the corrupt leaders of CDC and NIH , the 'media assets'. If justice is ever really done, then *Osler's Web* together with *Emerging Viruses: AIDS and Ebola* [See below-Dr. Leonard Horowitz] will come to be seen as the two most important books of our times.

1996: Dr. Leonard Horowitz published *Emerging Viruses: AIDS and Ebola*. CFIDS has been called the 'mirror image' of AIDS. In his dramatic record of his search for truth, Horowitz leads his readers through the labyrinth of military/CIA/medical hierarchy research, development, testing and deployment of AIDS.

Taken together, *Osler's Web* and *Emerging Viruses* can be seen as the record of Dr. MacArthur's June 9, 1969 [See above-1969: MacArthur] promise to Congressmen that two biological weapons were being developed by the Pentagon: one to kill (AIDS) and one to disable(CFIDS).

1997: Richard Rhodes published *Deadly Feasts*, which purports to tell the story of kuru and the Fore tribe of New Guinea; of the intrepid American medical researcher, Carleton Gajdusek; of Creutzfeldt-Jakob and mad-cow disease; and, of Prusiner's prion. In a note 'To the Reader', Rhodes writes:

> *"Nothing that you are about to read is fiction. No names have been changed. However harrowing, every word is true."*

However, Rhodes had preceded this assertion with an even more significant 'note':

"The author gratefully acknowledges a grant for travel from the Alfred P. Sloan Foundation."

And there's the rub. Every word in Rhodes book may, as he says, be 'true'. However, it's the words that are not in his book that loom large. There is no mention of Japan's 1942 occupation of New Guinea; no mention of a Japanese biological warfare test camp in New Guinea; no mention of Japanese scientists being recruited into the American biological weapons development program; no mention of the Rockefellers anywhere in the book; no mention of AIDS. And, of equal significance, there is no mention of his patron's role with Cold Spring Harbor Laboratory; population control studies by Planned Parenthood-World Population, New York; funding of the Community Blood Council of Greater New York and that organization's part in the 1979 hepatitis-B vaccine experiments.

'Truth' is not merely the accurate depiction of reality. Truth is the full depiction of that reality, and in this, Richard Rhodes is a liar. His book might be marketed as 'The Unthinking Person's Guide to Biological Research.'

1998: Senior Canadian Military medical doctor (Major Cook) sent a superficial, error-ridden MEMO to his Commanding Officer, General Baril, wherein he dismisses the mycoplasma and Gulf War Illnesses. Then he sends a copy of his MEMO prepared for his CO to "Craig Hyams." Craig Hyams is actually Captain Kenneth Craig Hyams of the United States Naval Research station at Bethesda, Maryland. Questions as to why a dishonest MEMO within the Canadian Forces should be sent to a ranking biowar American facility were not answered by the Military. Canadian Military Medical personnel are either very poorly informed about the 'pathogenic mycoplasma' or they are intentionally covering up the truth at the expense of Gulf War Veterans who are told by the Military and by Department of Veterans Affairs to pay for their own tests and treatment or to do without either. Hundreds of sick veterans are thus left twisting in the wind. Many die (including Captain Terry Riordan of Halifax) or commit suicide. Others, like Lt. Louise Richard, RN, are denied treatment for their diagnosed mycoplasma infection.

Major Cook also denigrated Dr. Garth Nicolson in the Memo to General Baril. Apparently Dr. Cook did not know that Dr. Nicolson had been a Nobel Prize nominee, and the Major also seemed unaware that in August of 1995 Dr. Nicolson had been invited to Washington, D.C. to speak to a closed meeting of representatives of the Department of Defense, the Department of Veterans Affairs, the National Institutes of Health, the U.S. Army Medical Corps and others about the mycoplasma.

1998: Angela H. DePace, *et al.* publish "A Critical Role for Amino-Terminal Glutamine/Asparagine Repeats in the Formation and Propagation of a Yeast Prion". [*Cell*, Vol. 93. June 26] This article draws together elements of the work done by Gajdusek [amyloid formation]; Prusiner [prion]; Gallo [foreign nucleic acids]; and Lennette [nucleic particles]. It may be relevant that of these four all, except Prusiner, are listed as contributors in the *Special Virus Cancer Program*, Progress Report # 8.

2000: On Monday, February 7 Dr. Charles Engel reported to the National Institutes of Health that he had come to the conclusion that "...mycoplasmas are the probable cause of Chronic Fatigue Syndrome and Fibromyalgia." Then he made the startling recommendation that "...funding should be withheld from civilian studies until the VA study is completed in two years."

2001: Christopher Hitchens published *The Trial of Henry Kissinger* wherein he purports to tell the story of the great crimes against humanity committed by Henry Kissinger while serving his equally criminal leader, Richard Nixon. While acknowledging that "...it will not do to blame the whole exorbitant cruelty and cynicism of decades on one man", Hitchens goes ahead and does so and is shockingly deficient in telling the full story (and hence the real truth) about the United States' crimes against humanity from 1942 until the present.

Nowhere does Hitchens mention Dr. Donald MacArthur's June 9, 1969 meeting with twelve Congressmen to whom he promised two new biological weapons: one which would disable and one which would kill. Nowhere does he mention NSSM 200, and the need to 'solve the world's population problem'. Nowhere worth mentioning does he tell of Lyndon Johnson's complicity, although he had obviously read Johnson's boast in *Vantage Point* about taking action on biological weapons and population growth.

The author does manage to mention George

Bush Sr. *once,* and Nelson Rockefeller *three times;* but, all of these references are bland, inconsequential remarks made *en passant.*

There are two categories into which one can fit Mr. Hitchen's book. First, it can be seen as what Jim Garrison has described as a 'limited hangout'. That is, to put an end to any growing search for the truth about any criminal and his accomplices, admit to most of those crimes and condemn them strongly. With eighty percent of the story told, the searchers for truth will forget the other twenty percent.

Second, it can be seen as scapegoating.

"And Aaron shall lay both his hands upon the head of the live goat, and confess over him all the iniquities of the children of Israel, and all their transgressions in all their sins, putting them upon the head of the goat, and shall send him away by the hand of a fit man into the wilderness: And the goat shall bear upon him all of their iniquities unto a land not inhabited: and he shall let go the goat in the wilderness." [Leviticus 16; 21-22]

Neither of these choices is sufficient. Only the whole story will do. There is no doubt that Henry Kissinger is a criminal who committed great crimes against humanity. However, Kissinger was only the most significant executor of the will of the Rockefellers, of the Council on Foreign Relations, of Richard Nixon and Gerald Ford and George Bush, Sr.

All the world now knows that Kissinger was involved in the crimes that Hitchens mentions such as the murder of Salvador Allende, and the plans to murder the head of state in Cyprus and the genocide in East Timor. And, for those who can read the entrails of the slaughtered goat, the CIA/Suharto/Freeport McMoRan/Bre-X scandal. Except for the latter, the world knows all about the crimes of Mr. Kissinger.

But the world doesn't know about the role of the others mentioned two paragraphs above, and all of the hundreds if not thousands who translated the June 9, 1969 decision of twelve Congressmen to fund a program to develop a "new microorganism, one that does not naturally exist and for which no immunity could have been acquired" into testable and ultimately deployable pathogens.

Aids!

The world doesn't know because the decisions were made in deep secret; the perpetrators served a different master than the government which paid their wages; and the media only disseminated what the 'establishment' approved. As George Bush said "I am what I read" and the public hasn't read about what Dr. MacArthur told the Congressmen on June 9, 1969.

Summary

Since 1942 over one million Americans and Canadians, in and out of the military, have been targeted by biowar researchers or biowar weapons used in Iraq. There is no doubt that such a large number could not help but have a great impact on the health of all citizens. Yet the medical profession remains poorly informed about the pathogens employed, and the victims plus those who catch the air-borne, insect vector or food chain pathogen from them are left under-diagnosed or dismissed as neurotics.

And, every day for the foreseeable future, 6,000 innocent persons die tragic deaths from AIDS.

AIDS: created in a laboratory to reduce the rate of the world's population growth. It had to have been conceived by someone, planned by someone, financed by someone, researched by someone, tested by [and on] someone, and deployed by someone.

The evidence shows who many of these 'someones' are. We have mentioned some; there are others.

Now its up to you.

What have you done about AIDS today?

CHAPTER THIRTEEN

BEGIN WITH BRUCELLOSIS

Myalgic Encephalomyelitis as New Variant Brucellosis

As our research continued, we kept encountering the question of where the 'brucellosis' pathogen with which the biowar researchers started their efforts in 1942 left off and the 'crystalline' bacterial disease particle (which we believe is that pathogen now referred to as a 'mycoplasma')reported by George Merck in 1946 began. Were some of the outbreaks of 'mystery' diseases which shared several characteristics (fatigue, nausea, headaches, etc.) sites where actual brucellosis bacteria were being tested, or were they sites where just the disease agent in crystalline form were being tested?

We concluded that although there was a period between the testing that went on from 1946 (in Akureyri, Iceland) and 1979 (in Southampton, England) where the pathogen employed could well have varied from the brucella bacteria to the crystalline disease agent of Merck, by 1984, the biowar researchers were employing the latter exclusively. However, whether the pathogen was the bacteria or the isolated disease agent of that bacteria, the presenting disease was essentially 'chronic brucellosis', later labelled 'chronic fatigue syndrome' and now more appropriately known as 'myalgic enecphalomyelitis', the consequences for the victim were the same. We therefore, feel that it is appropriate at this point to summarize the history of chronic brucellosis cum CFIDS.

In 1946 Dr. Alice C. Evans made a remarkably prescient observation:

> *"Evans advanced the opinion that the great adaptability of Brucella may bring about at any moment 'canine strains' and even 'human strains'".[1]*

Twenty-three years later Dr. Evans' prediction was demonstrated to be accurate in at least one respect:

> *"Explosive and widespread abortions have occurred in the beagle canine species in the United States since 1966. A new brucella species has been defined, **Brucella canis.**"[2]*

Does this mean that Dr. Evans was only half right in her forecast, having accurately anticipated a canine strain of brucella while a human strain had apparently failed to present itself?

No.

New Variant Brucellosis

It is the thesis of this chapter that the "human strains" of brucella that Dr. Evans had envisioned in 1946 did indeed present soon after she had voiced her prediction at the Congress on Brucellosis in Mexico City. However, the outbreaks of what came to be known as 'myalgic encephalomyelitis' or inappropriately as 'chronic fatigue syndrome' and which have been labeled 'the disease of a thousand names'[3] are better identified in the interests of scientific precision and more productive research as new variant *Brucellosis*.

The protean range of illnesses which had their epidemic onset in Iceland in 1946 and which continued on a sporadic basis until the Elkgrove, California outbreak in 1990[4] were not recognized for what they actually were for reasons which we have already alluded to and which we will enlarge upon in this chapter. At the time the different labels for the unrecognized disease entity including Iceland disease, Akureyri disease, Coventry disease etc. were applied in different locales.[5]

The confusion arose because no virus or bacteria could be isolated from those infected. Basically, all that could be noted were the patients' subjective description of their symptoms.

This confusion was largely but inappropriately resolved in 1988 when Gary P. Holmes, MD., Division of Viral Diseases, Centers for Disease Control, Atlanta, GA., published *"Chronic Fatigue Syndrome: A Working Case Definition"*[6], signed by himself and fifteen colleagues.

Holmes' label was rejected by many medical practitioners and researchers in several countries including Canada, Great Britain and the Netherlands because of its dismissive focus upon just one symptom of a disease which actually presents in every body system with a range of symptoms, of which 'fatigue' was just one. Although to a considerable extent the

CDC label of Chronic Fatigue Syndrome (CFS) has now been largely replaced by the label Myalgic Encephalomyelitis (ME) in the latter countries, it has been retained with an almost missionary zeal in the United States.

Brucellosis

Brucellosis,[7] variously known as undulant fever, Malta fever, Gibraltar fever, Cyprus fever, Mediterranean fever and Bang's disease, is a zoonotic disease caused by bacteria of the genus Brucella. It has apparently plagued animals and humans since the days of the cave men.[8] It is characterized by symptoms markedly reminiscent of those cited by Holmes, *et al.* [9]: "...great weakness, extreme exhaustion on slight effort, night sweats, chills, remittent fever, and generalized aches and pains."[10]

"Brucellae are aerobic, non-spore-forming, facultative intracellular gram-negative rods that do not ferment carbohydrates or form a capsule in vivo."[11]

Despite the symptomatic similarity between brucellosis and Holmes, *et al.*'s "chronic fatigue syndrome", no mention of the former is made in Holmes' list of " Other clinical conditions that may produce similar symptoms..." as cited on page 388 of the Annals article. In view of the evidence that was available to Holmes and his colleagues at the time, this oversight is remarkably unscientific.

Instead of considering the characteristic symptoms of brucellosis, and the marked similarity of these to patient symptoms as shown by (for example) the victims of the Incline Village epidemic of 1984[12] Holmes focuses upon "chronic Epstein-Barr virus syndrome" and mononucleosis. This total neglect of brucellosis as a possible diagnosis is more than passing strange when one notes the fact that at first review the two diseases present in almost identical fashion. In fact, *The New England Journal of Medicine* had once made it a point to editorialize: "Because of the similarity in the clinical manifestations of undulant fever [brucellosis] and infectious mononucleosis, one may easily be confused with the other."[13]

Brucellosis presents in many ways in its human victims, and is very insidious in its ability to escape objective detection. This is especially true of 'chronic' brucellosis about which Davies had observed:

"Acute brucellosis is a disease entity the clinical picture of which is fully described in all standard textbooks of medicine.[14] Only in recent years, however, has it become recognized that brucellosis may present and persist for many years in a more chronic form. Evans et al (1938) and Evans (1939) emphasized that many cases of brucellosis were overlooked because of the chronic and insidious nature of the disease."[15]

It is appropriate at this point to summarize the symptomatology of brucellosis as presented by three well-accepted specialists in the field, and then to compare these with the symptomatology of Holmes, et al's "Chronic Fatigue Syndrome: A Working Case Definition".[16]

1. "The cardinal symptoms of chronic brucellosis noted in this series of cases were: (1) muscle weakness with easy fatigability and generalized lassitude; (2) muscle pains and joint pains; (3) sweats and chills; (4) abdominal symptoms, chiefly of pain and flatulence; (5) neurological symptoms."[17] [Davies]

2. "In this study we have classified as having 'chronic brucellosis' all patients with complaints of malaise, fatigue, myalgia, arthralgia, backache, or feverishness for a period of one year or longer beyond the acute illness, unassociated with bacteremia, changing serological titer, or physical abnormalities."[18] [Trever, et al]

3. "Fever occurs in almost all patients with acute brucellosis and less often in chronic disease. The majority of patients also experience weakness, malaise, shaking chills, profuse sweats, anorexia, and weight loss averaging 15 to 20 pounds in the first 2 to 3 weeks. Approximately one fourth of patients also describe arthralgia of the large joints (true arthritis is rare), myalgias, cough, back pain, and headache. Constipation, diarrhea, nausea, retroorbital pain, tinnitus, insomnia, and impotence are also seen."[19] [Buggy & Fekety]

These three depictions of chronic brucellosis obviously vary in minor details and length, but all are apparently describing the same or a very closely related illness. It is useful at this point to compare these summaries with the description of "Chronic Fatigue Syndrome" as given by Holmes, *et al.*:

"As it was described (1-4) in four groups of patients, the syndrome [CFS] consists of a combination of nonspecific symptoms- severe fatigue, weakness, malaise, subjective fever, sore throat, painful lymph nodes, decreased memory, confusion, depression, decreased ability to concentrate on tasks, and

various other complaints- with a remarkable absence of objective physical or laboratory abnormalities."[20] [Holmes, et al.]

With such an obvious similarity between the four descriptions cited, the question must occur: how could Holmes and his fifteen colleagues have overlooked chronic brucellosis as possibly the disease they were looking at? Even in their "Other clinical conditions that may produce similar symptoms..." which they suggest "must be excluded", they don't mention the most obvious one: brucellosis. Instead, they cite "chronic or subacute bacterial disease (such as endocarditis, Lyme disease, or tuberculosis)..."

Why such an almost studied neglect of the most obvious possible diagnosis: brucellosis?

One might suggest that their oversight reflected a profound ignorance of brucellosis. Since all the sixteen signatories were medical doctors, such a suggestion must be dismissed out of hand.

Furthermore, one of the signatories was Stephen E. Straus who was apparently quite familiar with brucellosis. In the same month (March, 1988) that he signed "Chronic Fatigue Syndrome: A Working Case Definition", Straus also published "The Chronic Mononucleosis Syndrome". In that article he cited as brucellosis authorities, A.C.Evans, E.D. Acheson, L.E. Cluff and others.[21]

In 1991 he was to again cite brucellosis authorities such as A.C.Evans, W.W.Spink, J.B.Imboden, A.Canter, L.E.Cluff and R.W.Trever in an article he wrote for *Reviews of Infectious Diseases*.[22] But more of that Straus article later.

There can be no logical explanation for Holmes, *et al.*'s failure to include brucellosis as one of the principal possible causes of the "syndrome of unknown cause" which they purported to be studying.

Both Trever, *et al.* [Definition '2' above] and Holmes, et al refer to the absence of 'physical abnormalities'; Trever in reference to chronic brucellosis and Holmes in reference to the so-called chronic fatigue syndrome.

It is, therefore, pertinent at this point to refer to Gray's observations about bacterial *exotoxins* by quoting two paragraphs in full:

"(a) *Exotoxins in Disease. There is a tendency to divide bacterial exotoxins into specific and non-specific types, although the validity of this classification is open to question. The specific types include those with pharmacological activity, causing clinically recognizable signs, symptoms and lesions, even in the absence of the organism that produced*

them.[emphasis added] The paralytic action of tetanus and botulism toxins on experimental animals, and the rash of scarlet fever are classical examples. Each of these toxins has its specific cell targets. Diptheria toxin, a protein-synthesis inhibitor, affects a wider range of body cells, but again the targets are clearly defined, viz., suprarenal glands, cardiac muscle, diaphragm and the central nervous system. All of these toxins are slow-acting; so that symptoms develop over several days.

(B) "The so-called non-specific exotoxins do act specifically as haemolysisn, leucocidins, lecithinases, collagenases, lipases, mucinases, deoxyribonucleases, proteases, necrotizing agents, erythrogenic factors and emetics. They are non-specific only in the clinical sense and their effects will not unequivocally identify the infecting organism. [emphasis added] This simply means that certain of their activities, such as haemolysis, may be shared by several different organisms, including haemolytic streptococci, staphylococci, clostridia, corynebacteria and haemophils. Unlike the specific exotoxins, the damage inflicted on the host by non-specific exotoxins, while it may be serious, should be regarded merely as supplementary to other pathogenic activities of the organism. It is recognized, for example, that streptococcal invasion can persist even in the presence of antitoxic immunity in the patient. [emphasis added]

Emphasis has been placed upon the facts that: (1) exotoxins can present with recognizable signs, symptoms, and lesions even in the absence of the organism that produced them; (2) with their effects not unequivocally identifying the infecting organism; and, (3) this even in the presence of antitoxic immunity in the patient, because all are characteristic of the bacterial toxin of all brucellae species and because the victims of myalgic encephalomyelitis demonstrate these same characteristics.

These characteristics point to a further misleading aspect of the Holmes, *et al.*'s focus upon mononucleosis as the likely etiological basis of their so-called 'chronic fatigue syndrome'. When a patient presented with signs and symptoms which could equally well be interpreted as either 'chronic mononucleosis syndrome' or as 'chronic brucellosis', and a blood test showed the Epstein-Barr virus but no sign of the brucella bacteria, the answer would seem to be obvious and logical. Because Epstein-Barr is so ubiquitous and easily detected while the exotoxin from gram negative brucella is so difficult to detect, the answer would usually be a diagnosis that the patient had the so-called 'chronic fatigue syndrome'.

Thus the effect of the Holmes, *et al.* 'Case Definition' was to turn the attention of disease victims, their families and medical care givers, and researchers to chronic fatigue syndrome and direct continuing research onto the path of the Epstein-Barr/mononucleosis explanation for the epidemics to the almost total neglect of the most likely etiological factor: brucellosis.

The attribution of the illness to the Epstein-Barr virus also set off the 'search' for a name, which led to the totally inappropriate label of "Chronic Fatigue Syndrome".

Is it reasonable to suggest that perhaps the sixteen medical doctors who signed the Case Definition just did not know enough about brucellosis to be aware of their oversight?

Such a suggestion is untenable. Not only had signatory Steven Straus cited several brucellosis authorities in his concurrent article, but investigators of the Berlin, Punta Gorda and Bethesda Hospital epidemic outbreaks had reported upon their consideration of brucellosis as the etiological factor[23] and such reports were available to the signatories.

There were also hundreds of articles available in the literature. One landmark work by Buchanan, Faber and Freeman[24] in 1974 cited symptoms and signs which merit direct comparison with those cited by Holmes, *et al.*:

Table 1:
Symptoms and signs of brucellosis and chronic fatigue syndrome

Brucellosis[25]	Chronic Fatigue Syndrome[26]
malaise	malaise
chills	(mild fever) or chills
weakness	(muscle) weakness
arthralgias	(migratory) arthralgia
headache	(generalized) headaches
anorexia/weight loss	—
cough	—
lymphdenopathy	palpable or tender lymph nodes

The blatant and total failure of the principal American Public Health Agencies to acknowledge a possible and even most likely role of brucellosis in the etiology of the subject epidemics probably did not go unremarked by informed medical practitioners and researchers. However, few if any demurrers found their objections published. Intentionally or otherwise, Holmes, *et al.* had focused attention upon mononucleosis to the almost total neglect of brucellosis.

Despite the fact that there was little if any published suggestion that brucellosis meritted careful evaluation as a possible etiological factor, Stephen Straus was apparently well aware of such claims. In 1991 he returned to the field with an article titled "History of Chronic Fatigue Syndrome."[27] He had a personal stake in having his earlier thesis validated.[28]

Straus' second article moved his position one step further along in an attempt to discount brucellosis as a possible etiologic factor in the subject epidemics. Instead of continuing the original policy of benign neglect of brucellosis, Straus purported to evaluate the possiblity. However, in a very unscientific move, he selectively edited his authorities to create an impression that these upheld his original position.

For example, Straus pretends to cite Dr. W.W. Spink as follows:

> *"It was Spink's belief, then, that 'patients bordering on a personality disorder or emotional disturbance may be tipped over into a functional state of chronic ill health by an attack of acute brucellosis'". [p.S4]*

What Spinks had actually done was to present three possibilities, of which the one quoted by Straus was only a part. Spinks had also suggested:

> *" Third, Apter and his associates have studied with psychometric tests a small group of patients having chronic brucellosis, and have suggested that the behaviour patterns may be due to organic damage to the cerebral cortex. This possibility should be explored further."[29]*

Such selective editing by Stephen Straus is misleading.

The possible damage to the cerebral cortex suggested by Apter, *et al.* is another example of informed prescience such as that demonstrated at the outset of this chapter by Alice Evans. By 1991 Straus undoubtedly knew of the presence of punctate lesions shown by magnetic resonance imaging in the brains of eighty percent of myalgic encephalomyelitis patients.[30] And, he should have known of the cerebral damage to chronic brucellosis victims as described by researchers such as Kyger and Haden who linked neurobrucellosis to multiple sclerosis.[31] However, he gives no hint of having reviewed this literature before publishing his article.

The question must be asked: what reason might the representatives of the National Institutes of Health and the Centers for Disease Control, together with fourteen medical colleagues, have in first ignoring the evidence that suggested brucellosis as an etiological factor in the so-called 'chronic fatigue syndrome' and then moving to blatant misrepresentation of data to support their untenable hypothesis?

A likely answer is available to us in the statement by George Merck in 1946 and moving us in ten key steps to the present with the fraud of Dr. Brian Mahy (to be discussed below). And that ten-step answer supports the thesis that myalgic encephalomyeitis is actually better classified as 'new variant Brucellosis.'

From Brucellosis to Chronic Fatigue to nvBrucellosis in Ten Easy Steps

Step One: In 1946, George Merck, then biological warfare consultant to the Pentagon, reported to the Secretary of War that his researchers had for the first time, isolated and produced a crystalline bacterial toxin.[32] That is, it was no longer necessary to deliver living bacteria carrying an exotoxin to its target. The bacteria which was subject to destruction by temperature, aging, or other factors was no longer a problem. The bacterial toxin in crystalline form could be diffused by aerosol, insect vector, or in the food chain. There is compelling evidence that the principal bacteria involved was brucellosis, and that the 'crystalline form' referred to is actually that nucleic particle now known as the mycoplasma.

Step Two: Evidence of the emphasis on brucellosis can be deduced from two key articles in the literature; one from 1947 and one from 1959. The first is titled "Acute Brucellosis Among Laboratory Workers"[33] and reviews the onset and progress of acute brucellosis in 17 military laboratory workers at Camp Detrick,[34] Frederick, Maryland in the previous two years (i.e. 1945-7).

The second article was titled simply "Brucellosis", and appeared in three parts in the A.M.A. Archives of Internal Medicine.35 It reviews the onset and progress of 60 "personnel of a bacteriology laboratory engaged in studies of brucella melitensis and brucella suis" who became ill with the disease. The authors of this three part article are less forthright than the authors of the article by Howe, *et al.* and make no mention of the fact that the laboratory is the same one in Fort Detrick.

Step Three: By 1951 the U.S. Military had weaponized "the *brucella suis* biological bomb, which thus became the official American biological weapon."[36]

Step Four: "The Joint Strategic Plans Committee of the Pentagon summed up the position of research and development by August 1953, saying that the usefulness of biological warfare had received the "attention of many of the best scientific minds in the United States" and had been "the subject of applied research with the attendant expenditure of considerable sums of money." The effort from 1951 to 1953 had cost almost $350 million."[37]

Step Five: It is significant that the article by Trever, *et al.* referenced above, was published in 1959 and it revealed that sixty laboratory workers at Fort Detrick had contracted acute brucellosis. This is a startling figure when one takes into account the fact that the workers had all been vaccinated when they started to work; they wore protective clothes and face masks; and, they worked through sealed laboratory cabinets.

Even with such precautions, the infection rate is very high and demonstrates the extreme volatility of the brucella agent.

However, two other features of the Trever, *et al.* article merit comment. First, in the face of the reality that a significant proportion of the victims developed a condition of *chronic* brucellosis, the authors introduce the concept that such victims are psychologically ill rather than physically ill. A theme to be taken up by Straus and his cohorts twenty-five years later. Second, it has to be placed on the record that the medical researchers who prepared the three part article were faculty of the Johns Hopkins Hospital and University. The latter institutions had held several contracts with the Department of Defence in biowar weapons development and hence cannot be regarded as disinterested third parties.[38]

Step Six: On June 9, 1969, as we have seen, the Director of Biological and Chemical Warfare for the Pentagon, Dr. D.M. MacArthur, met with twelve U.S. Congressmen to explain the Pentagon's Budget requirements for the year 1970. In that meeting, several key points emerged including the fact that in addition to researching 'lethal' weapons involving 'a new microorganism, one which does not naturally exist and for which no natural immunity could have been acquired' [Hearings, p.129] the Pentagon was working upon biological weapons which would disable, not kill their targeted victim.[Hearings, p.114][39]

Dr. MacArthur stated that the disabling weapon would be infectious by primary aerosol, but would not be contagious by secondary aerosol. That is, targeted victims could be administered an effective level of pathogen and become diabled; however, such individuals, it was theorized, could not pass the pathogen on to others by secondary exposure.

It is important to note that Congressman Flood did not accept this claim and said: "I doubt that. I doubt that."

The capabilities, limitations and secondary hazards of the disabling weapon under development would have to be tested on someone, somewhere.

In respect to the latter key point, Dr. MacArthur told the Congressmen that in all testing of biological weapons on unsuspecting guinea pigs, the Department of Defense was monitored by the Public Health Agencies: the Centers for Disease Control and the National Institutes of Health.

Thus, in the event that scientific projections such as the belief that secondary infection would not occur were proven to be wrong, and if the new pathogen was found to be infectious and contagious to the extent that brucellosis in the wild is known to be, the CDC and the NIH would be anxious to obscure the reality of any new disease.

Step Seven: In the summer of 1984 the Tahoe-Truckee High School in northeast California was visited by a group of workmen who removed the heating/air-conditioning system and replaced it with a unique new system. The new system had ducts to and from each room to the heater/air-conditioner which were designed in such a way that the air from each room was individually removed, heated or cooled, and then returned to the room it had come from. Except for incidental air exchange in the hallways, there was no effective mixture of air between the other rooms of the school. Thus, occupants of one room re-breathed the same air all day long. In addition, the windows, which previously could be opened, were shut and bolted and sealed. Teachers were strongly directed not to open the windows.[40]

One of the rooms was a teacher work room to which eight teachers were assigned. Within days of their September return to school, these teachers were discussing the poor quality of the air in their work room. One of the eight refused to use the room and parked a camper trailer near the school to use as his work room.

Within the next few months seven of the teachers in that room had become ill with one of the major epidemics of myalgic enecphalomyelitis [CFIDS]. The only teacher not taken ill was the one who had refused to use the room!

However, there were other teachers and some students in the school who became ill with the new 'mystery' disease which had so many features in common with chronic brucellosis. There were also student family members and baby-sitters who became ill.

Two local doctors soon became the medical professionals of choice for the persons ill with the new disease: Drs. Paul Cheney and Dan Peterson who had located in the out-lying community just months before the High School heating system had been replaced. Also, both doctors had been to medical school at the expense of the U.S. Government and were obliged by their contracts to serve a period of time at a place designated by the Department of Defense.

The circumstantial evidence is very compelling that the Department of Defense had remodelled the school heating system so that eight teachers would be exposed to primary aerosol, while the remainder of teachers and the students would be exposed only to secondary aerosol.

According to Dr. MacArthur's theory, which had been challenged by Congressman Flood, those exposed to the primary aerosol in the staff room would be disabled, while those exposed to secondary aerosol would be spared.

Congressman Flood was apparently proven to be right. The new disease agent, quite likely based upon the brucella bacterial exotoxin, was contagious by secondary aerosol. The disease spread to the community and then to travellers visiting the community.

It was a 'mystery' to those who encountered it, since no bacteria could be recovered from victims. They were ill with a bacterial disease, but without any bacteria detectable.

This new disease drew the interest of Dr. Holmes of the CDC and of Dr. Straus of the NIH and it was they who came up with the suggestion that it was a variant of chronic mononucleosis.

Step Eight: By 1987 there had been several other outbreaks of the 'mystery' disease. One, also in 1984, had been in the St.Lawrence Valley, Canada, and had apparently been carried by an insect vector such as a mosquito.

In respect to the latter point, it is important to note that America's ally, Canada, had established the Dominion Parasite Laboratory in Belleville, Ontario. Here they bred 100 million mosquitos a month and then shipped them to Queen's University in Kingston. Let Endicott and Hagerman take up the story:

"Detrick scientists also worked closely with the developments in the use of insect vectors of the Canadian biological warfare program, where Dr. G.B. Reed, a pioneer in this sector, remained in charge of the Defense Research Laboratory at Queen's University in Kingston, Ontario, through the Korean War era. Reed continued his World War ll work on mosquito vectors; like the U.S. researchers, he was conducting extensive work on mosquito vectors and encephalomyelitis, a project in which Canadian records indicate that there was close cooperation between the two programs. Reed continued his work on the mass production of mosquito colonies, which he was sharing with the Americans as a joint project."[41]

It is relevant at this point to go back to June 9, 1969 and Dr. MacArthur's briefing of the Congressmen. At that time MacArthur claimed that the new disabling weapon that his researchers were developing, would only be contagious by "primary aerosol or the insect vector, a mosquito for example."

Step Nine: By 1991, the 'mystery' disease that left no hint of a viral or bacterial origin in the blood of its victims, but which had all of the characteristic of chronic brucellosis, was spreading world wide. The Holmes, *et al.* Case Definition had stuck in the U.S.

thanks to media asset support, but there was a growing call for an explanation of the so-called 'chronic fatigue syndrome.' It was at this point Straus came up with his dishonest and unscientific article on the disease wherein he advanced the claim that there was no real physical disease. There was, instead, a psychological condition, mainly limited to middle aged women, who could not stand the stress of modern life. The world of psychobabble was born.

Step Ten: On August 13, 1998, William Reeves, the Director of the Viral Exanthems and Herpesvirus Branch of the Centers for Disease Control reported under the protection of the Whistle Blowers' Act to a press conference that he had called for the purpose that millions of dollars voted by Congress to study Myalgic Encephalomyelitis had been misspent by Brian Mahy, Director of the CDC.[42]

An audit by the Inspector General for the Department of Health and Human Services reported that, yes, indeed, between 1995 and 1998, money voted by Congress for the study of ME/CFS had not been spent as directed by Dr. Mahy. Rather than do as he had been directed, Mahy had mis-directed $8.8 million and had lost track of another $4.1 million.[43]

The brucellosis wheel had come full circle. From the 1940's when brucellosis was the zoonotic bacteria of first choice for biowar researchers, through the isolation of the bacterial exotoxin in crystalline form, to the testing of the 'disabling' agent by aerosol, insect and food chain vectors , to the invention of the dismissive name (chronic fatigue syndrome) and to the effective sabotaging of honest research, the Centers for Disease Control and the National Institutes of Health in the United States had initiated and presided over one of the greatest crimes against humanity ever.

The new variant brucellosis had been set loose, and millions of people worldwide were now to pay the price.

SUMMARY

Millions of people throughout the world are now ill with new variant brucellosis. To offer them a hope for a cure and to prevent the continuing spread of the sub-viral pathogen, mycoplasma, the scientific community must do two things.

First, they must unite to demand that the Public Health Agencies of the United States, together with their partners in crime, the Department of Defense and the Central Intelligence Agency, release all records available on the research conducted to develop and test the 'disabling' weapon that official documents speak about. Only by knowing what has entered into the present health catastrophe, can the answers necessary to bring the disease under control be found.

Second, an international research and testing effort must be mounted wherein some one thousand patients diagnosed with chronic brucellosis, and one thousand patients diagnosed with myalgic encephalomyelitis, together with one thousand healthy controls participate in a five year program of evaluation and comparison to identify reliable markers for diagnosis of nvBrucellosis. Then, on the basis of such developed evidence, careful remedial protocols will have to be designed and tested.

There are many clues in the literature that could be further researched to establish the nvBrucellosis/ myalgic encephalo-myelitis linkage. For example, the following paragraph can be linked to the work of Dr. Lerner, et al.:

> "Brucellosis **without** endocarditis may be accompanied by electrocardiographic changes in the form of elevation or depression of the RS-T interval and low isoelectric or inverted T waves; however, these changes rapidly revert to normal as the fever and symptoms abate, though Friedberg (1949) has reported a case with inversion of T waves for two months."[44]

Dr. A. Martin Lerner, et al. has researched and reported upon the same phenomenon in chronic fatigue patients for many years. For example:

> "We have observed that abnormal oscillating T-waves (e.g., flattened and /or inversions) in one or both precordial leads (modified lead 1 or V5) at Holter monitoring are integral to chronic fatigue syndrome (CFS)."[45]

Dr. Lerner also reports in several places upon the high incidence of cardiac damage experienced by CFIDS patients,[46] noting in one instance that the fibrillary tangles and myelin deterioration resembled the same phenomenon seen in the brain of Alzheimer patients.

This cardiac involvement in CFIDS patients can also be re-examined in relation to the cardiac damage experienced by brucellosis victims. For example:

> "Endocarditis is the main cause of mortality associated with brucellosis. Until recently, prognosis of patients with endocarditis due to the **Brucella** organisms has been particularly poor..."[47]

There are many other examples in the literature, complemented by our own files, of dramatic parallels between myalgic encephalomyelitis and brucellosis.

In one instance a lady diagnosed with ME/FM by her general practitioner and confirmed by a rheumatologist, contacted our Foundation to discuss abscesses which had developed in the area of her ankles. Further examination revealed symmetrical suppurative ulcers on each leg near the medial malleoli.[48]

The ulcers bore a remarkable similarity to those of a patient with brucellosis reported by Trever, et al.[49] See illustration below. Such symptoms are extremely rare in both brucellosis and ME. However, the fact that they do occur on occasion supports the thesis of this chapter.

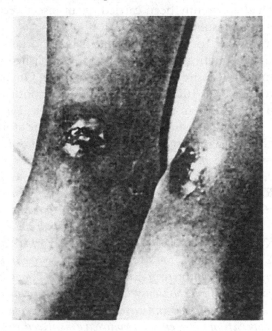

Symmetrical ulcers of the ankles in a patient with acute brucellosis.

The above examples of cardiac and abscess parallels in patients with brucellosis and ME are just two areas of many where a linkage can be seen between the two diagnoses.

This fact requires that we take a further look at the Holmes, et al. "Case Definition" of chronic fatigue syndrome, and consider further consequences for diagnosis of nvBrucellosis.

In the subject Case Definition Holmes and his colleagues are careful to include a long list of "clinical conditions" that may produce similar symptoms.[50] By this stratagem the authors manage to shut out of consideration most signs and symptoms that would lead an informed medical professional to diagnose brucellosis. By way of example, here are some of Holmes' 'exclusions':

1. 'localized infection (such as occult abscess)'. This exclusion relates to the case cited by Trever, *et al.* noted above.

2. 'chronic or subacute bacterial disease (such as endocarditis, Lyme disease, or tuberculosis)'. These exclusions relate to the cases cited by Lerner et al and Fernandez-Guerrero, *et al.* in respect to cardiac involvement as well as other studies such as that of Abernathy, et al who reported:

> *"While the majority of patients with brucellosis recover without residual effects, chronic localized infections may involve the bones, joints, bursae, meninges, endocardium, lungs, liver, spleen, epididymides, testes, and kidneys. **Such infections mimic tuberculosis and cannot be differentiated histologically from tuberculosis.**"[emphasis added][51]*

3. 'neuromuscular disease (such as multiple sclerosis or myasthenia gravis)'. These exclusions relate to the cases cited in the study by Kyger and Haden[52] wherein they linked multiple sclerosis to brucellosis. It also excludes the many studies which examine the links between MS and ME.

These and many more of Holmes, *et al.*'s 'exclusions' appear to be a concerted effort to turn attention from brucellosis as the etiologic factor in the so-called 'chronic fatigue syndrome'.

There is much more compelling evidence that Myalgic Encephalomyeitis (aka 'chronic fatigue syndrome') is actually new variant brucellosis, but space does not permit its inclusion.

The isolated bacterial toxin in crystalline form was a product of American, Canadian and British biowar weapons research, development and testing. Able to present bacterial disease without evidence of bacteria, the highly contagious pathogen was released into the human species in tests at Tahoe-Truckee, California ; the St. Lawrence Valley (Canada); Lyndonville, New York and other sites. Since the development and testing of the nvBrucellosis was at all stages monitored by the Centers for Disease Control and the National Institutes of Health in the United States, and by certain as yet unidentified military/ health officials in Canada and Great Britain, these 'health protection agencies' have felt obliged to misrepresent the truth of the disease.

The evidence is compelling: there is no such disease as myalgic encephalomyelitis or 'chronic fatigue syndrome.' There is new variant brucellosis.

ENDNOTES

[1]. "From a Special Correspondent"; (*Journal of the American Medical Association*. Vol. 133; No. 11 March 15,1947)

[2]. Morisset, Richard and Wesley W. Spink: "Epidemic Canine Brucellosis Due to a New Species, Brucella Canis." (*The Lancet*. November 8, 1969) pp.1000-1002

[3]. G.Parish, D. Bell, B.Hyde, H. Rubenstein: "The Disease of a Thousand Names". (Ottawa: The Nightingale Foundation. *The Clinical and Scientific Basis of Myalgic Encephalomyelitis/ Chronic Fatigue Syndrome*) p.3

[4]. There is an excellent summary of the 1946 to 1990 epidemics in Byron Hyde's (Editor): *The Clinical and Scientific Basis of Myalgic Encephalomyelitis/ Chronic Fatigue Syndrome.*(Ottawa: The Nightingale Foundation, 1992) pp. 176-186

[5]. A summary of such labels can be found in "A Bibliography of M.E./ CFS Epidemics" (Chapter 16) in *The Clinical and Scientific Basis of ME/ CFS*, Editor: Byron Marshall Hyde, MD. The Nightingale Foundation, Ottawa 1992)

[6]. Gary P. Holmes, MD. *et al., Annals of Internal Medicine.* 1988:108: pp.387-389

[7]. Brucellosis is named for Sir David Bruce (1855-1931) who, while serving with the British army on the Island of Malta, discovered the bacterial cause of undulant or Malta fever in 1886. He originally called the causal organism *Micrococcus melitensis*, but in 1920 the genus was renamed *Brucella* in his honour.

[8]. Arno Karlen: *Man and Microbes.* (New York; A Touchstone Book, 1995) p.19

[9]. Holmes, *supra*, pp. 388-9

[10]. Webster's *Medical Desk Dictionary,* (New York: Merriam Webster Ltd., 1986) p.88

[11]. Brian P. Buggy, MD. and Robert Fekety, MD."Brucellosis". *Current Diagnosis 8*; Editor: Rex B. Conn, MD. (Philadelphia; W.B. Saunders Company, 1996) pp. 177-9

[12]. The best account of the Incline Village epidemic symptomology is probably that developed by Hillary Johnson in her remarkable study: *Osler's Web.* (New York: Crown Publishers,

Inc. 1996). Johnson's careful scholarship is in marked contrast to the rhetorical style of Stephen E. Straus as demonstrated in his article: "The Chronic Mononucleosis Syndrome" published in *The Journal of Infectious Diseases,* Vol. 157, No. 3. (March, 1988) pp. 405-412

[13]. Editorial" Infectious Mononucleosis versus Brucellosis",(NEJM July 27, 1944) p.165

[14]. This observation may have been true in 1957, but is not true in 2002. It is pertinent to the thesis of this chapter that the latest edition of the *Johns Hopkins Family Health Book,* Editor-in-Chief, Michael J. Klag, MD., M.P.H. (New York: Harper Collins Publishers, 1999) omits all mention of one of the world's most ancient diseases: Brucellosis. However, it does have a two page reference (pages 877-8) to "Chronic Fatigue Syndrome". One might well ask of the editors: "Where has all the brucellosis gone?"

[15]. J.E. Davies, M.B., B.S. "Chronic Brucellosis in General Practice", (*British Medical Journal,* Nov.9,1957) p.1082

[16]. Holmes, *et al. supra*

[17]. Davies, J. E. *supra*

[18]. Robert W. Trever, MD.; Leighton E. Cluff, MD.; Richard N. Peeler, MD., and Ivan L. Bennett Jr., MD. "Brucellosis". (*A.M.A. Archives of Internal Medicine* Vol. 103, March,1959) p.62/390

[19]. Rex B. Conn, *supra* p. 178

[20]. Holmes, *et al. supra* p.387

[21]. Stephen E. Straus: "The Chronic Mononucleosis Syndrome". (*Journal of Infectious Diseases* Vol.157, No.3 March,1988) pp. 411-412

[22]. Stephen E. Straus: "History of Chronic Fatigue Syndrome". (*Reviews of Infectious Diseases,* Suppl.1 1991) S2-7

[23]. Byron Hyde,(Editor): *supra* p.148

[24]. Thomas M. Buchanan,MD., L.C. Farber, MD., and Roger A. Feldman. MD.: "Brucellosis in the United States, 1960-1972. (*Medicine,* Vol. 53, #6. In three parts. 1974)pp. 403-439

[25]. Buchanan, *et al.* p. 404

[26]. Holmes, *et al.* pp.387-389

[27]. Stephen E. Straus: "History of Chronic Fatigue Syndrome". (Bethesda, Maryland: National Institute of Allergy and Infectious Diseases. *Reviews of Infectious Diseases* 1991) p. 13 (Suppl 1):S2-7

[28]. Hillary Johnson in her marvellous book, *Osler's Web* recounts the following telling anecdote: Byron Hyde was sitting next to Straus at a 1987 meeting when a paper demonstrating some of the flaws in Straus' theory of E-B etiology for ME/FM was handed out. Hyde describes what happened this way:"Straus began talking to himself out loud as the scientific purport of the paper sank in...He held a monologue that lasted two minutes...I thought he was having a nervous breakdown. He kept saying ,'They've ruined me. What will my colleagues think? These goddamn patients!' He seemed to be taking it personally, and talked as if the patients had banded together to destroy him." (New York: Crown Publishers 1996) p.321

[29]. Wesley W. Spink, M.D. "What is Chronic Brucellosis?" *Annals of Internal Medicine* V.35 (1951) p. 373

[30]. See the several references to MRI in Johnson, *supra.*

[31]. E.R.Kyger, Jr., MD. and Russell L. Haden: "Brucellosis and Multiple Sclerosis". *The American Journal of the Medical Sciences* (Dec. 1949) pp. 689-693

[32]. Hearings before the Subcommittee on Health and Scientific Research of the Committee on Human Resources; United States Senate. Ninety-fifth Congress. (March 8 and May 23,1988) pp.72-3

[33]. Lt. Calderon Howe, (MC) U.S.N.R., Captain Edward S. Miller, M.C., A.U,S., Lt. (jg) Emily H. Kelly, H(W) U.S.N.R., Captain Henry L. Bookwalter, M.C., A.U.S., and Major Harold V. Ellingson, M.C.,U.S.A. "Acute Brucellosis Among Laboratory Workers". (*The New England Journal of Medicine,* V.236; No. 20 May 15,1947) pp. 741-747

[34]. The locale was known as 'Camp' Detrick, but was later elevated to the rank of 'Fort' Detrick. Henceforth the reference will be 'Fort' Detrick.

[35]. Robert W. Trever, MD.; Leighton E.Cluff, MD.; Richard N. Peeler, MD., and Ivan L. Bennett Jr., MD. "Brucellosis" Part One. (*A.M.A. Archives of Internal Medicine.* Vol.103 March, 1959) pp.53/381-69/397

Part Two: Leighton E. Cluff, MD,; Robert W. Trever, MD.; John B. Imboden, MD., and Arthur Canter, PhD pp.71/399-77/405

Part Three: John B. Imboden, MD.; Arthur Canter, PhD; Leighton E. Cluff, MD., and Robert W. Trever, MD.

[36]. Ed Regis: *The Biology of Doom,* (New York: Henry Holt and Company 1999) p. 139

[37]. Stephen Endicott and Edward Hagerman: *The*

United States and Biological Warfare. (Bloomington, Indiana: Indiana University Press 1998) p.79. It is to be noted that $350 million in this time period would be equivalent to over three billion dollars in the year 2002.

[38]. "Special Virus Cancer Program" *Progress Report # 8.* Program Staff, Viral Oncology, Etiology Area. National Cancer Institute. (July, 1971) Pp. 369-70.
"Biological Testing Involving Human Subjects by the Department of Defense." U.S. Senate, Subcommittee on Health and Scientific Research. (March 8 and May 23, 1977) On page 89 it is revealed that Johns Hopkins had received 12 Defense contracts between 1950 and 1971. Furthermore, the article by Trever, *et al.* was financed by the Department of Defense under contract "No. DA 18-064-404-CML-100 with Army Chemical Corps, Fort Detrick, Frederick, MD."

[39]. Hearings before a Subcommittee of the Committee on Appropriations: House of Representatives, Ninety-first Congress. "Chemical and Biological Warfare".

[40]. Hillary Johnson, *supra* p.26

[41]. Endicott and Hagerman, *supra*, p.75

[42]. Martin Enserik:"CDC Struggles to Recover from Debacle Over Earmark". *Science,* Vol. 287 #5450. (7 January 2000) p.22

[43]. June Gibbs Brown: "Audit of Costs Charged to the Chronic Fatigue Syndrome Program at the Centers for Disease Control and Prevention." Washington; Department of Health and Human Services. (May 1999) p.7

[44]. F.Dudley Hart, MD., Alan Morgan, M.B., and Brian Lacey, M.B., B.Sc.:"Brucella Abortus Endocarditis". *British Medical Journal* (May 12, 1951) p.1053

[45]. A. Martin Lerner, James Goldstein, Chung-ho Chang, Marcus Zeros, James T. Fitzgerald, Howard J. Dworkin, Claudine Lawrie Hoppen, Steven M. Korotkin, Marc Brodsky, and William O'Neil: "Cardiac Involvement in Patients with Chronic Fatigue Syndrome as Documented with Holter and Biopsy Data in Birmingham, Michigan, 1991-1993." *Infectious Diseases in Clinical Practice,* Vol.6, No.5. (1997) pp.327-333
Note that Dr. Lerner et al have several further reports on this subject.

[46]. Lerner, *et al. ibid* p. 331

[47]. Manuel L. Fernandez-Guerrero,MD.; Jorge Matinell,MD.; Jose Maria Aguado, MD.; Maria del Carmen Ponte, MD.; Julian Fraile, MD.; Gregorio de Rabago, MD. "Prosthetic Valve Endocarditis Caused by *Brucella melitensis.*" *Archives of Internal Medicine,* Vol.147 (June 1987) pp. 1141-1143

[48]. Personal files.

[49]. Trever, *et al. supra* p.64/392

[50]. Holmes, *et al. supra* p.388

[51]. Robert S. Abernathy, MD.; William E. Price, MD.; and Wesley W. Spink, MD.: "Chronic Brucellar Pyelonephritis Simulating Tuberculosis." JAMA, Vol. 159, #16. (Dec. 1955) p. 1534

[52]. E.R.Kyger, Jr. MD. and Russell L. Haden, MD.: *supra.*

CHAPTER FOURTEEN

THE MYCOPLASMA HYPOTHESIS

INTRODUCTION

Most people understand the word 'germ', although in precise medical language, its meaning is nebulous. Speaking more precisely, one talks about bacteria, which are one-celled animals, and viruses, which are bacterial nucleic particles in a protein coat.

However, another term for disease-causing organisms is gaining in notoriety: the mycoplasma. The mycoplasma lacks a cell-wall, and is composed of bacterial nucleic particles. Various mycoplasma species are known to be pathogenic to humans with diseases such as AIDS, chronic fatigue syndrome and even Alzheimer's being linked to certain species.

It is said of a wide range of neuro/systemic degenerative diseases that their etiology is unknown, there is no known cure, and the incidence of each is increasing dramatically. The 'mycoplasma hypothesis' considers whether it is more likely that each of over two dozen degenerative diseases has its unique disease agent and that each such agent has increased in incidence over the past three decades, OR whether there is a single pathogenic agent with an increased virulence which, like brucellosis, can affect every body system dependent upon the genetic predisposition of its victims and which presents in the protean range of degenerative diseases under review.

The mycoplasmas are defined as the 'smallest microorganisms known to be capable of reproduction outside of living cells; lack rigid cell wall and are pleomorphic.'[1] Their most critical characteristic is that although they '…require sterols for growth'[2] they lack the necessary organelles to process their own nutrients, and they must take up preformed sterols from their growth medium and incorporate such sterols into their cytoplasmic membranes.[3] As a consequence they ultimately kill their host cells, although this outcome is often delayed for significant periods of time:

"Mycoplasmas can attach to specific cells without killing the cells and thus their infection process can go undetected. No symptoms suggests no disease. In some people the attachment of mycoplasma to the susceptible cell membranes acts like a living thorn,

a persistent foreign substance, causing the host's immune defense mechanism to wage war."[4]

The latter hiatus may well be the 'chronic' phase of certain of the various diseases such as chronic fatigue syndrome that have been associated with the mycoplasma.[5] The association of the mycoplasma with chronic fatigue syndrome was made by Dr. Shyh-Ching Lo of the United States National Institutes of Health when on September 7, 1993 he applied for and received a United States Patent (# 5,242,820) for "Pathogenic Mycoplasma"! Dr. Lo stated in his Patent Application that:

"The M.fermentans incognitus pathogen is useful for the detection of antibodies in the sera of patients or animals infected with M.fermentans incognitus. Some of these patients who are infected with M.fermentans incognitus will be patients who have been diagnosed as having AIDS or ARC, Cchronic [sic] Fatigue Syndrome, Wegener's Disease, Sarcoidosis, respiratory distress syndrome, Kibuchi's disease, antoimmune [sic] diseases such as Collagen Vascular Disease and Lupus and chronic debilitating diseases such as Alzheimer's Disease."[6]

Further along in his Application Dr. Lo writes:

"Six patients from six different geographic areas who presented with acute flu-like illnesses were studied. The patients developed persistent fevers, lymphadenopathy or diarrhea, pneumonia, and/or heart, liver, or adrenal failure. They all died in 1-7 weeks.

"These patients had no serological evidence of HIV infection and could not be classified as AIDS patients according to CDC criteria. The clinical signs as well as laboratory and pathological studies of these patients suggested an active infectious process, although no etiological agent was found despite extensive infectious disease work-ups during their hospitalization.

"Post-mortem examination showed histopathological lesions of fulminant necrosis involving the lymph nodes, spleen, lungs, liver, adrenal glands, heart, and/or brain. No viral inclusion cells, bacteria, fungi, or parasites could be identified in these tissues using special tissue strains. However,

the use of rabbit antiserum and the monoclonal antibodies raised against M.fermentans incognitus…the pathogen shown to cause fatal systemic infection in primates…revealed M.fermentans incognitus antigens in these necrotizing lesions. In situ hybridization using a S labelled M.fermentans incognitus-specific DNA probe… also detected M.fermentans incognitus genetic material in the areas of necrosis."[7]

Certain of Dr. Lo's data merit emphasis: the six patients all died; there were no signs of any etiological agents such as viral inclusion cells, bacteria, fungi, or parasites; several critical body organs were affected by lesions of fulminant necrosis: lymph nodes, spleen, lungs, liver, adrenal glands, heart and/or brain; the necrotizing lesions all tested positive for *M.fermentans* incognitus.

The Mycoplasma Hypothesis, point one:
On the basis of these data we hypothesize that the *M.fermentans* incognitus was the causative etiological factor in all six cases cited; that certain mycoplasma strains are not only pathological, but their effects can be fatal; and, all major body systems are vulnerable to its damage.

Despite such *prima facie* evidence that the mycoplasma can do a protean range of damage to the victim, there is a puzzling lack of knowledge about this disease agent. We will cite just one example.

In August, 1998, Major T. Cook, Head Medical Services of the Canadian Military, addressed a Memorandum to his Commanding Officer, General J.M.G. Baril, titled "Gulf War Illnesses & Mycoplasma- Brief to CDS." The memo was in response to a request by General Baril who had asked for information about the mycoplasma because certain Gulf War Veterans (of whom Lt. Louise Richard, RN., was one) were very ill with some mysterious illness broadly labelled "Gulf War Illnesses" and a significant number had tested positive for the presence of the mycoplasma.

Major Cook's memo is superficial, dismissive of the dangers posed by the mycoplasma as described by Dr. Lo and as borne out in several peer-reviewed articles in professional journals, and is error-ridden, even in the most elemental details. For example, Major Cook states that "Mycoplasmas… were first identified and classified in the 1960's". However, Dr. Lo cites sources which show that the term was first used as far back as 1889[8], and in 1898 Nocard and Roux isolated the first mycoplasma species (now

known as M. mycoides var mycoides). By 1967 The *Canadian Medical Association Journal* stated that "The first human mycoplasma was isolated 30 years ago [ie. 1937] by Dienes and Edsall."[9]

Such errors in detail by Dr. Cook would not be worthy of comment were it not for the fact that a significant number of Canadian Gulf War Veterans have become ill, some fatally, since their period of service in the Gulf area, and that of this number, a large percentage have tested positive for mycoplasma infection. These facts, together with the fact that as Head Medical Services for the Military, Major Cook is the person primarily responsible for responding to the tragic disability of these young Canadians, one would expect him to be at the fore-front of those researching the Gulf War-Mycoplasma linkage. However. his memo clearly demonstrates that he has not met his obligation to those persons who were sent into the Gulf area in the service of their country, and that he has largely ignored the number of veterans who have died, apparently as a consequence of such service.[10]

How does one account for the fact that the Head Medical Services is so derelict in his duty to those whose health he has an obligation to protect?

The answer is probably to be found in the fact that Major Cook copied his memo for General Baril to a 'Capt. Craig Hyams" of the United States Naval Research Institute, Rockville, Maryland. Aside from the propriety of an officer in the Canadian Military sending a copy of a memo that he has prepared for his Commanding Officer to an officer in a foreign military institution, one must require an explanation as to why a superficial assessment of the mycoplasma would be deemed worthy of Captain Hyams' attention. After all, the Department of Microbiology of The Uniformed Services University of the Health Sciences (a medical facility operated by the U.S. Department of Defence for medical personnel of all four of the U.S. armed services…including the U.S. Navy) had a three page course unit on "Mycoplasma Infections" listed in its Calendar of the 1993-1994 Academic Year.[11] In this three page course unit it is stated (among other critical details) that:

"The most serious presentation of M.fermentans infection is that of a fulminant systemic disease that begins as a flu-like illness. Patients rapidly deteriorate developing severe complications including adult respiratory distress syndrome, disseminated intra vascular coagulation, and/or multiple organ failure.

"The organs of patients with fulminant infection exhibit extensive necrosis. Necrosis is most pronounced in lung, liver, spleen, lymph nodes, adrenal glands, heart, and brain."[12]

In view of such evidence that the mycoplasma is a very dangerous pathogen, one can infer that Major Cook of the Canadian Armed Forces sent a copy of his superficial and dismissive memo to Captain Craig Hyams of the United States Navy because they were anxious to keep their stories about the mycoplasma straight. His memo was not an exchange of critical or sophisticated scientific insights about a disabling and in some instances a deadly pathogen. The memo was an attempt to ensure that in-so-far as possible, the true danger posed by the mycoplasma had to be kept hidden from General Baril, from the pathogen's victims, their personal physicians and certain other military persons and from the public at large. Therefore, Major Cook in his memo to his Commanding Officer did not quote from the United States Uniformed Services University of the Health Services Calendar because to do so would be to face up to the reality that the mycoplasma for which so many Gulf War Veterans had tested positive, was extremely pathogenic and potentially fatal.

The question arises: What is the true nature of the mycoplasma and why must the true nature be obscured by persons such as Major Cook and Captain Craig Hyams? And, how does the mycoplasma figure in the range of neuro/systemic degenerative diseases that are under review?

The Mycoplasma Hypothesis, point two:
The mycoplasma is a naturally occurring pathogen which has, over the history of humanity, caused a variety of neural/systemic degenerative diseases. The human species has over time, acquired a significant degree of immunity to this naturally occuring pathogen; however, in the early decades of the twentieth century, biological warfare researchers, including United States Naval Research (which includes personnel such as Captain Craig Hyams) and the Canadian Military have succeeded in mutating [13] the pathogen to make it more contagious and infectious, and to make it refractory to the human immune system upon which we depend 'to maintain our relative freedom from infectious disease.'[14]

From the Hearings cited in Endnote 14 as well as from other official documents, it is now known that the United States Congress had approved huge appropriations of money to develop biological weap-

ons. Such research had begun during World War One, and was continued into the 1930's. In 1942 the United States entered into a tripart agreement with Canada and Great Britain to accelerate and coordinate their efforts. Under this agreement Great Britain turned over its research into the use of brucellosis to the United States Researchers at (then) Camp Detrick, Frederick, Maryland.[15] "From the moment of its birth in the highest levels of government, the fledgling biological warfare effort was kept to an inner circle of knowledgeable persons. George W. Merck was a key member of the panel advising President Franklin D. Roosevelt..."[16] Thus the direction of biological warfare research was clearly established: a joint military-industrial effort by Canada, Britain and the United States would in absolute secrecy research, develop and test biological pathogens in North America. We are still learning the consequences.

One of the consequences of this research, development and testing program was the threat to the health of the researchers and the long-term consequences for the health of the usually unwitting test victims. However, a more serious consequence could mean "... a worldwide scourge, or a black death type disease that would envelop the world or major geographical areas if some of these materials were to accidentally escape."[17]

The threat to the health of the researchers was evident very early, when in May, 1947, a group of military medical professionals published a report in *The New England Journal of Medicine* about acute brucellosis among laboratory workers.[18] It comes as no surprise to learn that the laboratory workers were from the Station Hospital, Camp Detrick, Frederick, Maryland! And, it also comes as no surprise that the report was written by medical professionals in the same Naval Research Institute that today employs Captain Craig Hyams to whom Major Cook of the Canadian Military apparently feels an obligation to report upon what he is telling his Commanding Officer.

In March, 1959, another group of Medical Professionals published a further report upon laboratory workers in (now) Fort Detrick. The report revealed that:

"From 1945 to 1957 sixty cases of acute brucellosis occurred among personnel of a bacteriology laboratory engaged in studies of Brucella melitensis and Brucella suis."[19]

It is significant to note that the report was written

by medical professionals from The Johns Hopkins University School of Medicine, and The Johns Hopkins Hospital under Contract No. DA 18-064-404-CML-100 with Army Chemical Corps, Fort Detrick, Frederick, MD. It is also significant to know that the same School of Medicine had been given several biological warfare research grants by the United States Military.

These two reports make it clear that medical professionals at the highest levels of their profession were working with the military-industrial professionals in their joint efforts to translate the naturally occurring brucellosis pathogen into a biological weapon. Further evidence suggests that they succeeded. By the time of the Korean War, the U.S. Military had a stockpile of weapons armed with *Brucella suis* and *Brucella melitensis.*

> *"Brucella suis, code US, which causes undulant fever in people- an incapacitating disease with a mortality rate of 3 percent. It is mainly a disease of animals, but can cause acute and chronic illness in humans; its distribution is worldwide. Flies, mosquitoes, ticks, and other insects can be infected and transmit the disease by biting animals or people. Brucella can be inhaled [ie 'aerosol' transmission- Ed] or it can enter the body through the digestive tract or through skin infections. The patient suffers from aches and pains, drenching sweats, rapid swings of temperature, and a loss of appetite, and complains of great weakness and fatigue. Severe depression, anxiety, irritability, restlessness, and apathy are typical of the illness."[20]*

Besides the fact that these symptoms are strikingly similar to those of the late Capt. Terry Riordan [See Endnote #10] this passage must be read against the background of two critical facts. First, in 1946 George Merck reported to his Pentagon superiors that the biological warfare researchers had for the first time succeeded in extracting the 'bacterial toxin in crystalline form' from the bacteria.[21] The significance of this statement cannot be over-emphasized. What it states is that the toxin which usually spread from detectable bacteria was now available to the biowar researchers independent of its original carrier. One could have the bacterial toxin without any trace of the bacteria. Since Mr. Merck specified that the toxin was in 'crystalline form' and since the mycoplasma which is known to be molecular fragments of bacterial nuclei is also crystalline, is it possible that George Merck's pathogen was the original free-form mycoplasma? We'll return to this possibility.

The other critical fact which must be held in mind as one studies the above passage is the reference to two of the principal methods of pathogen diffusion: aerosol and insect vectors. One needs to know that after World War Two the Government of Canada and its Military agreed with its United States research partner to continue with its biowar research and to open the Dominion Parasite Laboratory in Belleville, Ontario, Canada. In this Laboratory one hundred million mosquitoes a month were to be bred and transferred to Queen's University where they were to be contaminated with various disease agents and then trans-shipped to the American and Canadian military to be tested upon unwitting civilian guinea pigs at various sites in Canada, the United States, and other sites under US-British control such as South Africa and Iceland.[22]

Between 1940 and 1974 the United States used at least 500,000 of its own citizens as unwitting test subjects for various radiation, biological and chemical experiments.[23] The number of citizens used after 1974 is still kept top secret because the period from 1974 to the present was the time frame for testing the pathogens designed to disable or kill its victims using the 'new infectious agent' promised on June 9, 1969 by Dr. MacArthur to the Congressional Subcommittee. This was the pathogen for which, said Dr. MacArthur, "...no immunity could have been acquired" (AIDS) and its 'mirror image' which would disable its victims but not kill them (CFIDS).

In addition to these tests upon American citizens, the United States military received permission from the Government of Canada to test a new carcinogen on the whole City of Winnipeg,[24] and from the Government of South Africa the U.S. Military and CIA received the okay to test a variety of pathogens, both disabling and fatal, upon the Black population of that country.

Thus, in Canada and the United States between 1942 and 1974, over 1,000,000 people received a variety of pathogenic agents without their knowledge or consent. Since 1974 conservative estimates indicate that at least another million people in the two countries have served as unwitting guinea pigs.

Since such tests were conducted with the full knowledge and agreement of certain key persons in the health bureaucracy and the military/intelligence community of both countries, these same people now have a strong vested interest in keeping secret what was going on and their role in it. Sufficient reason for people such as Stephen Straus of the U.S. National Institutes for Health and Captain Craig Hyams of the U.S. Navy to mislead the public about the mycoplasma. After all, if the military/ health bureaucracies were to reveal the full story of their brucellosis - mycoplasma biowar research, development, testing and deployment they would likely help make it clear why so many neuro/systemic degenerative diseases are today increasing dramatically and taking such a heavy toll of victims diagnosed as specified above in Dr. Lo's Patent Application.

The mycoplasma hypothesis, point three:
The various species and strains of the mycoplasma are derived from the nucleic acids of various bacteria and the particles of each species or strain have a particular aptitude to penetrate specific host cells dependent upon the protein secretion system that had evolved to deliver bacterial effector proteins into host cells that then modulate host cellular functions. It is to be noted that this is not simply the usual bacterial-host interaction such as occurs when the complete bacterium delivers protein from its cytoplasm into the host cell cytosol[25], but hypothesizes that the nucleic acid particle (ie the mycoplasma) is able, using the same 'common protein secretion pathway', to enter a new host and function according to its specific capabilities, especially its capacity to uptake preformed sterols from its host.

The Brucellosis Antecedent

Brucellosis is an anthropozoonosis with a worldwide distribution. It has a high degree of morbidity with the brucella capable of surviving and even multiplying, within the cells of the mononuclear phagocytic system. Infection by organisms of the genus brucella has a wide clinical polymorphism, and almost every organ can be affected, with bone and joint involvement; genitourinary, neurological, cardiac, and gastrointestinal complications. It can persist as a diffuse chronic condition or as a disease of one or more focal points.[26]

As early as 1946 Benning [27] reported brucella characteristics which anticipated the later biowar research. For example, Benning reported a brucella culture filtrate 'without bacterial cells' wherein the 'active principle' seemed to be a nucleoprotein. This at about the same time that George Merck was reporting upon the success of his researchers in extracting the disease principle from selected bacteria in a crystalline form.

The Mycoplasma Derived

If our hypothesis can be sustained, then a specific species of the brucella could have been processed to yield a cell wall-less nucleic particle which could penetrate certain host cells and begin to uptake preformed sterols which it incorporated into its own cytoplasm.

Such research was clearly being done in the late 1960's and early 1970's. For example, in 1979 Robert Gallo made a report to a special symposium sponsored by the North Atlantic Treaty Organization wherein he discussed "...several possible mechanisms prompting the 'entry of foreign nucleic acids' into lymphocytes"[28] The question that naturally arises is what interest did NATO, a military alliance, have in medical/scientific research? And the answer is self-evident: it was all part of their efforts to develop new biological weapons.

The title of the symposium says it all: "The NATO International Symposium on Uptake of Informative Molecules by Living Cells".[29] The 'informative molecules' are the amino acid particles that have the power to carry a message to its new host. The 'living cells' are those targeted for destruction by the biowar researchers. The likelihood that the nucleic acid particles are the cell wall-less mycoplasma [30] which carries its 'information' to take up preformed sterols from its host is compelling.

The fact that Robert Gallo was engaged in this biowar research on the development of the mycoplasma explains his later disingenuous dismissal of the mycoplasma as a pathogen:

"Scientists have sometimes been embarrassed by reporting their role in one or another disease, only to learn later that mycoplasmas were accidental bystanders."[31]

The evidence suggests that one should give this position as much credence as one gives Gallo's claim to be a co-discoverer of the human immunodeficiency virus (HIV).

How did Gallo and his colleagues solve the problem of getting the target cell to admit the 'informative molecules'? Probably by establishing what the 'normal pathway' was and then by utilizing that pathway to secure the passage of the pathogenic particle. For example, from the *B. melitensis* bacterium which in the wild is capable of entering respiratory cells, causing a wide spectrum of pulmonary complications including "...unilateral or bilateral bronchopneumonia, cavitated pneumonia, pulmonary nodules, hilar lymphadenopathy, and emphysema" there could be extracted the *M.pneumoniae* particle which presents with "...pneumonia, pleural effusion, bronchitis, bronchiolitis, croup, exacerbations of chronic bronchitis, lung abscess,[32] and which have the necessary qualities to access the 'normal pathway' of its antecedent bacterium.

The former disease agent would be detectable (but often with some difficulty) by blood and tissue tests, while the latter, a 'bacterial disease without the bacteria', would only be readily detectible by polymerase chain reaction test which would keep most medical professionals from knowing of its existence, a desirable consequence in a biological weapon.

The Mechanics of the Mycoplasma

The mycoplasma, as a mere particle of its former bacterial antecedent, lacks the cellular organelles to process the nutrient requirements of a living cell. As a consequence it takes up the preformed sterols from its host and incorporates these into its own cytoplasm. This is the essential dynamic of cellular degeneration. Steroid by steroid the host cell, whether in the brain, the spinal column, the genito-urinary tract, or other body system loses its being to its parasitic intruder until it, the host cell, is killed.

Support for this hypothesis can be found by reviewing the nature of the signs and symptoms presented when the mycoplasma uptakes the preformed sterols from its host, and by determining what would cause such signs and symptoms.

The first fact that must be recognized is that, regardless of the organ cell from which the steroid is taken up, the structure of the steroid is basically the same: the three hexagons and one pentagon molecule of carbon, hydrogen and oxygen atoms of the "steroid nucleous". Around this basic pattern all the variants are built and present as hormones, cholesterol, and vitamin D. And all of these variants are subject to the ability of the mycoplasma to wrest them from the host cell and incorporate them into its own cytoplasm.

Hence the 'degeneration' of the host cell whether in the brain, the digestive system, the uterus or prostate, the bone marrow, the spinal column, the adrenal gland...wherever in the body that the steroid nucleus and its variants perform their metabolic duties. And when the host cells have a threshold level of their steroidal being taken up by the mycoplasma and die there occurs a primary, secondary and tertiary level of damage. At the primary level, the dead cell, of course, ceases to function. Secondarily it ruptures and dumps its remaining nucleic acids into the blood and presents with a range of symptoms. At the tertiary stage of the latter nucleic acid release, the glutamate is free to seize the ammonium ion from molecules of urea and so liberate the cyanate ion to do another range of damage.[33]

Thus the mycoplasma pulls cholesterol, testosterone, progesterone, cortisol, aldosterone etc. from its host cell and incorporates such molecules into its own being. The host cell is diminished and ultimately killed, while its parasitic intruder extends its being by the uptake of the steroids.

The latter scenario is strongly reminiscent of the activity of the 'amyloid' about which Nobel Laureate and Biowar researcher, Dr. Carleton Gajdusek has written:

"Amyloids are insoluble deposits of polymerized fibrils of crossed beta pleated sheet configuration of host precursor proteins which, under appropriate conditions of concentration and with appropriate nucleation, convert to this lower energy state conformation. If the nucleating amyloid is of identical amino acid sequence to the normal precursor which is not in beta pleated configuration, the process can mimic the replication of a microorganism, and the nucleant appears to behave like a very small virus but devoid of nucleic acid. When this nucleation catalyses the production of further identical nucleants by inducing the infectious beta pleated conformational change in host precursor molecules to amyloid molecules, themselves nucleating; and this process, in turn, proves to eventually kill cells; the resulting disease appears as an infectious amyloidosis."[34]

This statement takes on an added significance in the consideration of the mycoplasma hypothesis in the light of further points made by Dr. Gajdusek. First, he points out that the amyloid can "...clearly cause infectious disease, even epidemics, with an infectious chain, as in the kuru epidemic, the CJD outbreak from contaminated *human growth hormone*..."![35] Furthermore, Gajdusek suggests that the 'amyloid' is the same infectious agent as the 'prion' purportedly 'discovered' by Stanley B. Prusiner of the University of California at San Francisco. Gajdusek writes:

*"Since the unconventional and atypical viruses of SSVE (kuru-CJD-GSS-scrapie-BSE) have been identified as infectious amyloid **molecules**, our laboratory has slowly switched to designating them as **infectious amyloids** instead of **unconventional viruses**. Others have accepted the term **PRIONS** for these agents."* [36]

By thus classifying the prion as another name for the amyloid which he in turn defines as an 'infectious molecule' Gajdusek opens the door to the possibility that all are the same infectious particle...the mycoplasma. Finally, it is important to know that Gajdusek has entertained the possibility that the amyloid (and hence by extension the prion)studies:

"...have accumulated that suggest that multiple sclerosis and Parkinson's disease, disseminated lupus erythematosus, juvenile (type 1, insulin-dependent) diabetes, polymyositis, some forms of chronic arthritis, and even schizophrenia may be slow virus infections with a masked and possible defective virus as their cause."[37]

A list strongly reminiscent of Dr. Shyh-Ching Lo's Patent Application list!

Testing the Hypothesis

There are a number of phenomena which when considered in the light of the mycoplasma hypothesis, become more readily understandable. For example, most victims of chronic fatigue syndrome, fibromyalgia, lupus, multiple sclerosis and similar diseases experience a more marked degree of photophobia than do normal controls. If the mycoplasma hypothesis is correct, then such photophobia must be capable of logical explanation, and this is indeed the case.

If the mycoplasma is already wresting steroids from the cells of its victims, then the latter are more likely to be unable to sustain additional steroidal loss without increased discomfort. Thus, if they venture into sunlight where the ultra violet rays pull cholesterol to the surface of the skin and convert it into vitamin D, certain parts of their body will be painfully affected. Since cholesterol, although present in all tissue, is primarily present in the spinal chord, the brain, and gallstones, then the victim who is already suffering from the cholesterol uptake by the mycoplasma, losing even more to the creation of vitamin D, will experience an increased discomfort in the brain (migraine-like headaches) and the spinal column (pain which would suggest disk prolapse).

The cholesterol links to the gallbladder also suggest a promising subject for study in testing the mycoplasma hypothesis. As with photophobia, a significant number of persons diagnosed with myalgicencephalomyelitis (chronic fatigue syndrome), fibromyalgia and multiple sclerosis present with 'irritable bowel syndrome.'[38] Although Dr. Goldstein's emphasis is upon the limbic system, a case can be made for the mycoplasma's uptake of cholesterol in the digestive tract as a causative factor of IBS, and, quite possibly for the development of Crohn's-colitis. According to Makoto Makishima and his colleagues:

"The enzymatic conversion of cholesterol to bile acids is regulated through feed-forward activation by oxysterols and feedback repression by bile acids."[39]

This fact, together with the fact that:

"Bile acids are usually conjugated to glycine or taurine, a derivative of cysteine. Cells require the presence of an active bile acid transporter for uptake of these conjugated derivatives."[40]

If the above digestive functions are limited by the uptake of the necessary cholesterol by the sterol-dependent mycoplasma, then the digestive system is subject to damage and dysfunction which can present as irritable bowel syndrome.

A final area that could merit study in relation to the mycoplasma hypothesis is the use of squalene as an adjuvant for the anthrax vaccine given to many Gulf War Servicemen and women. Since squalene not only acts as an adjuvant, but is also the base for cholesterol production, questions might well be asked about its use.

At any rate, the role of the mycoplasma in potentially upsetting the complex workings of steroids and hormones merits further careful study in relation to the damage done within affected cells when such steroids are up taken by the invading pathogenic mycoplasma. This pathogen pulling cholesterol from the genetically predisposed brain cells could kill its host cell while creating its own neurofibrillary tangles of the Alzheimer brain. This would be a possible explanation for Dr. Lo's identification of Alzheimer's in his Patent Application.

Similar speculation can account for the protean range of symptoms associated with the other degenerative diseases. For example, glucocorticoid pulled from the adrenal glands by the sterol dependent mycoplasma can present with fatigue, weight loss, nausea, dizziness, anorexia, and hypotension.[41] A list of symptoms reminiscent of those seen in the my-algicencephalomyelitis (chronic fatigue syndrome) victim.

SUMMARY

The mycoplasma hypothesis postulates that the active principle of certain bacteria can maintain their essential dynamic even after its antecedent has been destroyed and that this particle can access certain cells and uptake preformed sterols into itself. The latter process ultimately destroys the host cell by a process of degeneration. Because the nucleic particle can access cells in any body system it is possible that it is the common pathogen in diseases as apparently varied as those listed above by Dr. Lo or Dr. Gajdusek. It is further postulated that such dynamic has existed since the earliest evolutionary times, but mankind has evolved an immune system that has largely kept the incidence of many degenerative diseases to a minimum. However, biological warfare experimenting as described in currently available government documents, has resulted in the increased incidence and virulence of the pathogenic mycoplasma. Since such research, development and testing of new infectious microorganisms refactory to the immune system by the governments and military establishments were monitored by the National Institutes of Health and the Centers for Disease Control, these latter public health agencies have failed to rigorously explore the role of the mycoplasma during the past three decades.

If this mycoplasma hypothesis can be sustained by rigorous scientific review it could well offer the prospect of arresting the dramatic increase in the incidence of these neuro/systemic degenerative diseases such as Alzheimer's; bi-polar depression; multiple sclerosis; Crohn's-colitis; diabetes type one; endometriosis; Parkinson's; and others and possibly slow the onset of many of them by appropriate antibiotic protocols.

ENDNOTES

[1]. Volk, Wesley A, and Jay C. Brown: (*Basic Microbiology,* Menlo Park, CA. Addison Wesley Longman, Inc. 1997) p.759

[2]. Jawetz, Ernest et al, 1989 *Medical Microbiology* (18th Edition) (Norwalk, Connecticut: Appleton & Lange) p.255

[3]. Volk & Brown, *supra,* p.17

[4]. Quoted in Leonard G. Horowitz: *Healing Codes for the Biological Apocalypse* (in press) from: Clark HW. What is a Mycoplasma and how does it work? In: *The Intercessor,* Summer, 1993, published by The Road Back Foundation, 4985 N. Lake Road, Delaware OH 43015-9249. Our thanks to Dr. Horowitz for his making his galley proofs available to us.

[5]. Shyh-Ching Lo: *Pathogenic Mycoplasma,* (United States Patent #5,242,820) September 7,1993 p.20

[6]. *Ibid,* p.20

[7]. *Ibid,* p.43

[8]. *Ibid,* p.2

[9]. Editorial:"Human Illness Due to Mycoplasmas". (*The Can. Med. Assoc. Journal,* Vol. 97, July 8,1967) p.84

[10]. A recent victim of Gulf War Illness who had tested positive for the *M.fermentans* was Captain Terry Riordan of Yarmouth, Nova Scotia. Capt. Riordan died on Thursday, April 29,1999. He had suffered since his return from the Gulf from migraines, memory loss, severe joint and muscle pain, shortness of breath, blurred vision, mood swings, muscle spasms and chest pain…all symptoms which can be associated with the *M.fermentans.* Capt. Riordan was largely ignored by the military which he had served and by the Dept. of Veterans Affairs who left him to carry the expense of many of the drugs and much of the medical care he needed. Reported on Saturday, May 1,1999 in the *Globe and Mail.*

[11]. Photocopy in author's files.

[12]. *Ibid,* p.91

[13]. On June 9, 1969, Dr. D.M. MacArthur testified before a secret meeting of the Subcommittee of the Committee on Appropriations of the House of representatives as to the objectives of the biological warfare researchers as follows: "6. Research in biological agent and munition systems -…whether viruses and bacteria can be mutated to new forms resistant to vaccines." *Hearings,* ninety-first Congress p. 144

[14]. From a statement by Dr. D.M. MacArthur, Deputy Director (Research and Technology) Chemical and Biological Warfare, the United States Department of Defense, to The Subcommittee on D. o. D. Appropriations for 1970 of the House of Representatives, Ninety-first Congress. June 9, 1969, p.129

[15]. A brief history of Fort Detrick titled Cutting Edge, can be had by writing to Public Affairs Office, Headquarters, U.S.Army Garrison, Fort Detrick, MD., U.S.A. 21702-5000.

[16]. Norman M. Covert, *Cutting Edge*. Address in footnote 15, above.

[17]. *Congressional Hearings*, June 9, 1969. Statement by Dr. D.M. MacArthur, p. 121.

[18]. Lieutenant Calderon Howe, (MC) United States Naval Reserve, et al "Acute Brucellosis Among Laboratory Workers". (*New Eng. Jour. of Med*. Vol.236, No.20. May 15,1947) pp.741-747

[19]. Robert W. Trevor, MD., et al. "Brucellosis".(*A.M.A. Archives of Internal Medicine*. Vol.103 March,1959). In three parts: pp. 381-397; 398-405; 406-414

[20]. Stephen Endicott and Edward Hagerman, *The United States and Biological Warfare*. (Indiana University Press: Bloomington and Indianapolis 1998) p.68

[21]. Information originally classified 'Top Secret'. Unclassified on Feb. 24,1977 and reported to the Senate *'Subcommittee on Health and Scientific Research'*. p.70

[22]. Iceland had been occupied by Britain at the outbreak of World War Two. Following the Pearl Harbour attack of 1941, the United States replaced Britain as the occupying force and remained there for over two decades. It was in 1947 that the first significant epidemic of chronic fatigue syndrome (CFIDS) occurred in Akureyri, Iceland.

[23]. Karen MacPherson"GAO lists government experiments on 500,000, 1940-1974. *Delaware State News*, (September 29,1994)

[24]. Robert Russo "Winnipeg germ tests were safe, report says". Canadian Press. *The Toronto Star*, (May 15,1997)

[25]. Jorge E. Galan and Alan Collmer, "Type lll Secretion Machines: Bacterial Devices for Protein Delivery into Host Cells." (*Science*, Vol. 284, # 5418 May 21,1999) pp.1322-8

[26]. Adapted from J.D. Colmenero *et al.*, "Compli-

cations Associated with *Brucella Melitensis Infection:* A Study of 530 Cases." (*Medicine*, Vol.75, # 4 1996) pp.195-211

[27]. Henry M. Benning, "Chronic Brucellosis: Success of Treatment with Brucellin". (*JAMA,* Vol. 130, # 6. Feb.9,1946) p.322

[28]. This reference and the ones which follow, are adapted from the information in Dr. Len Horowitz' critical study : *Emerging Viruses: AIDS & Ebola*. (Rockport, MA Tetrahedron, Inc. 1996,1997) p.72

[29]. *Ibid*.

[30]. Dr. Horowitz presents a very convincing case for the manufacture of AIDS-like viruses based upon bovine leukemia and sheep visna viruses. However, we are primarily concerned for the disabling pathogen that causes diseases such as fibromyalgia rather than the lethal virus which causes AIDS.

[31]. Robert Gallo: *Virus Hunting: AIDS, Cancer, & the Human Retrovirus*. (A New Republic Book,1991) p.45

[32]. James D. Cherry, *et al.* "Mycoplasma Pneumoniae Infections of Adults and Children" (*The Western Journal of Medicine*, Vol.125. July 1976) p.48

[33]. Wayne M. Becker and David W. Deamer: *The World of the Cell*. (The Benjamin/Cummings Publishing Company, Inc. 1991) p.10

[34]. Carleton Gajdusek, MD., "Infectious Amyloids: Subacute Spongiform Encephalopathies as Transmissible Cerebral Amyloidoses". (*Field's Virology*, Third Edition. Philadelphia: Lippincott-Raven Publishers, 1996) p.2853

[35]. *Ibid*, p.2854

[36]. Gajdusek, *Ibid* p.2862

[37]. Gajdusek, *Ibid* p.2888

[38]. Jay A. Goldstein, *The Limbic Hypothesis* (New York: The Haworth Medical Press 1992) pp. 71-72; 102;141;146

[39]. Makishima, *et al.*"Identification of a Nuclear Receptor for Bile Acids" (*Science*, Vol.284, # 5418) pp.1362-1365

[40]. Derek J. Parks, *et al.*, "Bile Acids: Natural Ligands for an Orphan Nuclear Receptor (*Science*, Vol. 284, # 5418) pp.1365-1368

[41]. Rex B. Conn, MD. (Editor) *Current Diagnosis 8*. (Philadelphia; W.B.Saunders Company, 1991) p.867

CHAPTER FIFTEEN

SPECIAL VIRUS PROGRAM, PROGRESS REPORT NUMBER NINE

With special thanks to Ms. Shirley Bentley,
President of the United States Chapter of the
Common Cause Medical Research Foundation

The Circle Opens...
Diane Martel, Chronic Fatigue Syndrome; Boyd (Ed) Graves, Acquired Immunodeficiency Syndrome; Lt. Louise Richard, Gulf War Illnesses

The Circle Now Closes...
Biological Warfare Research, Brucellosis, Mycoplasmas, Sterols, the Endocrine System, the Immune System...

Seven years ago the authors set out on a quest after we had been asked by 'chronic fatigue syndrome' victim, Ms. Diane Martel of Sudbury for our help. We had agreed to help her with her tragic disabling disease, but we also wanted to find the source of this terrible disease, chronic fatigue syndrome... more appropriately called myalgic encephalomyelitis. We knew nothing about the disease nor about its source and history. However, we had quickly become aware of the fact that the victims of this disease were very often victims in more than a health sense. In addition to their physical disabilities, the CFIDS/ME patients were often exposed to medical neglect, employment discrimination, insurance company and government social security benefits denial and even the loss of family and friends who to an amazing degree held a warped and cruel view of the disease.

We now believe that we have closed the circle around the truth and that the closing came about because of what a document called the "Special Virus Cancer Program, Progress Report Number Nine", has revealed to us.

SETTING OUT ON A QUEST

As we began our quest, we received initial help from two important sources: Hillary Johnson's magnificent book, *Osler's Web,* and from a survey we personally made of several ME/FM/CFIDS victims.

From *Osler's Web,* which must be ranked as one of this or any centuries most important books, we learned where the trouble started. Essentially, the United States Public Health Agencies turned out to be the primary source of both the medical neglect and the warped view held by so much of society. Essentially, the CDC and the NIH were the chronic fatigue victims' worst enemy. Then, from these so-called public health agencies there emerged a steady stream of prejudicial psychobabble that was picked up, popularized and disseminated by certain media assets such as *Time, The New York Times,* and psychobabble writers such as Edward Shorter and Elaine Showalter.

The fundamental and totally dishonest message wafting from this literary cesspool was the canard that ME victims were not really ill. According to the psychobabble school of critics, the victims' disability existed solely in the head of (mostly) stressed-out women who could not cope with the stress of our modern world. Blame the victim became the mantra of CDC/NIH and their media assets.

From our small, but genuine survey, we learned the truth of myalgic encephalomyelitis. Its victims were ill with a physical disease characterized by extreme fatigue, non-restorative sleep, nausea, initial weight loss often followed by weight gain, headaches, diffuse body aches and pains, benign cysts, cardiac problems characterized by a flat or inverted T wave, endocrine dysfunction, and many related signs and symptoms including restless leg syndrome, irritable bowel syndrome, carpal tunnel syndrome, endometriosis, and Sjogren's syndrome.

We read and considered all of the literature that we could access and found more puzzles than answers. But we did reach one very solid conclusion: the victims of ME were physically ill. They were not as the Stephen Straus, Edward Shorter, Elaine Showalter side show would have it: disabled by a disease that was all in their head. Now our goal became to identify the source of that physical illness.

We got another good boost from Hilary Johnson's *Osler's Web.* In several places in that magnificent book we found references to ME as a 'mirror image' of AIDS! And in many places, sometimes together with the AIDS references, sometimes separately, there were several references to cancer.

As our research progressed, the three...ME/FM, AIDS and cancer... were to be dramatically linked for us when Ms. Bentley sent us a very rare document: the "Special Virus Cancer Program: Progress Report #9".

AIDS

First, in response to the references to AIDS, we turned to a document that dealt with that subject. It was the minutes of secret Hearings held in Washington, D.C., on June 9, 1969 between Dr. Donald MacArthur of the Pentagon and twelve right-wing Congressmen. In these Hearings which were devoted to deciding how much money Congress would vote for the development of biological weapons during the year 1970, there occurred this startling statement:

*"MacArthur:...eminent biologists believe that within a period of 5 to 10 years it would be possible to produce a synthetic biological agent, an agent that does not naturally exist and for which no natural **immunity** could have been acquired...it might be refractory to the **immunological and therapeutic processes upon which we depend to maintain our relative freedom from infectious diseases."***

"Refractory to the immunological process"? That's one of the major characteristics of AIDS and ME/FM/CFIDS!

In this official U.S. Government document, Dr. MacArthur told the Congress of the United States: give us 5 to 10 years and $10 million dollars and the military/CIA of the U.S. will provide you with a biological weapon that will compromise or reduce the effectiveness of the human immune system and leave the victims open to all manner of infectious diseases.

The whole Congress, unaware of the top secret details that their sub-committee of their full Committee on Appropriations had learned, voted blindly and, as they were asked to do, to go ahead with the creation of AIDS.

Get this straight. We are not going to be mealy-mouthed about what MacArthur asked for and what the Congressional Sub-Committee voted for and then foisted off onto the whole of the Congress. Plain and simply, if you understand the English language, MacArthur had asked for money, time and approval to develop AIDS and his request had been

granted. From that day forward the official, albeit secret, policy of the United States National Security Agencies included the research, development, testing, and deployment of a biological weapon that would kill millions of innocent people because it would be refractory to the human immune system.

It is important to note that earlier in the same Hearings (p. 121) MacArthur had warned the Congressmen that as a consequence of their research some scientists worried "...that there will be a worldwide scourge, or a black death type disease that will envelop the world or major geographic areas if some of these materials were to accidentally escape."

He uses the qualifier 'accidentally' when speaking about the disease escape, but, as we have learned, he should also have said 'or is intentionally allowed to escape'. He was asked to provide a list of the lethal disease agents that the Pentagon was working on and he submitted the following list:"...Yellow fever virus; Rabbit fever virus; Anthrax bacteria; Psittacosis agent; Rickettsia of Rocky Mountain spotted fever; Plague". He could have mentioned two other deadly disease agents which we now know the Pentagon was working on: the so-called "unconventional lentiviruses (ie 'slow' viruses)" such as the visna and maedi retroviruses in sheep and various mycoplasma species. Why did he neglect to mention these?

We now know why Dr. MacArthur neglected to mention the two most important deadly disease agents that the Pentagon was working with, and we explain why.

But as we were to learn from our several re-readings of these Hearings, there was more to Dr. MacArthur's presentation on June 9, 1969. During those same Hearings there was something we had never noted before in our reading. In several places Dr. MacArthur revealed to the Congressmen that besides working to develop a lethal biological weapon, the Pentagon was also working to develop disabling biological weapons! Weapons which would not kill their victim but would disable them!

MacArthur told the Congressmen that to achieve these disabling biological weapons his researchers were working with "...Rickettsia causing Q-fever; Rift Valley fever virus; Chikungunya disease virus; Venezuelan equine encephalitis virus." He should have included another disease agent...the brucella bacteria, for the record shows that it was the most important disabling disease agent that the Pentagon researchers were working on. Why did he also neglect to mention these?

Dr. MacArthur did not mention the work being done with either the lethal visna/maedi retroviruses or the mycoplasmal species nor did he mention the disabling brucella bacteria because the Pentagon was *already* working covertly with these deadly and disabling agents! We know of his duplicity because we have learned that just ten days after these Hearings (on June 19, 1969) the National Institutes of Health renewed a Contract # 69-2053, originally awarded as far back as 1963, to Dr. Leonard Hayflick of Stanford University to (among other things) establish a Central Mycoplasma Diagnostic Laboratory. And we now know that the brucella bacteria were being weaponized by the Pentagon because as far back as 1951 the U.S. Air Force had taken *Brucella suis* biological bombs into inventory!

Thus, our initial research into the origins of myalgic encephalomyelitis had led us to parallel research into AIDS, and we found from an official (but hitherto top secret) U.S. government document that both the disabling disease [ME/FM/CFIDS] and the lethal disease [AIDS] were the major foci of Military biological warfare weapons development!

This is a good point to mention something else that needs to be recognized and emphasized. In several places in his testimony Dr. MacArthur makes it clear to the Congressmen that in all of the Pentagon's biological weapons development programs, the U.S. public health agencies *worked with* the Department of Defense. As you will see, the CDC and the NIH later would have ample reason to downplay the tragedy of myalgic encephalomyelitis: both of these public health agencies had co-operated in the development of the AIDS and ME/FM/CFIDS pathogens!

It was at this point in our research that we had the great good personal fortune to meet a wonderful lady: Lt.(RN) Louise Richard, RCN (Ret'd.)

Louise Richard was a brilliant registered nurse who had served with Canada's military contingent in Desert Storm. During her active service in the battle zone her unit came under Iraqi SCUD-missile attack and soon afterwards Lt. Richard's health began a precipitous decline. She presented with most of the symptoms of myalgic encephalomyelitis, plus a protean range of other signs and symptoms. She was totally disabled from pursuing her nursing career in the military and had to resign her commission in Canada's armed services.

Because of the very marked parallel between Lt. Richard's Gulf War Illness [GWI] symptoms and the symptoms of myalgic encephalomyelitis, it was evident to us that somehow, GWI and ME/FM/CFIDS were related and we extended our research to include GWI and the relation of all three to what the U.S. military had been doing. We found two significant sources of information: Senator Donald Riegle's Senate Report on Gulf War Illness (May 25,1994) and the articles being written by Drs. Garth and Nancy Nicolson.

From Senator Riegle's Report we learned that between 1985 and 1990 the Reagan/Bush Administrations had sold several batches of various brucella bacterial agents to Iraq.

Furthermore we learned that a weaponized brucella could induce symptoms of: " ...chronic fatigue, loss of appetite, profuse sweating when at rest, pain in joints and muscles, insomnia, nausea, and damage to major organs." All of these symptoms matched those of Lt. Richard!

It seemed apparent that Lt. Richard had a variant of brucellosis and brucellosis was one of the diseases weaponized by the U.S. military and sold to Iraq. Furthermore, brucella could be delivered by missiles and Lt. Richard had endured a missile attack while serving in the Gulf War.

Then we came to recognize another striking parallel. Just as the very real physical disease, myalgic encephalomyelitis had been mockingly denied by the CDC/NIH, through Stephen Straus, Edward Shorter, Elaine Showalter and the psychobabble crowd, Gulf War Illness was denied as a 'real' illness by everyone from the Canadian Minister of Defense through the Commanding General Baril to the military medical doctors such as Lt. Col Ken Scott and Major Tim Cook. And in this they took their lead from the U.S. military whose principal 'denier' was a Captain Kenneth Craig Hyams of the United States Navy.

The result: Lt. Louise Richard and many of her fellow military who were suffering from Gulf War Illnesses were betrayed and left to a diminished life of agony and even death by the Canadian military hierarchy and by extension, they were betrayed by their fellow Canadians whom they had served.

But the question arose, how could brucellosis be communicated to its victims and there be no sign of it in ordinary blood and tissue tests?

We found that there were two contributing factors that accounted for this apparent anomaly.

First, we learned that generally speaking little or no effort was made by the military medical services to test the GWI patients for any traces of the brucella bacteria.

But, secondly, and of greater significance to us, we learned from a study of U.S. Senate documents, that in 1946, the then Director of biological warfare research for the Pentagon, Dr. George Merck, had reported to the Secretary of the Army that his researchers had managed "...for the first time to *isolate* the disease agent from bacteria in *crystalline* form." Note that Dr. Merck said "isolate the disease agent". He was not, as some researchers claim, referring to 'freeze drying' the bacteria. The researchers were actually able to *isolate* the disease agent and then dispose of the rest of the bacteria.

In effect, the U.S. military could diffuse a crystalline brucella, infect target victims with a bacterial disease, but leave no obvious trace of the bacteria itself! And, we were later to learn, the 'disease agents' were probably nucleic acid disease particles.

Thus, the next question that began to occupy us was: Just what form did the crystalline disease agents take biologically?

We found a likely answer in the work of Drs. Garth and Nancy Nicolson who were beginning to report that forty-five to fifty-five percent of the Gulf War Illness patients that they were seeing had tested positive for one or more species of a mysterious and little heard of microorganism: the mycoplasma.

The mycoplasmas, we learned, were a group of eubacteria, phylogenetically related to gram-positive bacteria but retaining the rather unique position as the smallest self-replicating procaryotes devoid of cell walls. The current view among scientists is that they have degenerated from walled bacteria.

Our next question became: did the mycoplasma degenerate from walled bacteria naturally, or were they given a helping hand by military researchers?

Was this what Merck had reported in 1946? Had his researchers learned how to take normal walled bacteria and extract from them certain of their qualities harboured in their nucleic acids in the form of crystals? And were these crystals the repository for the disease symptoms certain bacteria could engender in a victim?

And, if these crystals were reduced to an infinitely small particle could they be diffused to target populations through the air, or by way of an insect vector, or in the food chain, or even by way of contaminated vaccines? And, if so diffused, would they go into solution in the victims' body fluids and re-gain their capacity to induce disease?

These questions took us back to Dr. MacArthur's briefing of the U.S. Congressmen. On page 120 of the Hearings, he has this to say about a particular biological weapon that the Pentagon was working on: "... would be used as a primary aerosol and infect people inhaling it. After that they could be carried from me to you, say, by an insect vector - a *mosquito* for example."

A mosquito?

This reference took us back to something else we had learned some time earlier. We had learned that after the Second World War, Canada had agreed to continue its wartime biological warfare research with the United States, and that one of the tasks that Canada had undertaken was to breed one hundred million mosquitoes a month at the Dominion Parasite Laboratory in Belleville, Ontario. These mosquitoes were then delivered to the care of Dr. G.B. Reed of the biology department of Queen's University, in Kingston, Ontario. Dr. Reed's job was to contaminate the mosquitoes with undisclosed pathogens and then turn them over to the Canadian and U.S. militaries for testing upon unsuspecting human guinea pigs.

Was one of the pathogens a crystalline form of a brucella disease agent which could be diffused on contaminated mosquitoes? And was one of the U.S. test sites Punta Gorda, Florida in 1956? We had learned that Punta Gorda had suffered an epidemic of myalgic encephalomyelitis in that year starting just a week after an unusually huge influx of mosquitos. These were the first cases of myalgic encephalomyelitis ever seen in that community!

And was one of the test sites in the St. Lawrence Seaway Valley of Canada in 1984 when after an influx of mosquitoes nearly 700 people became ill with a 'mystery' disease?

And aerosol diffusion? Could it have been that in Incline Village in Nevada an epidemic of myalgic encephalomyelitis apparently centred in the local Tahoe-Truckee High School occurred in 1984 after the High School heating system had been torn out and a new system installed? The new system was designed to take the same air from a room, heat or cool it as required, and then send it back to the *same* room. Was one room, a staff room for eight of the staff, exposed to a crystalline pathogen re-circulated in the system? After all, seven of the eight staff in that room became ill with myalgic encephalomyelitis over the next six months and some are still disabled. The only one of the eight teachers who did not become ill had been a teacher who refused to use the staff room because he felt that the air 'smelled strange.'

We turned back to Dr. MacArthur's briefing of the Congressmen and noted that he had wanted 18 million dollars in 1970 for "testing"! How much was spent in 1984 on testing? Where were the test sites? Who were the test subjects? What was being tested?

Our research had taken us from chronic fatigue syndrome to AIDS to Gulf War Illness to biological warfare weapons to brucellosis and then to the mycoplasma.

At about this point in time (1999) we had added another source to our research: Dr. Leonard Horowitz' startling book *Emerging Viruses: AIDS & Ebola.* Dr. Horowitz, trained initially as a dentist, had approached the problem of AIDS from an entirely different perspective than we had. He began his study after another dentist, Dr. David Acer, a homosexual infected with AIDS, had passed the disease to six of his patients. Actually, we had had Dr. Horowitz' book since 1996, but our focus had been on ME/FM/CFIDS and we had not made sufficient use of the dramatic details that the book contained. Then, by bringing Dr. Horowitz back into our efforts to find our way through the labyrinth of ME, AIDS, GWI, several things suddenly took on much greater significance. Of these, the most important was the reproduction of sections of a document called "The Special Virus Cancer Program; Progress Report #8."

The circle was beginning to close.

Before we were able to devote our best attention to the SVCP, Progress Report #8, an interesting coincidence occurred.

In August of that year we organized our first Conference of the Common Cause Medical Research Foundation in Gananoque, Ontario. We were coming to understand that there was a 'common cause' of ME/AIDS/and GWI. At that Conference of the Common Cause Medical Research Foundation our Director of AIDS Concerns, Mr. Boyd (Ed) Graves had provided a copy of the full Progress Report Number Eight to Ms. Sue Oleksyn who passed it to our United States Chapter President, Ms. Shirley Bentley. Ms. Bentley in turn provided us with a copy and a whole new world opened to our research. The Progress Report brought together in a very tantalizing way elements of AIDS, chronic fatigue, biowar research, and those mysterious disease agents, the mycoplasmas.

But the latter was to be a puzzle within an enigma wrapped in a mystery for us. We began piecing together the clues that slowly emerged, while at the same time engaging in a multitude of other Foundation activities: maintaining Foundation records and business; attending and participating in professional conferences; serving as interview guests on many radio and TV programs; editing and publishing and mailing our new *Journal of Degenerative Diseases;* helping sick victims with pension plan applications and appeals...

Then another important document came to us. It was a copy of a United States Patent, number 5,242,820, dated September 7, 1993. And what was being patented by whom? It turned out that a U.S. government researcher named Dr. Shyh-Ching Lo had patented a "Pathogenic Mycoplasma."

There was the mystery microorganism that Drs. Garth and Nancy Nicolson had been finding in sick Gulf War veterans, and with which, when she had herself tested, Lt. Louise Richard had found that she was infected! Here it was being patented by a government scientist as if he were patenting a new type of handgun! And not only had this U.S. government employee patented the 'Pathogenic [ie disease causing] mycoplasma' but on pages 19-20 of his patent he listed several of the diseases which, he claimed, infected patients with *Mycoplasma fermentans* incognitus strain. The list shocked us for it read as follows:

"AIDS or ARC, Chronic Fatigue Syndrome, Wegener's Disease, Sarcoidosis, respiratory distress syndrome, Kibuchi's disease (sic), autoimmune diseases such as Collagen Vascular Disease and Lupus and chronic debilitating diseases such as Alzheimer's Disease."

We returned to the Special Cancer Virus Program, Progress Report #8 with greater care, and there we found it! There on pages 255-6 as we have mentioned above, was the mycoplasma! We learned that as early as 1963, the NIH had awarded a contract to Dr. Leonard Hayflick to establish "...a Central Mycoplasma Diagnostic Laboratory." We re-read the details and now several things became clear about the Special Virus Cancer Program and its role in the research, development, testing and ultimately the deployment of the AIDS and CFS pathogens and apparently according to Dr. Lo's Patent, their corollary diseases.

The circle closed even further for this is what our careful analysis of the SVCP Progress Report #8 also made clear to us: the AIDS/CFIDS pathogens had been the subject of a secret CIA/military biological research program for several years before Congress had been asked to approve it! How did we come to realize this? We found our clue on page 282 of the Progress Report:

"4. MK-SVLP, 2/66 - 3/67 This study was initiated by Drs. Manaker and Kotin..."

First, the significance of the title "MK-SVLP". We knew that the CIA assigned code names to their covert projects. We were aware of 'Project BLUEBIRD' and 'Project EARSHOT' and 'Project IRIDIUM'. However, we were also aware of 'Project MK-ULTRA' and 'MK-NAOMI' and 'MK-DELTA'... and we knew some things about the three latter projects, but we never knew what the 'MK' had signified.

Now SVCP, Progress Report #8 made it clear that the 'MK' in MK-SVLP stood for Drs. Robert Manaker and Paul Kotin.

And the interesting thing about MK-SVLP was the fact that after the June 9, 1969 Hearings, when the Congressmen approved the task of developing the AIDS pathogen, the covert MK-SVLP project became a mainstream Defense Department project buried within cancer research and the 'MK' designation could be dropped. In other words, the covert research already being done was retroactively incorporated into the new 'Special Virus *Cancer* Program' [SVCP] which became the public front for President Nixon's great political triumph...his 'Great War on Cancer'.

We noted that the MK-SVLP program had included activities from May, 1962 through June, 1971. Someone had been doing something to someone else during that period in the research for new biological weapons. What we now had to include in our research was the who, what, and why of those activities.

Next, we realized that the 'eminent biologists' to whom Dr. MacArthur had referred would undoubtedly include those already in Defense Department activities...including "MK-SVLP." We decided to check out each of those mentioned. We wanted to know who they were, where they did their research, what scientific papers had they published, how their diverse activities might relate to each other... and any other question that needed to be asked.

We hit the jackpot!

The Gallo Jackpot!

One of the names that we noted was that of Robert Gallo! Here, in this 1960's work, was the scientist who two decades later would 'discover' the so-called

'AIDS virus'-HIV. According to Progress Report #8, Gallo had engaged in research in such esoteric areas as "RNA- and DNA-dependancy polymerases"; "physiology of human leukemic leukocytes"; "Reverse transcriptase in type C virus *particles*" [emphasis added]; "DNA polymerases of human normal and leukemic cells".

From another source we learned that Gallo had served on an SVCP Committee which was chaired by none other than Dr. Robert Manaker who, as we have mentioned, had lent his initial to the "MK-SVLP" Program, and who was also Gallo's senior at NIH. However, there was something bothersome about this latter fact because in the book Gallo wrote [*Virus Hunting*] he has apparently forgotten a number of details. First, he referred to the SVLP cum SVCP as the 'Virus Cancer Program'. Then, he apparently forgot just when the Program under any name had begun and ended. He reported that it had begun in 1970 and had ended in 1977 yet he had done work under the program as far back as 1962! Finally he had apparently forgotten that while serving as a servant of the American people for the National Institutes of Health, he had found the time to lend his considerable talents to Litton Bionetics, Inc.

The latter enterprise was at the time, engaged in some activities clustered under the SVCP Progress Report #8 as : The Inoculation Program" [p. 276] and all of these elements figure in the tragedy of AIDS/ME/FM and GWI. But that must wait until we have seen the evidence in the Special Virus Cancer Program, Progress Report Number *Nine*.

The Gajdusek Beginnings

Another name in the SVCP Report #8 that quickly drew our attention was Nobel Laureate, Dr. D. Carleton Gajdusek. We learned that in 1966 and 1967, Gajdusek and his long-time associate, Dr. C. Joseph Gibbs, had spent some of the MK-SVLP money trying to infect certain primates [initially chimpanzees, later monkeys] with human diseases such as kuru and encephalomyelitis! Why?

We were particularly interested in Gajdusek because in 1996 one of the authors [DWS] had conducted a one hour telephone interview with him. During that interview we advised him that we believed that he was one of the scientists who had been engaged in biological warfare weapons development.

He offered to send us some of his research and told us "If you can find any evidence of biowar activities you're welcome to them." We did indeed find some of that evidence in those documents. However before reporting what we found we decided to re-check the research of Gajdusek and Gallo as co-workers in the SVCP. We returned to Gallo's *Virus Hunting* and there we had another of what Edward Hooper calls a 'Eureka moment.' Gallo had this to say:

" We have learned about iatrogenically induced (medically caused) prion diseases from the earliest studies of Gajdusek and his co-workers on kuru..."
What's that you say? 'Medically caused?'

Kuru is a degenerative brain disease, the most important characteristic of which is the fact that the victim's brain turns to mush. Something of a young person's Alzheimer's. It was first recorded in an official document by an outsider among the Fore tribe of New Guinea by an Australian government Patrol Officer

(J.R. MacArthur) on December 6, 1953. Earlier visitors to the Fore tribe including Luthern missionaries in 1949, had made no mention of it.

Four years after Patrolman MacArthur had encountered the victim of Kuru in New Guinea Dr. D. Carleton Gajdusek turned up to study the disease on behalf of his United States sponsors. His principal sponsor was Dr. Joseph Smadel of the Walter Reed Army Institute of Research. We learned that Gajdusek had written a letter to Smadel on March 15, 1957 wherein he stated:

"(Kuru) has been the major disease problem of the region, as well as a social problem for the past *five years.*"

In other words, kuru wasn't an ancient disease and social problem; it had only been such for *five* years! From 1952, that is. Now, given that it is caused by what was then called a lentivirus which can take from five to fifteen years to present as an illness, it is apparent that the disease pathogen had been introduced into the Fore tribe sometime in the early 1940's. Kuru had then began appearing in the late 1940's and was seen by Patrolman MacArthur in 1953. By 1957 when Gajdusek arrived in New Guinea, it was the major social and disease problem of the Fore tribe. Where had it come from? What was the disease agent? Let us continue our research summary.

Gajdusek's study led him to the realization that the disease was transmitted from one generation to the next by the Fore tribe's burial practise of the women and children of the tribe eating the diseased brain of the victims being prepared for burial. They had been doing this for thousands of years, but there had been no Kuru reports until Patrolman MacArthur's 1953 observations. And eating the brain was how the disease was transmitted... not how, as Gallo put it, the Kuru was caused! Where had Gallo gotten the idea that Kuru was a 'medically caused' disease.

We think we know the answer both to Gallo's strange comment and to the mystery of the disease itself.

Our research demonstrated that in 1942 when most of New Guinea had been occupied by the Japanese army, their biowar medical research team under Dr./Gen. Ishii Shiro had singled out a primitive and remote tribe to test a new biological weapon. We believe that biological weapon was an inoculant developed by Japanese scientists from either visna-infected sheep brains, or from the brains of Japanese victims of Creutzfeldt-Jakob Disease.

It is our hypothesis that the Japanese had initiated this ghastly experiment when they laboured under the illusion that their 'Co-Prosperity Sphere' of most of Asia would last for hundreds of years. They hadn't counted on the Australian Army stopping them just north of Port Moresby, and then, with the help of arriving Americans, driving them out of New Guinea over the next few months. And when they left, they left behind the group of Fore tribesmen whom they had inoculated.

The 'lentivirus' in the brains of the infected did not begin to present as a Kuru variant of C-JD until about 1947. *That* was the 'medically caused' part! That's what Gallo was talking about when he inadvertently let slip the truth in his book *Virus Hunting*. Then, the ancient practise of eating the brain of the tribes' dead continued to *transmit* the disease, *not cause it*, and as Gajdusek suggested, became their major medical problem by 1952.

Upon what do we base our claim? We have created this hypothesis based upon knowing that: (i) the Japanese were very actively engaged in biowar weapons research (ii) they had occupied New Guinea and had established a 'biological test site' (iii) when the war was over the Americans spared the lives of the Japanese researchers on condition that these researchers told all of their secrets (iv) we know that General Ishii Shiro revealed that they had established the New Guinea test site, but the Americans have never revealed what the Japanese said they were testing at that site. As mentioned above: our hypothesis is that the site was a test of the fore-runner of

AIDS... the visna 'scrapie' virus, and that Gajdusek had been sent to New Guinea to reap the benefit of the Japanese experiment.

We also hypothesize that the active disease agent of the visna virus is quite possibly the same as the nucleic acid particle of the brucellosis bacterium. We base this possibility upon the idea suggested by Gajdusek and extended by us that "The possibility that the viruses of all four of the subacute spongiform virus encephalopathies are not just closely related agents, but different strains of a single virus which has been modified in different hosts." And we hypothesize that the same disease agent presents as Parkinson's Disease, multiple sclerosis, Crohn's-Colitis and even Diabetes Type One and other of the degenerative diseases.

We developed much more information about Gajdusek, but that has to be the subject of its own report. We must return to the SVCP, Progress Report #8, and the people therein, as background for the startling evidence to be revealed in Progress Report #9.

Besides finding Gallo and Gajdusek in the shadows of the covert MK-SVLP antecedent to its SVCP successor, we noted another name of great interest: Dr. Hilary Koprowski.

Dr. Koprowski was of interest to us for several important reasons. First, he had been reported upon in several passages of Johnson's *Osler's Web!* This was odd, because the latter book was a chronicle of the myalgic encephalomyelitis epidemic... not of the AIDS epidemic. And what he was doing in the covert MK-SVLP program was also odd: he was trying to infect some primates with Adenovirus 7! The "easy transmissibility" of the adenoviruses according to Gallo, "made possible a local epidemic among groups at high risk for AIDS."

Why was Gajdusek busy trying to infect a primate species with it? And, we had learned privately but from a highly placed and very reliable scientist, that Koprowski and former director of the CDC, Brian Mahy, had quite possibly sabotaged the research of Wistar researcher, Dr. Elaine DeFreitas. Then we learned that Koprowski had been hired in 1940 by the Rockefeller Foundation to work in Brazil, and the many links of the Rockefellers and their institutional extensions into the realm of world population growth rate reduction made any employee suspect. Later Koprowski had moved to the United States where he again went to work for the Rockefellers. We also knew that Koprowski had worked exten-

sively with none other that Dr. Leonard Hayflick who was the one signed to a contract renewal by SVCP on June 19, 1969, to continue a *mycoplasma* laboratory!

Then, just recently from Edward Hooper's great book *The River*, a study into the origins of the AIDS epidemic, we note that Koprowski merits fifteen centimetres of Index citing!

On a brief tangent: we have recently had the opportunity to read Hooper's book *The River*. It is a magnificent book, thoroughly researched by an obviously intelligent, careful, fair-minded and moral person. However, his research has not yet sufficiently factored in the role of the U.S. military researchers in the development and deployment of the AIDS pathogen. Mr. Hooper at this point believes that the AIDS epidemic had its origins in the attempts to develop and test polio vaccines in Africa. Given Mr. Hooper's exemplary qualities as a researcher, we anticipate his movement on the question as he continues his work.

Thus, from SVCP Progress Report #8, we have noted the presence of Gallo, Gajdusek, Koprowski, Hayflick and many others whom we cannot list in this short space. But we'll conclude this part of our summary by noting the fact that many key players in the SVCP are also to be found playing critical parts in *Osler's Web!* For example, Dharam Ablashi, a doctor of *veterinary medicine* has nine Index citations in Johnson's book and ten citations in MK-SVLP! Then, also in the SVCP Report, he turns up in 1970 trying to inoculate some primate species with the saimiri virus!

We puzzled: how do people like Robert Gallo and Leonard Hayflick and Dharma Ablashi, who, in the early 1960's, were all engaged in the early stages of AIDS and CFIDS research before such disease entities *even existed*, undergo a metamorphosis in the 1980's into experts in these very disease entities? We pose another hypothesis: these people were the experts in the 1980's precisely because they were the researchers developing the pathogens in the 1960's-1970's.

Our Eureka Moment

Our research had by this present point in time, brought us to the position of looking for the final closing of the circle. What was it that completed our research journey from chronic fatigue to AIDS to Gulf War Illness to biowar weapons research to brucellosis to the mycoplasma to the Special Virus Cancer Program?

And then we found it!

Not long ago our United States Common Cause Medical Research Foundation President and dear friend, Shirley Bentley, located a copy of none other than: *Special Virus Cancer Program: Progress Report Number Nine*. She photocopied all 425 pages and mailed it to us. We put aside our time-worn copy of Report Number Eight and turned to our new source…and there it was. Our closing link in the circle.

Here is what we read:

"We have for the first time demonstrated that the virogenic markers, group specific antigens (g.s.) and the RNA directed DNA polymerase, can be activated by alteration of the physiological endocrine balance."

Return briefly to 'The Gallo Jackpot' above. The very subjects of his studies in the 1960's appears in the Moloney revelation of 1972.

The mechanism by which the HIV retrovirus RNA can take over the DNA of its host is initiated by first altering the endocrine balance! Eureka! HIV does not cause AIDS…it only takes advantage of the loss of immunity caused by the alteration of the endocrine balance!

With the endocrine system disbalanced, the immune system does not have the capacity to prevent the process of RNA directed DNA polymerase. We must emphasize that this is a flat out conclusion stated by government researcher and NIH Director of the Cancer Institute, Dr. Moloney in the Special Virus Cancer Program…Progress Report Number Nine.

In other words, the new disease agent that Dr. Donald MacArthur promised the Congressmen on June 9, 1969, the one that would be "refractory to the immunological and therapeutic processes upon which we depend to maintain our relative freedom from infectious disease" had been achieved.

How Does It Work?

The endocrine system includes the hypothalamus, pituitary, pancreas, adrenal and other glands. They function in a finely balanced system of co-operation. And how can one alter their physiological balance?

That is just what Gallo and his AIDS - CFIDS creating cohorts learned to do and their secret lay in the mycoplasma species for which Dr. Leonard Hayflick was contracted to establish a "central diagnostic facility for the detection and identification" and, in collaboration with Drs. Todaro and Aaronson to do studies "on isotope labelling and density gradient separation of mycoplasma contaminants." Dr. Moloney then links the continuing Hayflick, Todaro and Aaronson research to the seminal work of Rottem, Pfend, and Hayflick on "The Sterol Requirements of T-Strain Mycoplasmas".

And that is the key!

They had learned that many of the mycoplasma species had an absolute dependance upon the uptake of pre-formed sterols from their host cells. And, they learned from the research of Rottem, Pfendt and *Hayflick,* financed by a grant within the Special Virus Cancer Program, and published in the January, 1971 issue of *The Journal of Bacteriology,* that the main source of sterols for the mycoplasma was cholesterol. Furthermore, cholesterol is an upstream factor in glandular hormone production. Pull the cholesterol out of the cycle and the endocrine balance is *drastically* altered. And when the endocrine balance is altered the way is opened for the RNA directed DNA polymerase.

In other words, HIV did not lead to endocrine disbalance. The endocrine disbalance induced by the mycoplasma compromised the immunocompetence of the victim and opened the door for the HIV and the opportunistic diseases to sicken and ultimately to kill him, if the concentration were sufficient by fluid exchange (blood, semen, vaccine, or mother's milk) infection, or disable him if the concentration were less by aerosol, mosquito or food chain infection.

Here is the mechanism for both AIDS and ME/ FM/CFIDS and GWI:

1. Mycoplasmal infection introduced into the target victim by body fluid transfer through blood, semen, vaccine or mother's milk to subject victim to high level concentration sufficient to present as the Acquired Immune Deficiency Syndrome; or, to introduce at a lesser level of concentration sufficient to present as chronic fatigue syndrome, fibromyalgia, multiple sclerosis, sarcoidosis, Wegener's Disease, collagen vascular diseases and others, including cancer, dependent upon the individual victim's genetic predisposition and his/her immune health status.

2. The sterol dependant mycoplasma begins the up-take of the pre-formed sterols in the host cells

that it accesses. The richest sources of such sterols are to be found in the blood, the brain, the gray matter of the brain and spinal column, the synovial cartilage and fluid of joints and spinal discs.

3. Since the endocrine glands depend upon the up-stream production of cholesterol, the balance of the endocrine system is upset, and the capability of the cellular immunity to prevent RNA directed DNA polymerase is compromised. This opens the way for the HIV enzyme reverse transcriptase to copy its viral genetic material from RNA to double stranded DNA, access and splice into the cell DNA and direct the making of proteins and RNA.

4. The newly made HIV RNA makes its way to the host cell surface where it buds and then breaks away, carrying with it a protein envelope of cell membrane. It encounters another cell, adheres to the cellular membrane, refractory to the disabled immune system, and accesses the interior of its new host, where the process of RNA directed DNA polymerase is repeated. And, as Dr. Moloney states in Progress Report #9... the process was activated by "...alteration of the physiological endocrine balance"!

Our research circle had been closed! Our review not only revealed what we have summarized above, but has led us to these further hypotheses:

First, the program to develop population growth rate limiting pathogens had been under way for several years; initially by the private eugenics fanatics such as the Rockefellers, and later by the incorporation of their research into U.S. Government biowar weapons research by Eisenhower Under-Secretary of Health and later Gerald Ford Vice-President, Nelson Rockefeller. The public health agencies at a covert level, became allies of the Military/CIA efforts.

Second, the initial testing had begun in central and eastern African nations in conjunction with or masked under, research into polio vaccine development. The consequences of the research were quite possibly discovered serendipitously from the polio vaccine tests. However, Progress Report #9 makes something else very clear. The study of the mycoplasma species by the biowar researchers began much earlier than previously known. On page 287 of the SVCP-PR #9 Dr. Moloney reveals that the NIH contract to Dr. Hayflick to procure and study mycoplasmas first noted by us in Progress Report #8, had been initiated in 1964 or even as early as the 1950's.

Third, when it was apparent that the kuru /C-JD disease agent was a mycoplasma or nucleic acid sterol dependent particle variously labelled as an amyloid or a prion, which worked by creating an endocrine system disbalance which in turn activated RNA directed DNA polymerase, the test stage of its development gave way to mycoplasma-laced smallpox vaccine in target countries. The mycoplasma-laced hepatitis-B vaccine program was probably initiated in American gay men to develop a strong public resistance to public funding of research.

Now all manner of questions have been answered for us.

The link between the hepatitis-B vaccine program of gay men in 1979 and the 1968 smallpox vaccine program in the 'lesser developed countries' was obvious. The former with a more virulent vaccine had been initiated to stem any public demand for research into the lentivirus-based AIDS vaccine program. The obvious linkage of AIDS/ME/GWI to the endocrine system was now explained. The early roles of Gallo, Hayflick, Todaro, Aaroson, Levine, Ablashi, and their relationship to each other became apparent. The outbreaks of ME/CFIDS in Incline Village and Lyndonville and the St. Lawrence Valley had been necessary to test the researchers' pathogens. The reason for Brian Mahy's diversion of CFIDS research money could now be seen in the light of the need to limit genuine research. The answers were already known! All now fit together.

Epilogue

Acquired immune-deficiency syndrome (AIDS), chronic fatigue immune-deficiency syndrome (CFIDS), Gulf War Illnesses (GWI) and a broad range of the neuro-systemic degenerative diseases such as Alzheimer's, bi-polar depression, Creutzfeldt-Jakob Disease, Parkinson's, multiple sclerosis, Crohn's-colitis and others are all the consequence of a common cause: a pathogen identified as a mycoplasma, a particle of a bacterial nucleic acid, which was researched, developed, tested and deployed by agencies of the United States government and, to an extent, its allies.

The authors hope that this work will contribute to a greater understanding of the role of the mycoplasma in the disease process, and lead to a more candid and complete exploration of this disease agent.

It is also our hope that the heavy burden of the political and economic factors will be set aside, and that the sole goal of all research will be the return to health of millions of its victims.

About the authors:

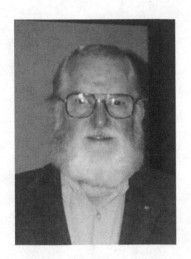

Donald W. Scott was born in Wiarton, Canada in 1924. He served in Canada's wartime navy and later graduated from the University of Toronto (BA), Guelph University (MSc) and Laurentian University (MA). He is the President of the Common Cause Medical Research Foundation and is an Adjunct Professor of the Institute for Molecular Medicine. He edits The Journal of Degenerative Diseases and **able** magazine. Mr. Scott married the late Edith Goody of Cobourg in 1946 and has eight children. He is presently married to Cecile Marie Courtemanche, and resides in Sudbury, Canada.

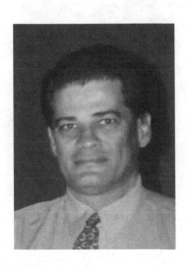

William L.C. Scott was born in Toronto, Canada in 1955. He graduated from Laurentian University in 1982 with a Double Honours Bachelor of Arts degree in History and Political Science. Mr. Scott lives in Ottawa where he is the founder and President of Executive Services Limited. He has two children, Krysten and Alexander. In addition to his researching the mycoplasma and its role in world health he is also very active with the shared parenting/shared grandparenting rights of children of divorce.

Printed in the United States
by Baker & Taylor Publisher Services